Informed Infection Control Practice

For Churchill Livingstone:

Senior Commissioning Editor: Ninette Premdas
Project Development Manager: Gail Wright
Project Manager: Joannah Duncan
Designer: Judith Wright

Informed Infection Control Practice

SECOND EDITION

Rozila Horton MPhil RGN
Infection Control Nurse Advisor/Director, edhitec Health Systems,
Harrogate; Formerly Clinical Nurse Advisor, Infection Control,
Harrogate Healthcare NHS Trust, Harrogate, UK

and

Lynn Parker MSc RGN
Clinical Nurse Specialist, Infection Control, Sheffield Teaching Hospitals NHS Trust,
Sheffield, UK

With a contribution by

Diane Thompson
Library Services Manager
Library and Knowledge Management Services, Hull and East Riding Health Authority,
Hull, UK

Foreword by

Sheila Morgan
Infection Control Consultant and Chair of the Infection Control Nurse's Association,
Newcastle upon Tyne Hospitals NHS Trust, UK

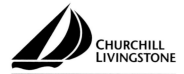

CHURCHILL
LIVINGSTONE

EDINBURGH LONDON NEW YORK PHILADELPHIA ST LOUIS SYDNEY TORONTO 2002

CHURCHILL LIVINGSTONE
An imprint of Elsevier Science Limited 2002

First edition 1997
Second edition 2002

ISBN 0 443 07102 0

British Library Cataloguing in Publication Data
A catalogue record for this book is available from the British Library

Library of Congress Cataloging in Publication Data
A catalog record for this book is available from the Library of Congress

Note
Medical knowledge is constantly changing. As new information becomes
available, changes in treatment, procedures, equipment and the use of
drugs become necessary. The authors, contributor and the publishers have
taken care to ensure that the information given in this text is accurate and
up to date. However, readers are strongly advised to confirm that the
information, especially with regard to drug usage, complies with the latest
legislation and standards of practice.

 your source for books,
journals and multimedia
in the health sciences
www.elsevierhealth.com

The
publisher's
policy is to use
**paper manufactured
from sustainable forests**

Printed in China by RDC Group Limited

Contents

Foreword

Prevention and control of infection are essential cornerstones of clinical care in all healthcare settings. The changing pattern of infection, together with the emergence of bacteria with multiple antibiotic resistance, emphasizes the requirement for all healthcare workers to have a sound knowledge of medical microbiology and a good understanding of infection control evidence-based practices. These are essential and important factors in the delivery of a quality patient-focussed service.

This edition of *Informed Infection Control Practice* discusses the developments and quality initiatives in healthcare that have been implemented in recent times. The inclusion of the chapter on *Knowledge Management* is a welcome addition and will be a valuable resource for all involved in infection control practice. The book is well referenced and uses simple yet clear diagrams to illustrate and clarify particular points highlighted within the text.

This second edition of the book continues to give a comprehensive overview of infection control which should confirm its appeal, relevance and value to all healthcare professionals: undergraduate or postgraduate, in primary, secondary or tertiary settings, and those colleagues wishing to develop, influence and provide support for infection control services in developing countries. The authors have drawn together the essential clinical, laboratory and quality elements of infection control in a language that is readily comprehensible. I am confident that this edition of *Informed Infection Control Practice* will prove to be the essential companion that its predecessor was for all healthcare professionals.

Sheila Morgan, 2002

Preface

With the current government drive to modernize the National Health Service it was appropriate to revisit the book *Informed Infection Control Practice* to ensure the content reflects the aims and goals of the modernization objectives.

This book is divided into two distinct sections: the first section explores the changing nature of infection control in the current political arena, core processes of infection control, management of infection control, knowledge management and infection control in developing countries; the second section is dedicated to essential infection control knowledge and its application to practice.

Infection control incorporates a vast number of topics with some or all being grounded in a number of healthcare disciplines. The chain of infection provides a template for discussion of topics in a structured format. Informed practice demands an insight into all areas in order to understand the complete chain. This book attempts to deliver material relevant to each link to enable the reader to understand how all the links are intricately connected in order to influence the infection outcome in people.

We hope this book becomes a prime resource for all infection control professionals and that it will find its place as a reference text in microbiology departments, wards, GP surgeries, Primary Care Trusts, medical libraries and colleges of nursing. The book should also appeal to healthcare workers abroad, as it provides a framework for the development of infection control practice in any country.

We would like to record here our gratitude to everyone who has helped us, in particular our family and colleagues for encouragement, support, help and patience. We owe a special thank you to Mrs Viv Duncanson, Senior Nurse Infection Control, Northern Lincolnshire and Goole Hospitals NHS Trust; Mrs Sue Ross, Infection Control Nurse, Wakefield and Pontefract Community NHS Trust, for reading the draft text; and a particular thanks to Mrs Diane Thompson, Library Services Manager, Library and Knowledge Management Services, Hull and East Riding Health Authority, for her contributory chapter on Knowledge Management.

We hope that the readers of this book will find both the content and the format suitable for their needs. Readers' feedback and evaluation of whether the book meets colleagues' needs would be welcome, and useful for future editions.

Rozila Horton
Lynn Parker

Harrogate and Sheffield 2002

Section 1
Strategic aspects of infection control

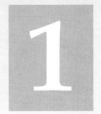

SUMMARY

The last few years have seen a much-needed and welcome interest in and awareness of healthcare-associated infections and infection control. Infection control is now integral to healthcare organizations' risk management (DoH 1993, 1999a), control assurance (National Health Service Executive (NHSE) 1995, 2001) and clinical governance (DoH 1995, 1998, 1999b) strategies. This high level recognition is owed to the following publications:

1. The socio-economic burden of hospital-acquired infection (Plowman et al 2000);
2. The House of Lords Select Committee on Science and Technology Report *Resistance to Antibiotics and Other Antimicrobials* (House of Lords Select Committee on Science and Technology 1998) and the Government's response to this report (DoH 1999c), and *Action for the NHS* (DoH 1999d) and
3. The National Audit Office Report on *The Management and Control of Hospital-acquired Infection in Acute NHS Trusts in England* (National Audit Office (NAO) 2000) and the report of the Auditor General in Scotland (Auditor General 2000).

The media attention that followed these publications helped raise public consciousness to the issue of infections and infection control.

It has to be recognized that, outside of these reports, infection control has always functioned within the constantly changing political and economic structure of the health service. This requires a level of educational preparation as well as a degree of political awareness on the part of all infection control personnel.

INTRODUCTION

This section explores various dimensions that allow infection control to function at a strategic level. These are contained in the following chapters:

Chapter 1 – The changing role of infection control

Chapter 2 – Essential infection control: a framework for practice

Chapter 3 – Management of infection control

Chapter 4 – Knowledge management

The increasing awareness of the struggles faced by infection control colleagues in the developing world are discussed in Chapter 5:

Chapter 5 – Infection control and developing countries

REFERENCES

Auditor General 2000 A clean bill of health. Aduit, Scotland

Department of Health 1993 Risk management in the NHS. National Health Service Management Executive

Department of Health 1999a Corporate governance in the new NHS: controls assurance standards 1999/2000: risk management and organisational controls. HSC1999/23. Available: http://tap.ccta.gov.uk/doh/rm5.nsf/Publications?Open View

Department of Health 1995 Clinical governance in the new NHS. HSC1995/065 Available: http://www.doh.gov.uk/nyro/clingov/links.htm

Department of Health 1998 Guidance on clinical governance MEL (1998) 75. The Scottish Office. Available: http://www.show.scot.nhs.uk/CRAG/TOPICS/CLINGOV/CLINGOV.htm

Department of Health 1999b Clinical governance: in the new NHS HSC1999/065. DoH, London. Available: http://tap.ccta.gov.uk/doh/coin4.nsf

Department of Health 1999c Government's response to the House of Lords Select Committee on Science and Technology 1998. Resistance to antibiotics, and other antimicrobial agents. Cm 4172. DoH, London

Department Health 1999d Resistance to antibiotics, and other antimicrobial agents Action for the NHS following Government's response to the House of Lords Select Committee Inquiry. HSC 1999/049. DoH, London

House of Lords Select Committee on Science and Technology 1998 Resistance to antibiotics, and other antimicrobial agents. (HL Paper 81-1, 7th Report Session, 1997–98). Stationery Office, London

National Audit Office 2000 The management and control of hospital acquired infection in acute NHS Trusts in England. Report by the Controller and Auditor General. Stationery Office, London

National Health Service Executive 1995 Corporate Governance in the NHS: Controls Assurance Statements HSG(97)17. Available: http://tap.ccta.gov.uk/doh/rm5nsf/AdminDocs/CAStandards?OpenDocument

National Health Service Executive (NHSE) Control Assurance Standard in Infection Control 1999 (Revision 02). HMSO, London. Available: http://tap.ccta.gov.uk/doh/rm5.nsf/b7546ce4a0608579002565c4003bf709/9bd9b4beb414923100256a5400615b0b?OpenDocument

Plowman R, Craven N, Griffin M et al. 2000 The socio-economic burden of hospital acquired infection. PHLS, London

The changing role of infection control

SUMMARY

Infection control is evolving rapidly, with quality as the main focus of the service. This chapter considers the issues at the centre of this development and examines the core processes that are needed to deliver a high quality infection control service.

INTRODUCTION

The 21st century sees infection control at its pinnacle. It is now recognized and accepted as a service of importance in all healthcare establishments.

This recognition comes in part from the high-level media attention attracted by recent surveys by the Public Health Laboratory Service entitled *Socio-economic Burden of Hospital-acquired Infection* (Plowman et al 2000), the National Audit Office (NAO) survey report *The Management and Control of Hospital-acquired Infection in Acute NHS Trusts in England* (NAO 2000), and the Auditor General's Report, in Scotland, *A Clean Bill of Health* (Auditor General 2000). These publications highlighted the burden, both economic and human, attributable to infections acquired by patients in hospitals. There is now interest and awareness of, as well as support and commitment for, infection control from health service executives and the government. Infection control is now a high-priority service.

Looking back

Despite the well-documented value of infection control programmes (DHSS 1988, Haley 1986), the profile of infection control remained low until the publication of the reports mentioned above. A possible explanation for this is a lack of awareness on the part of health service executives, who might not have known what infection control personnel do on a daily basis, nor the value of the service to the organization. It is a service that could be seen as costing money to operate, as opposed to helping the organization save money – let alone generate revenue.

Without a systematized surveillance programme and dissemination of data and information, clinicians and managers have little indication of the size of the problem and cost of both preventable and non-avoidable infections within their specialty or organization. There is now a requirement on the part of individual health service organizations to carry out surveillance of bacteraemias, infections of wounds following orthopaedic surgery, and problems of antimicrobial-resistant microbes (DoH 1999a, 2000a,b). This programme will help identify the size of each problem, although its financial impact might not be easily measurable. According to Plowman et al (1997), the costs of infection are distributed amongst hospitals, community services, patients, their families and industry. Several studies have tried to calculate the direct and indirect costs of hospital-acquired infections but their true economic impact on the organization and community at large remains uncertain.

Nevertheless, the reporting of the results of the surveillance programme will help keep clinicians and health service executives firmly in the infection control loop. Infection control is important and should demand everyone's attention and commitment. The 42nd report of the Select Committee on Public Accounts on *The Management and Control of Hospital-acquired Infection in Acute NHS Trusts in England* (Select Committee on Public Accounts 2000) states that 'The NHS do not have a grip on the extent of hospital-acquired infection and the costs involved'.

HOSPITAL-ACQUIRED INFECTIONS

Hospital-acquired infections are infections that are not present or incubating on admission, but are acquired during a hospital stay. These infections can manifest themselves during the stay in hospital or in the period following the hospital stay (Haley 1986).

The latest PHLS/London School of Hygiene survey (Plowman et al 2000), identified around one in 11 hospital patients at any one time as having an infection caught in hospital, suggesting about 9% of inpatients with hospital-acquired infection at any one time; at least 100 000 infections per year. The cost of these infections is placed at around £1 billion each year, although the cost to the patient and family in pain, anxiety and possible prolonged or permanent disability cannot be measured. The key findings of this study, which was carried out in one hospital over a 13-month period, showed:

- 7.8% of patients acquired an infection during their stay in hospital
- A further 19.1% of patients reported symptoms of, and some received treatment for, an infection manifesting post-discharge, which could have been associated with their hospital admission
- Patients with one or more infection incurred costs that were on average 2.8 times higher than uninfected patients; an average additional cost of £2917 per case. The cost ranged from £1122 for urinary tract infections to £6209 for bloodstream infections
- Patients with hospital-acquired infections remained in hospital on average 2.5 times longer than uninfected patients; equivalent to 11 extra days.

A small proportion of deaths each year are primarily attributable to hospital-acquired infection. The Plowman et al (2000) survey indicated that patients with hospital-acquired infections were 7.1 times more likely to die in the hospital than uninfected patients.

The publicity that followed the publication of the Plowman et al (2000) survey and the Report by the Comptroller and Auditor General on the management and control of hospital-acquired infection in acute NHS Trusts in England (NAO 2000) focused on the fact that the number of deaths in the UK due to hospital-acquired infections, approximately 5000, was greater than the number of people killed in road traffic accidents. This figure is presented in the Department of Health's (DoH) guidance on the control of infection in hospitals (DoH/PHLS 1995) and is extrapolated from the findings of prospective hospital studies in the US (Haley 1986). These findings indicated that of those patients who acquire an infection in hospital, 10% will subsequently die in hospital and, therefore, hospital-acquired infection is directly responsible for 10% of hospital deaths, and is a major factor in a further 30%. Based on this American data, hospital-acquired infections in the UK in 1995 were estimated to be the primary cause of, or a major contributor to, death in 1% and 3%, respectively, of all fatalities in hospital (DoH/PHLS 1995).

Preventing hospital-acquired infection

In most instances, the outcome of an infection is governed by patient susceptibility; the very old, very young, those with suppressed immune system and those undergoing invasive procedures are particularly susceptible. It is therefore accepted that not all hospital-acquired infections are preventable, because there is an 'irreducible minimum' (Ayliffe 1986). Based on the American study (Haley et al 1985), DoH guidance from the Hospital Infection Working Group (DoH/PHLS 1995) is that a proportion of hospital-acquired infections are preventable:

It is possible that currently about 30 per cent of hospital-acquired infection could be prevented by better application of existing knowledge and implementation of realistic infection control policies.

The NAO survey report (NAO 2000), places the figure of preventable infections at 15%. This reduction rate of 15% is considered achievable by infection control teams from the 213 Trusts in England that took part in the survey, and puts the potentially avoidable cost at around £150 million a year.

The NAO survey report reiterates that this reduction is possible by better application of existing knowledge and realistic infection control practices. The 'existing' knowledge for safe infection control practice will be discussed in Section 2 of this book.

The delivery of safe infection control practice rests with individual healthcare workers. In considering the NAO (2000) report, the 42nd Report of the Select Committee on Public Accounts writes that:

> A root and branch shift towards prevention will be needed at all levels of the NHS if hospital-acquired infection is to be kept under control. That will require commitment from everyone involved, and a philosophy that prevention is everybody's business, not just the specialist.

Thus the responsibility for infection control is placed equally on health service executives and other members of staff.

Raising the profile

Infection control received an additional boost with the publication of two national priorities guidance documents for the modernization of the NHS (DoH 1998a, 2000b) and Health Service Circular 1999/049 (DoH 1999b). These guidance documents set out an action for the NHS following the government's response (DoH 1999c) to the House of Lords Select Committee Report on Antibiotic Resistance (House of Lords Select Committee on Science and Technology 1997–98). Health authorities, primary care groups, Trusts and NHS Trusts have an obligation to ensure:

> The continuing and effective protection of the public's health, with particular regard to the prevention and control of hospital infection, communicable disease, and antibiotic resistance.

The merging of issues surrounding antimicrobial resistance with those of hospital-acquired infection will help strengthen the profile of infection control in hospitals, as well as in the community.

Such a high-profile service requires resource commitment. Health service executives have the unenviable task of maximizing resources and allocating funds to all the services within the organization. The national priorities guidance documents provide an opportunity for infection control personnel to secure the support and funding needed to meet government objectives but, in order to do this, the core processes and activities of infection control have to be clearly defined.

DEFINING CORE PROCESSES WITHIN THE FRAMEWORK OF QUALITY

Every government initiative since the early 1990s has challenged NHS providers to deliver low-cost, low-risk and high-quality care. 'The new

NHS. modern·dependable' ended the internal market (DoH 1997) and put partnership, quality and performance at the heart of running the NHS. These quality issues are encompassed in government documents on risk management (NHS Executive (NHSE) 1993), clinical governance (DoH 1995, 1998b, 1999d) and controls assurance standards (NHSE 1995). There are 18 national controls assurance standards, including infection control, which cover risk management and organizational controls and are seen as firmly underpinning clinical governance and the government's modernization agenda. The standards provide a new system of quality improvement and, for the first time, a statutory duty of quality on all NHS organizations (DoH 1999d), which now have a statutory duty to seek quality improvements by ensuring that financial control, service performance and clinical quality are fully integrated at all levels (Masterton & Teare 2001). The value and quality elements of infection control activities now have to feature strongly in risk management, clinical governance and control assurance programmes.

The core processes and activities of infection control

The identification of risk factors for infection and the development and implementation of practices and policies to reduce these risks are the foundations of the core processes and activities of infection control. These planned actions, with measurable results, are clearly outlined in the DoH's *Controls Assurance Standard in Infection Control*: 'There is a managed environment, which minimises the risk of infection, to patients, staff and visitors' (NHSE 2001a).

Fifteen criteria support this standard and these are reinforced by the action plan (NHSE 2000), which is designed to strengthen prevention and control of communicable disease and infection control processes. The achievement and measurement of the standard will make infection control an integral part of an organization's risk and quality management programmes, and will help to meet the NHS priorities guidance objectives.

Risk management

Risk management (NHSE 1993, 1999) has been described by Roy (1996) as 'the timely identification and subsequent management of existing risk, in order to protect all parties concerned'. Farrington & Pascoe (2001) define risk management as a proactive approach that:

- identifies risks
- assesses those risks for potential frequency and severity
- eliminates the risks that can be eliminated
- minimizes the effect of those risks that cannot be eliminated.

Partly as a result of an increasing number of litigations and claims for clinical negligence and personal injuries, new regulations were introduced in the mid-1990s demanding a more formal approach to risk management. These included:

- The removal of Crown Immunity Cover. This made the NHS liable to prosecution with regard to the health and safety of staff, patients and visitors and environmental hygiene and food safety.
- The Clinical Negligence Scheme for Trusts (CNST), an insurance scheme designed to assist Trusts in meeting the costs of clinical negligence. Payment to the scheme is calculated on the basis of the level of actual claims and the clinical risk management policy, procedures and standards that are in place (Masterton & Teare 2001). The future discount awards of basic contributions by Trusts are determined by how well the individual Trusts meet these CNST risk management standards (CNST 2000a). Infection control was integrated into the CNST in July 2000 (CNST 2000b).
- The need by the NHS to demonstrate to commercial insurers of non-clinical risks that risks were being managed. This commercial insurance has now been replaced by the NHS non-clinical risk pooling scheme (Wilson 1997). This is a voluntary scheme enabling Trusts and health authorities to pool the cost of settlements each year in return for an annual contribution.
- Increasing awareness and expectations of NHS service users following the publication of *The Patients' Charter* (DoH 1996).
- Introduction of clinical governance and controls assurance guidance, which places the accountability for compliance with the principles of these guidances at Trust board level. Health service executives have to demonstrate formal compliance with the guidance.

Identifying and managing infection risks are essential to the Controls Assurance Standard and, therefore, have become one of the core processes of infection control.

Quality as a core process in infection control

Quality of care at all levels of the NHS is the driving force for the development of the health service (DoH 1998a). The tool to drive quality is clinical governance (DoH 1998b, 1999d). The NHS has a statutory duty to seek quality improvements through clinical governance and to '... transform the delivery of primary, hospital and community care so that consistently better outcomes are produced for patients' DoH 1999d p. 3). Clinical governance is defined as:

> *... a framework through which NHS organisations are accountable for continuously improving the quality of their services and safeguarding high standards of care by creating an environment in which excellence in clinical care will flourish. [DoH 1998c p. 33]*

The local clinical governance structure is responsible for delivering quality care based on clear national standards. The key elements of a clinical governance framework are described as:

> *Clear lines of accountability and responsibility for the quality of clinical care, a comprehensive programme of quality improvement activities, such as clinical*

audit clear policies aimed at managing risk procedures for identifying and remedying poor performance. [DoH 1999d]

The DoH clinical governance document, however, emphasizes the importance of '…moving away from a culture of "blame" to one of learning so that quality infuses all aspects of the organisation's work' (DoH 1999d p. 5).

Infection control: a means to quality improvement

The government's response (DoH 1999c) to the House of Lord's report on antimicrobial resistance states that infection control is at the heart of quality of clinical care. Demonstrating quality through effective risk management is one of the core processes in infection control. There is guidance in England, Wales, Northern Ireland and Scotland (DoH/PHLS 1995, DoH 1998d) on the structures necessary to deliver an effective infection control service but, despite clear data to support the importance of infection control (Emmerson et al 1996), the commitment of senior managers has often been poor. Clinical governance now provides an ideal framework to demonstrate the value of infection control to all healthcare workers; an infection control service is integral to clinical governance.

Educating the workforce – a core process to improve quality

Poor practices result in poor quality care. Apart from a formal programme of surveillance, under clinical governance, infection control services will be judged by infection outcomes in patients. If infection control is everyone's business, all staff members must be educated. The NAO survey report (NAO 2000) considers the provision of effective education and training to be a key measure in the prevention of hospital-acquired infection. Criterion 12 of the Controls Assurance Standard (NHSE 2001a) states 'Education in infection control is provided to all healthcare staff, including those employed in support services'. Included in the criterion is the 'Induction of all new staff as well as a programme of on-going education for existing staff'. Standard 7 of the CNST clinical risk management standard that covers induction, training and competence (CNST 2000a), requires 'management systems in place to ensure the competence and appropriate training of all clinical staff'.

Lifelong learning is considered crucial to clinical governance. Lifelong learning, the DoH states 'will give NHS staff the tools of knowledge to offer the most modern, effective and high quality care to patients' (DoH 1998c p. 9). Education of all healthcare workers about prevention and control, and teaching them ways to incorporate infection prevention and control measures into patient care practices, is a core activity of an effective infection control service.

Policies and procedure development

The production and dissemination of up-to-date infection control policies and procedures remain one of the core activities of infection control service.

The need for every hospital to have written policies, procedures and guidelines for the prevention and control of infection is reaffirmed in the control assurance guidance (NHSE 2001a), which also recommends a regular review of these policies. This is a time-consuming activity and must be identified as such in the business plan. An alternative approach, which avoids every organization developing and reviewing their own policy manual, was put forward in the NAO survey report (NAO 2000), which supports the Scottish Office initiative of a single infection control manual, produced, amended and issued centrally (DoH 1998d). All health boards and hospitals in Scotland are expected to conform to this.

Whether the policies are produced locally or centrally, the infection control team carries the responsibility for ensuring that they fulfill local requirements and are understood by all staff members. This is one of the core processes of an infection control service.

Audit – a core process in quality management

If risk management is integral to infection control, audit is the mechanism for ensuring that risks are identified and managed. The national Controls Assurance Standard in Infection Control (and the criteria contained within this) provides an effective framework to measure achievements and/or to improve performance. Criterion 7 recommends 'an annual programme for the audit of infection control policies and procedures'. The 1995 *Guidance on the Control of Infection in Hospitals* (DoH/PHLS 1995), considers the following to be some of the main components of an effective infection control programme:

- setting and auditing standards of own work
- contributing to the standard-setting and audit processes in other clinical and support services to ensure compliance with infection control policies and procedures, and monitoring of hospital hygiene.

High quality experience for patients is classed as one of the indicators of performance standard (DoH 2000c). However, there is little evidence to suggest that most patients can recognize the quality element of infection prevention and control measures practised; the exception is patients in isolation. Isolation precautions can create stress for patients and their families. An audit of actions to decrease stress can help determine if patients and their families are satisfied with the infection control service. The aspects of an effective service, such as easy-to-understand leaflets, explanation of the reason for isolation, what to expect (e.g. aprons, gloves, masks) and the anticipated duration of isolation, can form an audit of patient satisfaction.

This core process of audit in clinical areas can be very resource intensive, often requiring time from hard-pressed colleagues and leading to resentment. However, clinical managers also have to illustrate risk management and quality improvement as part of their own clinical governance responsibility. Prioritizing audit activities with the help of these senior managers will help overcome many obstacles.

Surveillance

Surveillance is needed to understand the extent, cost and effects of hospital-acquired infection. According to the NAO survey report (NAO 2000), surveillance is the foundation for good infection control practice and improving patient care. The role of surveillance in infection control has been illustrated by the American SENIC study (Haley et al 1985), which showed that hospitals with infection control programmes that included surveillance and feedback of results to clinicians reduced infections by 32%. This is resource intensive and requires careful consideration of the risk and cost of every infection. The DoH directive (DoH 2000a) stipulates monitoring of three types of infection:

- infections of wounds following orthopaedic surgery
- bacterial bloodstream infections
- hospital-acquired infections that become apparent after the patient is discharged from hospital.

The high morbidity and mortality associated with bloodstream infections make these high-risk infections, and the excess cost associated with post-operative joint replacement infections make these high cost infections also.

Miscellaneous core processes of infection control

Numerous other core processes support the infection control programme, including:

- daily monitoring of alert microbes
- implementation of intervention measures such as the isolation precaution system
- outbreak investigation and management
- participation in committees (e.g. infection control, health and safety, risk management, clinical governance, product procurement and evaluation, employee health)
- participation in benchmarking and performance indicator initiatives
- research
- membership of national and regional professional groups
- own professional development.

CONCLUSION

The main message to the health service executives who are responsible for ensuring that there are effective arrangements for infection control within hospitals (as set out in criterion 1 of the Controls Assurance Standard) is that infection control can affect the quality of service given to patients. This argument has to be supported by a strong business case. Quality of infection control care is dependent on risk identification and management. The infection control standards within the Controls Assurance Standard are ideal tools to use to determine the risk that hospital-acquired infection poses for an organization (Wilcox & Dave 2000). A system of audit and surveillance can determine the cost effectiveness of the programme but the health service executives and other stakeholders need to understand the essence of the core processes of infection control if they are to secure both resources and support for infection control services, whether these are in hospitals, community healthcare establishments or the private sector.

REFERENCES

Auditor General 2000 A clean bill of health. Scottish Audit office, Edinburgh

Ayliffe GAJ 1986 Nosocomial infection – the irreducible minimum. Infection Control 7(2):92–95

Clinical Negligence Scheme for Trusts (CNST) 2000a Risk management standards and procedures manual of guidance. CNST, Bristol. Available: http://tap.ccta.gov.uk/doh/rm5.nsf/AdminDocs/CNSTReview?OpenD

Clinical Negligence Scheme for Trust (CNST) 2000b News update. Infection control to be added to CNST assessment. CNST, Bristol

Department of Health (DoH) 1989 Working for patients. HMSO, London

Department of Health (DoH) 1995 Clinical governance in the new NHS (HSC1995/065). Available: http://www.doh.gov.uk/nyro/clingov/links.htm

Department of Health (DoH) 1996 The patients' charter (H51/006 0870 2RP 500K Nov 96(23)EP). HMSO, London. Available: http://www.doh.gov.uk/pcharter/patientc.htm

Department of Health (DoH) 1997 The new NHS. Modern·dependable. HMSO, London

Department of Health (DoH) 1998a Modernising health and social services: national priorities guidance for 1999/00–2001/02. HMSO, London

Department of Health (DoH) 1998b Guidance on clinical governance (MEL(1998)75). The Scottish Office, Edinburgh. Available: http://www.show.scot.nhs.uk/CRAG/TOPICS/CLINGOV/CLINGOV.htm

Department of Health (DoH) 1998c A first class service: quality in the new NHS. HMSO, London

Department of Health (DoH) 1998d Scottish infection manual. Guidance on core standards for control of infection in hospitals, health care premises and the community interface. The Scottish Office, Edinburgh

Department of Health (DoH) 1999a Hospital-acquired infection: a framework for a national system of surveillance for the NHS in Scotland. The Scottish Office, Edinburgh

Department of Health (DoH) 1999b Resistance to antibiotics and other antimicrobial agents – action for the NHS following government's response to the House of Lords Select Committee Enquiry (HSC 1999/049). HMSO, London

Department of Health (DoH) 1999c Government's response to the House of Lords Select Committee on Science and Technology Report: resistance to antibiotics, and other antimicrobial agents (Cm 4172). HMSO, London

Department of Health (DoH) 1999d Clinical governance: in the new NHS (HSC 1999/065). HMSO, London. Available: http://tap.ccta.gov.uk/doh/coin4.nsf

Department of Health (DoH) 2000a All hospitals to monitor hospital-acquired infection (2000/0584). HMSO, London

Department of Health (DoH) 2000b Modernising health and social services: national priorities guidance 2000/01–2002/03. HMSO, London

Department of Health (DoH) 2000c The NHS plan. HMSO, London

Department of Health and Social Security (DHSS) 1988 Hospital infection control. Guidance on the control of infection in hospitals, prepared by the Joint DHSS/PHLS Hospital Infection Working Group. HMSO, London

Department of Health/Public Health Laboratory Service (DoH/PHLS) 1995 Hospital infection control. Guidance on the control of infection in hospitals (prepared by the Hospital Infection Working Group of the Department of Health & Public Health Laboratory Service). HMSO, London

Emmerson AM, Enstone JE, Griffin M, Kelsey MC, Smyth ETM 1996 The second national prevalence survey of infections in hospitals – an overview of results. Journal of Hospital Infection 32:175–190

Farrington M, Pascoe G 2001 Risk management and infection control – time to get our priorities right in the United Kingdom. Journal of Hospital Infection 47:19–24

Haley RW 1986 Managing hospital infection control for cost-effectiveness: a strategy for reducing infectious complications. American Hospital Publishing, Chicago, IL

Haley RW, Culver DH, White JW et al 1985 The efficacy of infection surveillance programs in preventing nosocomial infections in US hospitals. American Journal of Epidemiology 121:182–205

House of Lords Select Committee on Science and Technology Report. Resistance to antibiotics, and other antimicrobial agents. House of Lords 7th Report, 1997–98. HMSO, London

Masterton RG, Teare EL 2001 Clinical governance and infection control in the United Kingdom. Journal of Hospital Infection 47:25–31

National Audit Office (NAO) 2000 The management and control of hospital-acquired infection in acute NHS Trusts in England. NAO, London

National Health Service Executive (NHSE) 1993 Risk management in the NHS. HMSO, London

National Health Service Executive (NHSE) 1995 Corporate governance in the NHS: controls assurance statements (HSG(97)17). Available: http://tap.ccta.gov.uk/doh/rm5.nsf/AdminDocs/CAStandards?OpenDocument

National Health Service Executive (NHSE) 1999 Corporate governance in the new NHS: controls assurance standards 1999/2000: Risk management and organisational controls. HSC 1999/23. HMSO, London. Available: http://tap.ccta.gov.uk/doh/rm5.nsf/Publications?Open View

National Health Service Executive (NHSE) 2000 The management and control of hospital infection. Action for the NHS for the management and control of infection in hospitals in England (HSC 2000/002). HMSO, London

National Health Service Executive (NHSE) 2001a Controls assurance standard in infection control 1999 (Rev 02). HMSO, London. Available: http://tap.ccta.gov.uk/doh/rm5.nsf/b7546ce4a0608579002565c4003bf709/9bd9b4beb414923100256a5400615b0b?OpenDocument

Plowman RM et al 1997 Hospital acquired infection. Office of Health Economics, London

Plowman RM et al 2000 The socio-economic burden of hospital acquired infection. PHLS, London

Roy S 1996 Risk management. Nursing Standard 10(18):50–56

Select Committee on Public Accounts 2000 Forty-second report on the management and control of hospital-acquired infection in acute NHS Trusts in England. HMSO, London

Wilcox MH, Dave J 2000 The cost of hospital-acquired infection and value of infection control. Journal of Hospital Infection 45:81–84

Wilson J 1997 The clinical negligence scheme for trusts. British Journal of Nursing 6:1166–1167

Essential infection control: a framework for practice

2

■ CONTENTS

SUMMARY

The fundamental principle of infection control is the creation and mainten-ance of a safe environment, which ensures the safety of patients, their relatives and healthcare workers. The practice of infection control demands knowledge, skills and attitudes appropriate to each situation. The identifi-cation of the what, when and how of practice rests with the infection control personnel, who are responsible for developing a framework for infection control practice, be it writing policies and protocols, provision of education to ensure safe care or producing data showing rates of infection. Both man-agers and practitioners rely on these individuals to provide them with expertise and a learned platform from which to draw advice and guidance. This chapter examines the role and contribution of individuals who are charged with this function.

INTRODUCTION

The core business of an infection control service is to identify and manage risks of infection to patients, staff and visitors. The outcome of the service contributes to an organization's overall strategy for delivering low-risk, high-quality care. It is essential to achieving the Department of Health (DoH) objectives set out in the National Priorities Guidance 1999/00–2001/02 and 2000/01–2001/03 (DoH 1998a, 2000).

The high profile afforded to infection control is illustrated in the DoH publication *Guidance on the Control of Infection in Hospital*, which was released as DoH policy on infection control (DoH/PHLS 1995) and as an infection manual in Scotland (Scottish Office Department of Health (SODH) 1998). This guidance placed the responsibility for ensuring that effective infection control arrangements are in place, and are subject to regular review, on the chief executive of every NHS Trust. It makes infection control a core management responsibility.

INFECTION CONTROL MANAGEMENT FRAMEWORK

The key management forum for infection control within NHS Trusts is the Infection Control Committee (ICC). The day-to-day issues are addressed by the Infection Control Team (ICT), which has a primary responsibility for all aspects of surveillance, prevention and control of infection. The ICT consists of infection control nurses (ICNs) and practitioners, and infection control doctors (ICDs). The roles and responsibilities of each practitioner, including the Consultant in Communicable Disease Control (CCDC) and Consultant in Public Health Medicine (CPHM), are addressed in the guidance documents mentioned above (DoH/PHLS 1995, SODH 1998).

The infection control committee (ICC)

The operational duties of the ICC include:

- endorsing all infection control policies, procedures and guidelines
- supporting the implementation of policies
- participating in the development of the annual infection control programme and monitoring its progress.

The membership of the ICC is usually (Fig. 2.1):

- the ICT
- a representative of the Chief Executive Officer
- occupational health personnel
- senior clinical representative(s)
- the CDCC (this would be the CPHM in Scotland) (SODH 1998)
- other identified representatives.

The key components of infection control

The DoH guidance document and SODH infection manual (DoH/PHLS 1995, SODH 1998) identify the main components and principal objectives of an effective infection control programme as:

- surveillance of infection
- education and training of staff
- production, review and dissemination of written policies, procedures and guidelines

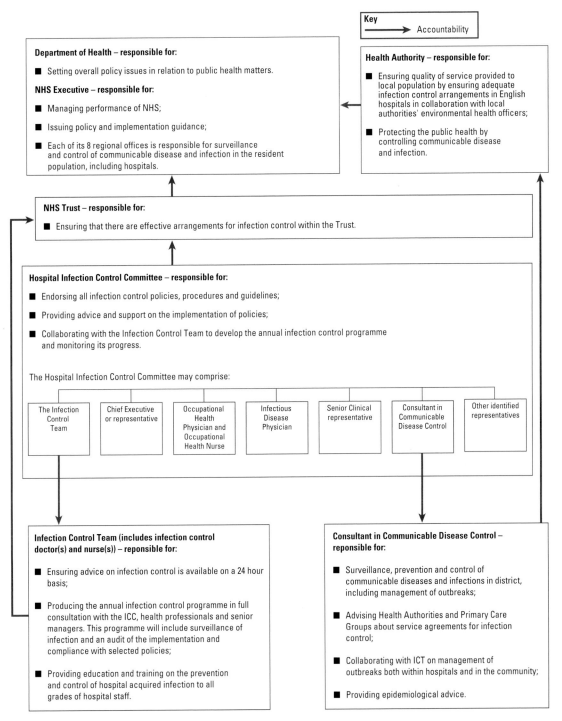

Key
——→ Accountability

Department of Health – responsible for:

■ Setting overall policy issues in relation to public health matters.

NHS Executive – responsible for:

■ Managing performance of NHS;

■ Issuing policy and implementation guidance;

■ Each of its 8 regional offices is responsible for surveillance and control of communicable disease and infection in the resident population, including hospitals.

Health Authority – responsible for:

■ Ensuring quality of service provided to local population by ensuring adequate infection control arrangements in English hospitals in collaboration with local authorities' environmental health officers;

■ Protecting the public health by controlling communicable disease and infection.

NHS Trust – responsible for:

■ Ensuring that there are effective arrangements for infection control within the Trust.

Hospital Infection Control Committee – responsible for:

■ Endorsing all infection control policies, procedures and guidelines;

■ Providing advice and support on the implementation of policies;

■ Collaborating with the Infection Control Team to develop the annual infection control programme and monitoring its progress.

The Hospital Infection Control Committee may comprise:

| The Infection Control Team | Chief Executive or representative | Occupational Health Physician and Occupational Health Nurse | Infectious Disease Physician | Senior Clinical representative | Consultant in Communicable Disease Control | Other identified representatives |

Infection Control Team (includes infection control doctor(s) and nurse(s)) – reponsible for:

■ Ensuring advice on infection control is available on a 24 hour basis;

■ Producing the annual infection control programme in full consultation with the ICC, health professionals and senior managers. This programme will include surveillance of infection and an audit of the implementation and compliance with selected policies;

■ Providing education and training on the prevention and control of hospital acquired infection to all grades of hospital staff.

Consultant in Communicable Disease Control – reponsible for:

■ Surveillance, prevention and control of communicable diseases and infections in district, including management of outbreaks;

■ Advising Health Authorities and Primary Care Groups about service agreements for infection control;

■ Collaborating with ICT on management of outbreaks both within hospitals and in the community;

■ Providing epidemiological advice.

Source: Department of Health

Figure 2.1 Responsibilities in the NHS in relation to hospital-acquired infection. (After The Management and Control of Hospital Acquired Infection in Acute Trusts in England 2001, with permission of National Audit Office.)

- setting and auditing standards of own work and participating in standard-setting and auditing of other services of the organization to ensure compliance with infection control policies and procedures
- monitoring aspects of a safe environment
- contributing in decision making with regard to equipment purchase, external contract tendering, building and alterations of structures
- management of infections, outbreaks, targeted screening and isolation of patients.

The operational framework for infection control service is encompassed in the *Standards in Infection Control in Hospitals*, developed and issued in 1993 by the Infection Control Standards Working Group comprising the Association of Medical Microbiologists (AMM), Hospital Infection Society (HIS), Infection Control Nurses Association (ICNA) and Public Health Laboratory Service (PHLS). A new document *Standards in Infection Control in Acute NHS Trusts* was issued, under the aegis of the Department of Health, in November 1999 as the Controls Assurance Standard in Infection Control (NHSE 2001a).

Controls assurance standard

Controls assurance is a process whereby the NHS Trust boards can assure the public that the Trust operates an effective system of internal control covering key risks. The controls assurance standard operates within the core risk management standard:

> *A risk management system is in place which conforms with the generic principles contained in AS/NZS 4360:1999, and meets NHS and other requirements in respect of managing risks, hazards, incidents, complaints and claims. [NHSE 2001b]*

The core risk management standard requires the chief executive officer to sign a controls assurance statement to accompany the annual report.

The first controls assurance standard in infection control has been produced for acute hospital Trusts; the standard for community and primary care settings will follow in due course. The essence of the standard, however, applies to all healthcare situations – in hospitals as well as community settings. The standard states that 'There is a managed environment, which minimises the risk of infection, to patients, staff and visitors' (NHSE 2001a).

Fifteen criteria, which accompany the standard, reflect the components identified in the original 1993 standards. These criteria include:

- management structures and responsibilities
- education and training
- policies and procedures
- microbiology service
- surveillance.

These criteria form the basis of the programme of action, which is set out in the Health Circular HSC 2000/002 (NHSE 2000). The programme of action aims to meet the DoH objectives set out in the National Priorities Guidance

1999/00–2001/02 (DoH 1998a) and 2000/01–2001/03 (DoH 2000). One of its main objectives is to 'strengthen prevention and control of communicable diseases and infection control processes' (DoH 1998a).

Other controls assurance standards that strengthen the infection control service include decontamination of medical devices (NHSE 2001c), catering and food hygiene (NHSE 2001d) and waste management (NHSE 2001e).

Infection control professionals

The day-to-day responsibility for implementing infection control programmes rests with infection control professionals. These include infection control nurses (ICNs) and infection control doctors (ICDs). In most organizations ICNs are full time infection control practitioners, whereas ICDs invariably have other clinical responsibilities, usually as a consultant microbiologist.

The infection control nurse (ICN)

The role of the ICN has evolved since the appointment of the first nurse to undertake infection control responsibility (Bradbeer et al 1966, Gardner et al 1962, Moore 1969). There has been a gradual transition from 'on the job' training by the ICD to a dedicated and structured educational framework and an established professional body, the Infection Control Nurses Association (ICNA).

Educational framework for ICNs

The initial educational preparation of ICNs started at certificate level courses in infection control nursing. Three courses were accredited by the Joint Board of Clinical Nursing Studies (JBCNS) in the 1970s:

- course 326 (level 1) in 1974 (JBCNS 1974)
- a shorter course 910 in 1977, entitled 'Principles of Infection Control Nursing' (JBCNS 1977)
- a longer part-time foundation course in infection control nursing, course 329, in 1979 (JBCNS 1979). This course was designed to prepare newly appointed ICNs in the basic skills and knowledge of infection control.

The names of the courses changed to ENB 910 and ENB 329 when the JBCNS was replaced by the English Board for Nursing, Midwifery and Health Visiting (see ENB 1987, 1995a for details of the courses). Similar courses also exist in Scotland (ICNA 1998).

In 1986, the United Kingdom Central Council for Nursing, Midwifery and Health Visiting (UKCC) introduced Project 2000 – 'A New Preparation for Practice' – which was designed to raise the minimum educational level of pre-registration nurses. These changes reflected the education and training requirements specified in working paper 10 of *Working for Patients* (NHSME 1989). The schools of nursing moved to universities and the level of nurse training changed from that of certificate to a Diploma in Nursing.

Inevitably, this demanded a higher level of academic learning for registered nurses. Infection control nurses are now prepared at diploma, honours degree and master's degree level (Jenner & Wilson 2000).

Infection control nurses as specialist practitioners

The specialist practitioner was defined by the UKCC (1994a) as a practitioner who will:

> ... demonstrate higher levels of clinical decision making and will be able to monitor and improve standards of care through supervision of practice, clinical audit, the provision of skilled professional leadership and the development of practice through research, teaching and the support of professional colleagues.

ICNs with the ENB 329 qualification easily demonstrate the above characteristics. However, the changes in the professional registrable status of courses invalidated ENB 329 as a recordable qualification on the UKCC professional register (UKCC 1994b). The registering bodies – UKCC and the Scottish National Board (NBS) – now stipulate an academic degree to register as a specialist nurse practitioner (UKCC 1996, NBS/SCIEH 1999).

Infection control nurse consultant

In 1999, the British Prime Minister announced a plan to create nurse consultant posts in the NHS (DoH 1999a). This was part of the vision outlined in *Making a Difference: Strengthening the Nursing, Midwifery and Health Visiting Contribution to Health and Healthcare* (NHSE 1999a). The aim was to '...help provide better outcomes for patients by improving services and quality, to strengthen leadership and to provide a new career opportunity' (NHSE 1999b). The key component of the role, working through local arrangements for clinical governance, is to take responsibility for:

- promoting evidence-based practice
- setting, monitoring and auditing standards
- identifying measures to secure and evaluate quality improvement.

The principles for creating this consultant post (NHSE 1999b) emphasize leadership and change management skills of the highest order and a portfolio of career-long learning, experience and formal education, usually up to or beyond master's degree level. With regard to the professional accreditation, evidence of significant post-registration development in the relevant field and completion of a programme of study recordable with and approved by the UKCC is needed. The UKCC standard for a 'higher level of practice' is a suggested means of professional recognition. The qualification for a higher level of practice includes a relevant programme of study at a minimum of degree level and an equally relevant level of expertise (UKCC 1998, 1999a).

Role development and its relation to educational preparation

The role development in infection control progresses from role identification to becoming a change agent and finally assuming an advisory/consultancy

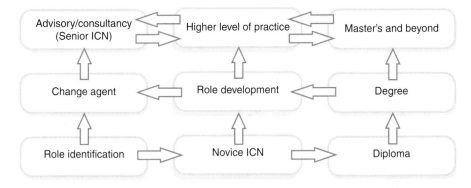

Figure 2.2 Ideal educational preparation for senior ICNs.

role. This role development structure can be easily married with the core functions of a nurse consultant as defined in NHSE (1999b). The functions are described as:

- an expert practice function
- a professional leadership and consultancy function
- an education, training and development function
- a practice and service development, research and evaluation function (NHSE 1999b).

The functions specified above are already integral to the role of a senior ICN, who must 'display leadership and change management skills of the highest order' (NHSE 1999b) in order to deliver an effective service. It can be argued that, for these qualities to be recognized within the framework of clinical governance, and to accord the professional standing deserved by the post, advanced learning as specified in a 'higher level of practice' programme (UKCC 1998, 1999a) is necessary for all higher-grade posts, whether the ICN wishes to be considered for a nurse consultant post or not (Fig. 2.2).

Competencies

Qualities of leadership and change management skills, plus the ability to deliver the above functions, have to be documented as evidence. This requires an assessment of clinical competencies. Assessment of clinical competencies is a requirement in all post-registration training courses and will form part of the new career framework for nurses (ENB 1995b, NHSE 1999b). The Glasgow group of the Scottish Group of Infection Control Nurses Association (ICNASG 2000) has developed areas of competency that are designed to be completed in association with the National Board of Nursing, Midwifery and Health Visiting for Scotland (NBS) portfolio route to enhanced competence (NBS 2000a) and embrace a framework for quality-assuring professional development in NHS Trusts in Scotland (NBS 2000b). The ICNA education sub-committee (ICNA 2000) has now produced the professional core competencies for ICNs and a document depicting a method of self-audit by ICNs is available. This will provide the practitioner, as well as

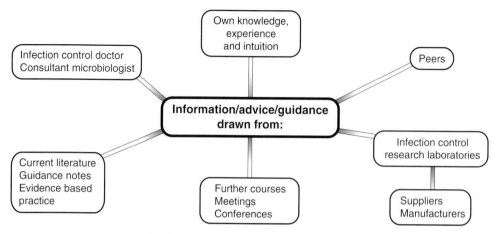

Figure 2.3 Sources of expertise for the infection control nurse.

the management, with evidence of how well the individual is meeting these clinical competencies.

The professional core competencies are divided into five domains and include key criteria designed to identify the elements of knowledge and practice necessary to meet each competency. The domains include:

- specialist knowledge of microbiology, immunology and epidemiology
- application of knowledge to practice and decontamination
- evidence-based practice: using research in practice and using audit to improve quality through audit skills and surveillance
- teaching and learning: facilitating learning in others by sharing knowledge, learning through appraisal and self-learning for professional development
- management, leadership and clinical research.

These competencies are acquired through formal education, lifelong learning opportunities (both formal and informal) and from practical experience and intuition (Fig. 2.3).

Evidence-based practice

Evidence-based practice remains one of the cornerstones of infection control practice. The classic example is Semmelweis's work (1861), which established a link between unwashed hands and cross-transmission of microbes resulting in puerperal sepsis in women following childbirth. Often, the evidence of and for best practice in infection control emerges from research studies, observation and, in many instances, adverse incidents. The evidence is not always clear-cut and it tends to differ between studies. This is overcome by identifying the strength of evidence as specified in the categories quoted in the revised guidelines for the control of methicillin-resistant *Staphylococcus aureus* (MRSA) infection in hospitals (Working Party Report 1998). These are based on the American guidelines for isolation precautions

(Garner 1996) and are described as:

- Strongly recommended and strongly supported by well-designed experimental or epidemiological studies
- Strongly recommended and viewed as effective by experts in the field and has achieved consensus of relevant professional bodies. The guidelines are based on a strong rationale and suggestive evidence, although definite scientific studies are not available
- No recommendation. An unresolved issue or there is insufficient evidence or consensus regarding efficiency.

A detailed discussion of the arguments for and against what can be classed as evidence-based practice in infection control is provided by Ayliffe (2000).

National evidence-based guidelines from the epic Project

The development of new national standards is one of the approaches identified by the DoH to improve quality of care (DoH 1999c). According to Grimshaw et al (1995), national guidelines can change clinical practice and lead to improvement in patient outcome.

The DoH has commissioned and funded a nurse-led multiprofessional project to develop national evidence-based guidelines for preventing healthcare-associated infections (The *epic* Project 2001). The group developing the guidelines is based at the Thames Valley University. The project describes evidence-based guidelines as:

> *Systematically developed broad statements (principles) of good practice which are driven by practice need, based on evidence and subject to multiprofessional debate, timely and frequent review, and modification.*

The process of producing nationally agreed, evidence-based and authoritative guidelines includes:

- reviewing national and international guidelines to extract key statements
- generating areas of importance for which a systematic search of the literature can then be carried out
- reviewing literature and the references from the original guidelines
- assessing and categorizing the quality of evidence
- an expert review of this technical assessment by members of a multidisciplinary professional panel.

In January 2001, the *epic* Project released three sets of guidelines:

- guidelines dealing with standard principles of environmental hygiene, hand hygiene, personal protective equipment and sharps
- guidelines for preventing infections associated with the insertion and maintenance of short-term indwelling urethral catheters in acute care
- guidelines for preventing infections associated with the insertion and maintenance of central venous catheters.

It is suggested that these guidelines can assist practitioners and managers to achieve sound clinical governance. The guidance also includes an implementation protocol (The *epic* Project 2001 pp. S69–S74).

Infection control practice through link practitioners

The implementation of evidence-based guidelines requires managerial and professional support and adherence by individual practitioners to guidance (The *epic* Project 2001). Many ICTs have introduced infection control link nurses (ICLN) within their Trusts to enhance infection control practice (Horton 1988). These are ward-based staff with sufficient clinical experience and standing to have authority with managers and colleagues. The link nurse programme allows both ICNs and ICLNs to work together to:

- identify the infection control educational requirement for staff in an individual workplace
- implement safe measures immediately on recognition of infection or patient susceptibility
- examine outbreaks of infection to establish avoidable and non-preventable elements of the outbreak
- evaluate the care given to patients with a hospital-acquired infection
- identify good practice and commend staff
- recognize aspects of care that could have been tackled differently, for future reference
- investigate outbreaks of infection without producing negative reactions amongst colleagues
- develop a programme of audit of knowledge and practice.

The concept of a link/liaison nurse system has been found to be very effective in raising infection control profile and changing practice in clinical areas (Teare & Peacock 1996). They become a good resource for their own work colleagues and a valuable asset to the ICT.

Preparation of link nurses for practice

The programme for ICLN role preparation varies from locally organized courses to an ENB-validated course (ENB 1995a).

The ENB has described the link nurse scheme as providing 'an excellent example of a partnership approach to clinical effectiveness' (ENB 2000). However, the success of these training programmes in equipping ICLNs to influence clinical effectiveness or change practice is difficult to judge. Cooper (2001) argues against a traditional model of link nurse training, stating that it does not 'encourage staff to explore attitudes and deeply held beliefs' and suggesting that implementing change requires the necessary clinical skills, knowledge and appropriate attitudes. A programme of role preparation should instead allow the ICLNs to explore their own attitudes in relation to topics that are of relevance to them. Cooper suggests a collaborative process involving both ICNs and ICLNs, where students are treated as equals in the learning partnership with the ICNs facilitating the learning process (Hinchcliff 1998). This approach is considered suitable because ICLNs are usually experienced nurses who attend the programme because they have an interest in infection control and have areas of practice they wish to learn more about. Cooper suggests that:

- ICLNs should have influence over the course curriculum so that their own personal learning needs are met
- The programme should include a system of 'guided inquiry' with the ICN guiding the ICLNs to topics and issues of importance and providing relevant information. The ICLNs should be supported as they select and explore the topic of interest
- This process will allow the ICLNs to feel ownership of the topic
- The resulting curriculum will have been designed by both parties.

Other important topics for inclusion in the programme include reflective practice and management of change (Cooper 2001).

Additional factors, which are thought to make the link nurse programme effective in clinical practice, are:

- a relatively stable workforce
- a hospital on a small number of sites
- ICLNs with recognized authority
- Allocation of time to attend meetings and training sessions (NAO 2000).

ICNs as educators

Provision of education and training is one of the main components of an effective infection control programme (DoH/PHLS 1995). An NAO report (NAO 2000), considers the provision of effective education and training to be a key measure in the prevention of hospital-acquired infection.

Criterion 12 of the Controls Assurance Standard in Infection Control states: 'Education in infection control is provided to all health care staff, including those employed in support services'. This is a huge mandate for the ICNs and ICDs. However, the standard does not place the sole responsibility for infection control education on the ICT. ICLNs and similar representatives from other professions allied to medicine can take on an educator's role. Nurses and other professionals undergo a programme of preparation for practice, and knowledge and skills in infection control practice should form an integral part of the curriculum for all healthcare professionals.

A collaborative approach to developing competency-based learning for nurses and midwives is the essence of the Peach Report (UKCC 1999b). The ICNA education sub-committee has produced recommendations for competence in infection control practice at key stages in pre-registration nurse education and training. Similar competences need to be recommended in education and training programmes for all healthcare professionals.

Infection control education through information technology

In most healthcare organizations, a percentage of the workforce will have received inadequate or inappropriate infection control education or training (Horton 1993). Addressing this gap can be resource intensive. Information technology offers a new way of delivering knowledge and skills both in educational establishments and clinical areas. A number of CD-ROMs and computer-assisted packages in infection control are now available. According to the NAO report (NAO 2000), these offer a cost-effective way of addressing weaknesses in training and education.

ICNs as expert witnesses

Expert witnesses are 'professionals who are recognized as experts in their field' (Carson & Montgomery 1989, Dimond 1995, Tingle & Cribb 1995) and ICNs, as specialists in their field, might be called upon to act as expert witnesses.

Two recent changes have been introduced by The Lord Chief Justice, Lord Woolf (Office of the Lord Chief Justice 1996) with regard to expert witnesses (Friston 1999):

1. Clinical experts will be appointed jointly instead of by one side or the other. This might be done either with both parties' agreement or at the direction of the court. Thus, the function of the expert witnesses changes from that of advancing the case of the side paying their fee to being responsible to, and helping, the court by being a 'neutral giver of opinions'. There are, however, provisions in the rules for both sides to use their own expert witness.

2. The clinical experts will be required to set out both their own professional views as well as those of any other 'relevant recognized body of opinion'.

Expert witnesses give factual and own-opinion evidence on the standard of care that a patient could have expected to receive. Standards of care are measured by the Bolam principle:

> When you get a situation which involves the use of some special skill or competence, then the test as to whether there has been negligence or not is ... the standard of the ordinary skilled man exercising and professing to have that special skill. [Bolam v. Friern Barnet Hospital Management Committee (1957) 2 All ER 118]

The standard that applies is the standard at the time that the incident occurred.

To meet the Bolam principle, the following criteria have to be answered:

- Was the situation forseeable?
- What were the indicators that the patient was at risk?
- How should the assessment have been carried out and by whom?
- What reasonable preventive action should have been taken?
- Who was responsible for the allocation of staff to ensure this action was taken?
- Were staff allocated?
- Could tests have been carried out as an additional measure?
- If all the above measures had been taken, would the 'problem' have been reasonably prevented?

- Once the 'problem' had been noted (e.g. infection, pressure ulcer), what action could have been taken to prevent deterioration and ensure the healing process?
- What was the recommended procedure?
- Who was responsible for ensuring that appropriate action was taken?

The expert witness will need to produce a clear, succinct report that defines the issues clearly and is based on a detailed reading of the literature surrounding the subject being considered by the court.

The infection control doctor (ICD)

Infection Control Doctors (ICDs), initially known as Control of Infection Officers, were first appointed following Ministry of Health advice on the control of staphylococcal infections in hospital (MoH 1959). In the UK, most ICDs are consultant microbiologists who spend part of their time in infection control activity. It is recommended that 50% of a consultant microbiologist's time should be spent on infection control (NAO 2000).

Educational preparation

The official infection control guidance in the UK (DoH/PHLS 1995, SODH 1998), recommends that ICDs should be trained in all aspects of hospital infection control, including epidemiology. As yet, there is no requirement for formal qualifications in infection control for ICDs. Instead, the knowledge and skills gained by microbiologists in their training for membership of The Royal College of Pathologists (RCP) is relied upon (Jenner & Wilson 2000), together with the experience gained working alongside the existing ICDs and ICNs (RCP 1998). The need to create a formal education programme in infection control for ICDs is now recognized and has resulted in the development of a diploma course in hospital infection control (Emmerson et al 1997, Masterton 1999).

Performance indicators in infection control

In addition to new national guidelines and dependable local delivery, improved monitoring and performance assessment is considered an important aspect of improving quality (DoH 1999b). The use of indicators is suggested as a means by which the NHS measures its performance in order to improve the service it provides.

An infection control service can be encompassed in two of the six areas covered in the Performance Assessment Framework (DoH 1999d). These are 'delivering effective healthcare' and 'health outcomes'. The commitment of the infection control service to improve quality is identified in criterion 13 of the Controls Assurance in Infection Control (NHSE 2001a):

> Key indicators capable of showing improvement in infection control and/or providing early warning of risk at all levels of the organisation, including the Board, and the efficacy and usefulness of the indicators is reviewed regularly.

Two levels of measurements are embedded in this criterion: performance of the service and effectiveness of risk management.

Types of indicator

The essence of various key indicators that can be used in the NHS is identified in a recent document by a working group comprising members of the Hospital Infection Society (HIS), the Infection Control Nurse's Association (ICNA), the Association of Medical Microbiologists (AMM) and the DoH (HIS, ICNA, AMM, DoH 2001). These are:

- *Structure indicators*: define organizational compliance with internal policies and guidelines that reflect statutory requirements
- *Process indicators*: define the methods used by workers within the organization to follow these internal rules and guidelines, such as how they acquire the knowledge about the rules and guidelines and how these are applied to practice
- *Outcome indicators*: define a link between a risk indicator and the progress of the patients. This allows the measurement of performance against certain standards. Examples include urinary tract infection in catheterized patients and surgical site infections in clean surgery.

The Audit Commission suggests that the information collected as part of indicator measurement can help assess progress towards achieving the organization's corporate objectives (Audit Commission 2000). It puts forward six principles to be considered when undertaking indicator measurement:

1. Clarity of purpose – who will use the information and how and why it will be used. This suggests that the indicators should be devised to help stakeholders make better decisions
2. The performance measurement system should focus the information on the priorities of the organization, its core objectives and areas in need of improvement
3. The performance measurement system should be linked with the objective-setting and performance review processes
4. The indicators should provide a balanced picture of the organization's performance. They should also reflect a balance between the cost of collecting the indicator and the value of information provided
5. The indicators should be refined on a regular basis to meet changing circumstances. A balance should be kept between having consistent information to monitor changes in performance over time, taking advantage of new improved data and reflecting current priorities
6. The indicators should be robust enough for their intended use. An independent scrutiny, internal or external, is recommended.

Regardless of whether criterion 13 of the Controls Assurance Standard in infection control is measured against national priorities or against the identification and management of infection risks at a local level, it needs to be linked with the organization's own risk management and clinical governance process.

Vested interests in achieving high performance

Support and commitment for achieving an effective infection control programme can come from stakeholders with vested interests. For instance:

- surgeons, operating room personnel and health service managers interested in preventing surgical wound infection
- physicians and staff in critical care units committed to preventing ventilator-associated pneumonia.

A successful outcome is as much a desire for these professionals as for the infection control personnel.

Other interested parties include individuals with an overall responsibility for risk management and clinical governance, who can often become champions or ardent supporters of the programme and increase the opportunity for success.

Colleague cooperation for achieving high level performance

Improvement in performance is achieved through work colleagues at every level of organization, although enlisting their support and commitment is often an uphill struggle. Apart from giving them a knowledge-base to deliver safe care, it is often necessary to use powers of persuasion. In a survey by Raven & Haley (1982), ICNs were asked to rate different categories of power that could be used to influence change in the behaviour of a nurse who 'repeatedly breaks technique and exposes patients to a high risk of infection'. The six categories of power were:

1. Coercive power: warning of possible disciplinary action or dismissal
2. Reward power: reminding of the influence carried by the ICN, which could be advantageous to the nurse's future
3. Legitimate power: emphasizing the ICN's position and the nurse's obligation to comply
4. Referent power: emphasizing that proper procedures are followed by other nurses in the hospital
5. Expert power: emphasizing the ICN's own expertise regarding infection control procedures
6. Information power: indicating the reason for infection control techniques, e.g. evidence, researches, available literature.

Information, expert and referent powers gained the majority support.

Another power, which places the responsibility on every individual, is the demand for healthcare workers to define the effectiveness of their own contribution to patient care.

Achieving essential infection control

National reports and government guidance help create a high profile for the infection control service but unless suitably resourced, the service cannot deliver. The minimum resource should include:

- a consultant microbiologist able to dedicate at least 50% of his or her time to infection control and, hopefully, with appropriate infection control training
- sufficient ICNs to reflect the changing nature of the work
- computers and office space
- strong clerical support
- educational textbooks and subscriptions to professional journals
- allocated funds and time to acquire appropriate qualifications and attend meetings, seminars and conferences.

CONCLUSION

Complex, organization-wide systems and personnel from many departments contribute to processes of care that reduce the risk of clinically acquired infections. These personnel own the processes of care but need help from the infection control staff to incorporate infection prevention measures into them. The time spent building relationships can affect the amount of active participation from colleagues in all areas of the organization in infection prevention efforts.

A good relationship is also needed with clinical managers, financial experts, educationalists and colleagues at the coalface, who also have much to offer.

REFERENCES

Audit Commission 2000 Management paper on targeting the practice of performance indicators. Audit Commission, London

Ayliffe GAJ 2000 Evidence-based practices in infection control. British Journal of Infection Control 1(2):5–9

Bradbeer TL et al 1966 Duties and status of an infection control sister in the Exeter Hospital Group. Monthly Bulletin Health & PHLS 25:269–276

Carson D, Montgomery J 1989 Nursing and the law. Macmillan Press, London

Cooper T 2001 Educational theory into practice: development of an infection control link nurse programme. Nurse Education in Practice 1:35–41

Department of Health (DoH) 1998a Modernising health and social services: National Priorities Guidance 1999/00–2001/02. DoH, London

Department of Health (DoH) 1998b A first class service: quality in the new NHS. HMSO, London

Department of Health (DoH) 1999a Making a difference. HMSO, London

Department of Health (DoH) 1999b Improving quality and performance in the new NHS: clinical indicators and high level performance indicators (HSC 1999/139). HMSO, London. Available: http://www.doh.gov.uk/indicat.htm

Department of Health (DoH) 1999c The new NHS. Modern · dependable. HMSO, London

Department of Health (DoH) 1999d Performance assessment framework in the NHS (HSC 1999/78). DoH, London

Department of Health (DoH) 2000 Modernising health and social services: National Priorities Guidelines 2000/01–2002/03. DoH, London

Department of Health/Public Health Laboratory Service (DoH/PHLS) 1995 Hospital infection control. Guidance on the control of infection in hospitals (HSG(95)10). DoH, London

Dimond B 1995 Legal aspects of nursing. Prentice Hall, London

Emmerson AM et al 1997 Diploma in infection control. Journal of Hospital Infection 37:175–180

English National Board for Nursing, Midwifery & Health Visiting (ENB) 1987 Short course in principles of infection control (number 910). ENB, London

English National Board for Nursing, Midwifery & Health Visiting (ENB) 1995a Post registration courses (Circular 1995/05/RLV). ENB, London

English National Board for Nursing, Midwifery & Health Visiting (ENB) 1995b Changes to regulations and guidelines relating to assessment (DCL/01/RLV). ENB, London

English National Board for Nursing, Midwifery & Health Visiting (ENB) 1995c Developments in infection control nursing for nurses, midwives and health visitors on all parts of professional register (course N26). ENB, London

English National Board for Nursing, Midwifery & Health Visiting (ENB) 2000 Infection control: results of a survey. ENB News, January: 35

Friston M 1999 New rules for expert witnesses (editorial). British Medical Journal 318:1365–1366

Gardner AMN et al 1962 The infection control sister. A new member of the control of infection team in general hospitals. Lancet ii:710–711

Garner JS 1996 Hospital infection practice advisory committee. Guidelines for isolation precautions in hospitals. Infection Control Hospital Epidemiology 17:54–80

Grimshaw J et al 1995 Developing and implementing clinical practice guidelines. Quality in Health Care 4(1):55–64

Hinchcliff S 1998 Practitioner as teacher. Baillière Tindall, London

Horton R 1988 Linking the chain. Nursing Times 84:44–46

Horton R 1993 Infection control in nurse education and practice. MPhil Thesis. University of Bradford

Hospital Infection Society, Infection Control Nurses Association, Association of Medical Microbiologists, Department of Health 2001 Key indicators. HMSO, London

Infection Control Nurses Association (ICNA) 1998 Educational opportunities in infection control for qualified nurses, midwives and health visitors, 2nd edn. ICNA

Infection Control Nurses Association Education Sub-committee 2000 Professional competencies for infection control nurses. ICNA, Edinburgh

Infection Control Nurses Association Scottish Group (ICNASG) 2000 A route to enhanced competence in infection control. ICNASG, Glasgow

Jenner EA, Wilson JA 2000 Educating infection control teams – past, present and future. A British perspective. Journal of Hospital Infection 46:96–105

Joint Board of Clinical Nursing Studies (JBCNS) 1974 Outline curriculum in infection control nursing for state registered nurses (course 326). JBCNS, London

Joint Board of Clinical Nursing Studies (JBCNS) 1977 Short course in the principles of infection control nursing (course 910). JBCNS, London

Joint Board of Clinical Nursing Studies (JBCNS) 1979 Foundation course in infection control nursing for state registered nurses (course 329). JBCNS, London

Masterton RG 1999 Worthwhile infection control information? Journal of Hospital Infection 42:269–274

Ministry of Health (MoH) Central Health Services Council Standing Medical Advisory Committee 1959 Staphylococcal infections in hospitals. Report of the Sub-Committee. HMSO, London

Moore B 1969 The infection control sister in British hospitals. International Nurse Review 17:84–91

National Audit Office (NAO) 2000 The management and control of hospital acquired infection in acute NHS Trusts in England. NAO, London

National Board of Nursing, Midwifery and Health Visiting in Scotland (NBS) 2000a Continuing professional development portfolio, a route to enhanced competence. NBS, Edinburgh

National Board of Nursing, Midwifery and Health Visiting in Scotland (NBS) 2000b Strength through partnership – a framework for quality assuring continuing professional development in NHS Trusts in Scotland. NBS, Edinburgh

National Board of Scotland for Nursing, Midwifery and Health Visiting and The Scottish Centre for Infection and Environmental Health (NBS/SCIEH) 1999 A collaborative Report 2. The findings of a review of current infection control educational opportunities for health care professionals in Scotland. NBS, Edinburgh

National Health Service Executive (NHSE) 1999a Making a difference, strengthening the nursing, midwifery and health visiting contribution to health and healthcare (HSC 1999/158). HMSO, London

National Health Service Executive (NHSE) 1999b Nurse, midwife and health visitor consultants. Establishing posts and making appointments (HSC 1999/217). HMSO, London

National Health Service Executive (NHSE) 2000 The management and control of hospital infection. Action for the NHS for the management and control of infection in hospitals in England (HAS 2000/002). HMSO, London

National Health Service Executive (NHSE) 2001a Controls assurance standard in infection control 1999 (Rev 02). HMSO, London. Available: http://tap.ccta.gov.uk/doh/rm5.nsf/b7546ce4a0608579002565c4003bf709/9bd9b4beb414923100256a5400615b0b?OpenDocument

National Health Service Executive (NHSE) 2001b Risk management – core standard (Rev 02). HMSO, London. Available: http://tap.ccta.gov.uk/doh/rm5.nsf/b7546ce4a0608579002565c4003bf709/4540eacc98d50a4d00256a5400623d18/$FILE/Risk+Management.PDF

National Health Service Executive (NHSE) 2001c Controls assurance standard – decontamination of single-use medical devices (Rev 02). HMSO, London. Available: http://tap.ccta.gov.uk/doh/rm5.nsf/b7546ce4a0608579002565c4003bf709/ed0073a14114f65200256a5400603d8b/$FILE/Decontamination.PDF

National Health Service Executive (NHSE) 2001d Controls assurance standard – catering and food hygiene (Rev 02). HMSO, London. Available: http://tap.ccta.gov.uk/doh/rm5.nsf/b7546ce4a0608579002565c4003bf709/c0085bd586edd66200256a54005f9b96/$FILE/Catering+and+Food+Hygiene.PDF

National Health Service Executive (NHSE) 2001e Controls assurance standard – waste management (Rev 02). HMSO, London. Available: http://tap.ccta.gov.uk/doh/rm5.nsf/b7546ce4a0608579002565c4003bf709/54a137c7413a83a200256a5400628536/$FILE/Waste+Management.PDF

National Health Service Management Executive (NHSME) 1989 Working for patients. Education and training, working paper 10 (Cmnd 555). HMSO, London

Office of the Lord Chief Justice 1996 Access to justice. Final report to the Lord Chancellor on the civil justice system in England and Wales. HMSO, London

Raven BH, Haley RW 1982 Social influence and compliance of hospital nurses with infection control policies. In: Eiser R (ed) Social psychology and behavioural medicine. John Wiley, Chichester

Royal College of Pathologists (RCP) 1998 Training record for medical microbiology. RCP, London

Scottish Office Department of Health (SODH) 1998 Advisory group on infection. Scottish infection control manual. Guidance on core standards for the control of infection in hospitals, healthcare premises and at the community interface. SODH, Edinburgh

Semmelweis IP 1861 The aetiology, the concept and the prophylaxis of childbed fever. CA Hartleben's Verlag-Expedition. Translated by FP Murphy, Republished Classics of Medicine Library, Birmingham

Teare EL, Peacock A 1996 The development of an infection control link-nurse programme in a district general hospital. Journal of Hospital Infection 34:267–278

The *epic* Project 2001 Developing national evidence-based guidelines for preventing healthcare associated infections. Journal of Hospital Infection 47(suppl):S1–S82

Tingle J, Cribb A (eds) 1995 Nursing law and ethics. Blackwell Science, Oxford

United Kingdom Central Council for Nursing, Midwifery and Health Visiting (UKCC) 1994a The future of professional practice – the Council's standards for education and practice following registration. UKCC, London

United Kingdom Central Council for Nursing, Midwifery and Health Visiting (UKCC) 1994b The Council's standards for education and practice following registration. Programmes of education leading to the qualification of specialist practitioner, Annex 1 to Registrar's Letter 20/1994. UKCC, London

United Kingdom Central Council for Nursing, Midwifery and Health Visiting (UKCC) 1996 Registrar's letter 15/1996, Annex 1. UKCC, London

United Kingdom Central Council for Nursing, Midwifery and Health Visiting (UKCC) 1998 UKCC CC/98/19 higher level practice (specialist practice project – Phase 11). UKCC, London

United Kingdom Central Council for Nursing, Midwifery and Health Visiting (UKCC) 1999a A higher level of practice. Report of the consultation on the UKCC's proposals for revised regulatory framework for post-registration clinical practice. UKCC, London

United Kingdom Central Council for Nursing, Midwifery and Health Visiting (UKCC) 1999b Fitness for practice. UKCC, London

Working Party Report 1998 Revised guidelines for the control of methicillin resistant *Staphylococcus aureus* infection in hospitals. Journal of Hospital Infection 39:253–290

Management of infection control

SUMMARY

This chapter considers public health issues and provides an outline of the theories that underlie the specialty of infection control. It considers the change to a new public health approach of focusing on the prevention of disease and discusses the emergence of new diseases and outbreak control measures. The importance of epidemiology, surveillance and audit is discussed.

INTRODUCTION

The *Health of the Nation* strategy

An ambitious plan of targets arising out of the theme of *Health for All by the Year 2000* (World Health Organization (WHO) 1978) and the Ottawa Charter was published in the *Health of the Nation* strategy (DoH 1992). The *Health of the Nation* is concerned with determining priorities and setting targets on the basis of an epidemiological assessment of health needs. Although this was an English initiative, strategies for health have also been developed in Northern Ireland, Scotland and Wales. Baggott (1994) considers that plans have attempted to follow the WHO approach to health for all by taking the context of people's lives into account. The *Health of the Nation* strategy has now broadened its scope, with many local and community initiatives taking place in an attempt to redress the initial failure of the document to address issues of poverty in relation to health. The strategy selected five key areas for action with regard to improving health:

1. coronary heart disease and stroke
2. cancers
3. mental illness
4. human immunodeficiency virus (HIV)/acquired immunodeficiency syndrome (AIDS) and sexual health
5. accidents.

Three criteria governed the selection of the key areas:

1. The area should be a major cause of premature death or avoidable ill health
2. Effective interventions should be possible, offering significant scope for improvement in health
3. It should be possible to set objectives and targets, and to monitor progress towards these.

Other areas for action were later developed to include other communicable diseases besides HIV/AIDS, and food safety was also added to the list.

A public health approach

Arising from these national and international resolves has been an increasing move among health professionals towards primary healthcare. Although the hospital and institutional setting is often characterized as secondary care, viewed as separate from primary healthcare in the community, in fact, people's needs are similar. A public health approach adopts a holistic, collective view of health with a seamless continuum between hospitals, institutions and the wider community.

The impact of these two recent publications ('Shifting the balance of power: the next steps' and 'Getting ahead of the curve' DoH 2002a,b) has yet to be determined. The government has stated that these publications will have a radical influence on the way healthcare is delivered in the 21st century.

■ **REFLECTIVE PRACTICE 3.1   The public health responsibilities of infection control nurses (ICNs)**

Consider the public health responsibilities identified below. How might they relate to the work of ICNs in the community as a whole – including hospital and institutional settings?

- Monitoring and describing the population's health
- Identifying those groups most in need of health support, guidance and treatment
- Identifying the social, economic and environmental factors that impact on people's health
- Taking health action to promote and protect the population's health
- Assessing the impact of healthcare on health (Billingham 1994).

Nurses can be involved in infection control at any point on the continuum in one-to-one teaching, counselling and advising, and in informing the whole community through pressure groups, campaigns or community programmes, as well as fulfilling their role in infection control within their specialty. For example, Stanford (1990) identifies the nurse's role in preventing the spread of HIV and AIDS (Box 3.1).

■ **BOX 3.1   The nurse's role in preventing the spread of HIV and AIDS**

- Learn about HIV/AIDS
- Follow guidelines on the prevention of infection
- Inform the public about HIV/AIDS and help dispel myths and prejudices
- Encourage people to accept responsibility for their sexual relationships and activities, and so protect themselves and their partners' health
- Encourage the use of condoms
- Encourage intravenous drug users to practise safer sex and not to share needles
- Inform the public about donating blood – there is no risk to the donor
- Allay anxieties about blood transfusions – the risk is negligible
- Encourage people with HIV to adopt a healthy lifestyle and tell them how to avoid infecting others
- Know where to refer patients for specialized help and counselling
- Promote a caring and responsible attitude towards people who have the virus.

The Acheson report

In 1988, a commission of inquiry reported on public health in England (DHSS 1988). Under its chairman, Sir Donald Acheson, then Chief Medical Officer at the DoH, it agreed a working definition of public health as: 'the science and art of preventing disease, prolonging life and promoting health through organised efforts of society'.

The committee of inquiry was set up in response to two major outbreaks of communicable disease: salmonella food poisoning at Stanley Royd Hospital in Wakefield in 1984 and Legionnaires' disease in Stafford in 1985; both of these outbreaks resulted in public inquiries (DHSS 1988). The main task of the committee was to do a thorough review of the state of public health medicine in England. The committee's report, known as the Acheson report, made 39 recommendations, representing a significant package of proposals designed to clarify and strengthen the implementation of public health functions. Specific infection control recommendations were that:

- district health authorities should make arrangements for the surveillance, prevention, treatment and control of communicable disease and infection
- executive responsibility was to be given to a named medical practitioner, who should be called the district control of infection officer
- a district control of infection committee should be established

- health authorities should include a section in their annual report on controlling communicable disease
- regional health authorities have a duty to monitor the performance of district health authorities, including adequate management arrangements for dealing with communicable disease and infection in hospital and in the general population
- the notification system of diseases should be reviewed regularly.

The new public health

The new public health is a development that recognizes that health problems are embedded not only in the physical but also in the social psychological aspects of the environment (Ashton & Seymour 1991). Its origins stem from a report prepared for the Canadian government about the health of the population (Lalonde 1974). This report argued that all causes of death and disease could be attributed to four separate elements:

1. inadequacies in current healthcare provision
2. lifestyle or behavioural factors
3. issues related to the environment
4. biophysical characteristics.

Besides a regeneration of public health, the Lalonde report has been associated with developments in health promotion and a world-wide focus on primary healthcare. These three major approaches are identified as:

1. public health
2. health promotion
3. primary healthcare.

These are all now recognized as being closely linked and interdependent, and are all relevant to the study and uses of epidemiology.

EMERGING INFECTIOUS DISEASES

In 1995, the World Health Organization (WHO) established its Division of Emerging and other Communicable Diseases Surveillance and Control to monitor and react to new events. This development reflects growing international concern about the emergence of apparently new and the re-emergence of old human infectious diseases worldwide.

Incidents included an outbreak of Ebola viral haemorrhagic fever infection in Zaire in May 1995, as a result of which 245 people died. Ebola virus is transmitted by direct contact with blood secretions or body fluids from an infected person. There is no specific treatment; control depends upon strict barrier nursing and infection control techniques for infected patients. Although no cases were reported outside the infected area in Zaire, appropriate agencies in the UK were alerted about the possibility of infection in anyone returning from the area, and how expected cases should be managed (DoH 1996).

The diphtheria epidemic in the former Soviet Union in 1995, and the evidence of the increase in tuberculosis in many countries (including the

UK), are examples of known pathogens that continue to cause concern (WHO 1995). A recent British report found a steady increase in tuberculosis in some inner London boroughs since 1987, with London overall having three times the national average of reported cases (Pearson et al 1996).

THE PREVENTIVE MODEL

Preventive health is concerned with improving public health not only by increasing life expectancy and reducing premature deaths, but also through adding life to years. This entails improving the quality of life by minimizing the effects of illness and disability, promoting healthy lifestyles and improving social and physical environments. For example, nurses need to use their knowledge and influence to address the complex needs of homeless people. A recent report about tuberculosis and homeless people (Griffiths-Jones 1997) highlights the need to:

- reduce the number of homeless people and improve available accommodation
- improve nutrition through health education and support
- identify tuberculosis in homeless people and provide prompt, successful treatment
- establish a thorough contact-tracing programme.

Preventive health has been classified as having three levels: primary, secondary and tertiary.

Primary prevention

Primary prevention means averting the onset of a disease or condition. For instance, good housing and nutrition help to prevent new cases of tuberculosis. Other examples are immunization programmes that protect children from infectious diseases and regulations to ensure that blood donations are free from infectious agents, including hepatitis B and C viruses. Health education, for instance, relating to hygienic food preparation and handling, helps to prevent food poisoning. Teaching people effective catheter care and management, both at home and in hospital, aims to avoid infection.

The Health and Safety Commission (1992) places responsibility on employers to ensure the health and safety of their employees by providing:

- safe plant and equipment, with maintenance, and safe systems of work
- safety in relation to use, handling, storage and transport of articles and substances
- information, instruction, training and supervision
- maintenance of a safe working place
- facilities and arrangements for welfare at work.

Managers of healthcare workers need to assess risks to their staff and then to plan, organize, control and monitor the necessary preventive and protective measures.

Secondary prevention

In secondary prevention the emphasis is upon early diagnosis and treatment – detecting disease in people sometimes before they are aware of a problem, such as through screening activities. Screening for tuberculosis, breast cancer and cervical cancer are current examples of such programmes. Criteria for justifying such a screening programme are given in Box 3.2.

■ BOX 3.2   Criteria for screening

- The disease must have a significant effect on the length or quality of life
- The disease must have a sufficiently high prevalence rate to justify the cost of the screening programme
- The disease must have been shown to have better therapeutic results if detected in the early stages, and worse results if detection and treatment are delayed
- The disease must have a significant symptom-free period, allowing an opportunity for detection and treatment that will reduce mortality and morbidity rates
- Screening procedures must be acceptable to those being tested
- Screening tests must be sensitive and specific in early detection, avoiding false positive and false negative results
- The disease must have an effective and acceptable method of treatment.

Tertiary prevention

The function of tertiary prevention is to prevent complications where disease already exists, promoting rehabilitation and preventing relapse so that the best level of health can be achieved. The development of primary nursing roles in both hospital and community, including nurses with a role in infection control, would facilitate tertiary prevention. Health education and counselling in this stage can help patients and their relatives, friends and carers to adjust to terminal illness with the goal of keeping the patient as comfortable as possible. Palliative care, which has developed out of the hospice movement, aims to maintain the patient's ability to function and maximize the quality of life.

OUTBREAK CONTROL

The management and control of outbreaks includes aspects of primary, secondary and tertiary prevention (Fig. 3.1).

Whatever the size of the outbreak, the same steps need to be followed:

- *Confirmation*: depending upon the disease, there might be an outbreak of just one case, such as rabies or botulism, or two or more patients presenting with the same symptoms, for instance food poisoning.
- *Identification of cases and characteristics*: a detailed history should be taken from all ill patients to decide whether they should be included as cases.

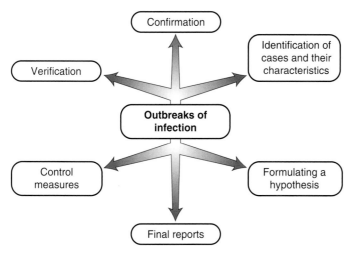

Figure 3.1 Outbreak control.

Laboratory testing could be used, or clinical diagnosis on its own might be sufficient.

• *Verification*: each patient's diagnosis should be verified to ensure that it matches the outbreak under investigation. For example, in a food poisoning outbreak, symptoms and clinical history should be compatible with the suspected organism's effects. Laboratory testing of specimens and of food samples are important aspects of the investigation.

• *Formulating a hypothesis*: after gathering the information, the investigating team should decide on a hypothesis identifying the likely source and spread of the outbreak.

• *Control measures*: once the hypothesis has been arrived at, appropriate precautions can be taken to stop further spread, e.g. quarantine measures, isolation, closing of food shops, surveillance of contacts. Control measures can be undertaken before all the information has been gathered in serious incidents.

• *Final report*: once the outbreak has been declared to be over, the outbreak team should send a written report to the chief executive. This should include details of the cause of the outbreak, control measures undertaken and their effectiveness, the number of cases, and recommendations to prevent future occurrences.

EPIDEMIOLOGY

The word 'epidemiology' is of Greek origin, and literally means 'studies upon people'. It involves studying patterns of health and illness in groups of people or in populations, rather than in individuals. Epidemiology provides a broader understanding of the causes, prevention and natural history of diseases and outcomes of treatment than can be gained from single cases.

Epidemiologists monitor trends in disease patterns. They seek to find out whether diseases are increasing or decreasing in frequency and monitor the disease distribution throughout a population before, during and after interventions are undertaken. They need to know how many people are affected by a particular condition, how many are likely to die from it and who in the population are most at risk of developing it. They ask questions such as:

- Why does a disease affect one person rather than another?
- Why does it occur in one country rather than another?
- Why does it occur in one season (e.g. winter) rather than another?

Epidemiology in Europe

'A blend of today's reality and tomorrow's dreams' was the vision of the 32 member states of the WHO European region, which was created in 1984. The region adopted the first set of European targets for health with the help of experts using the active and vital feedback of the member states in 1991. A decade later, the updated version (WHO 1993) is still serving as an inspiration to many nurses in their study of ways to control and prevent disease and promote health, with epidemiology seen as an integral component to help in their task.

Two of the revised European targets with particular relevance to infection control nurses are Targets 3 and 35:

- *Target 3 – reducing communicable disease*. By the year 2000, there should be no indigenous cases of poliomyelitis, diphtheria, neonatal tetanus, measles, mumps and congenital rubella in the region and there should be a sustained and continuing reduction in the incidence and adverse consequences of other communicable diseases, notably HIV infection (WHO 1993).

- *Target 35 – health information support*. By the year 2000, health information systems in all member states should actively support the formulation, implementation, monitoring and evaluation of health for all policies (WHO 1993).

The use of epidemiological data enables countries in the European region to share information by adopting regional targets and using regional indicators that result in regular, adequate monitoring and control of disease. For example, communicable diseases can be monitored by using the indicators of the number of cases of specific diseases such as:

- measles
- acute poliomyelitis
- tetanus
- neonatal tetanus
- congenital rubella
- diphtheria
- congenital syphilis
- indigenous malaria
- mumps.

Ways of controlling and reducing the incidence of such diseases can then be targeted effectively throughout Europe. How well these targets have been achieved is now being assessed as we start a new millenium.

Estimates of rates of transmission of HIV infection are collected on a European basis using each country's own figures and are used for planning healthcare.

Uses of epidemiology

Across the world, infectious conditions are responsible for about half of all known human diseases in the community and, in hospitals, hospital-acquired infections complicate illness and delay the recovery of large numbers of people. Clinical epidemiology applies epidemiological theories and principles to problems in groups of people in clinical medicine. This framework can be applied equally, although with a different emphasis, to nursing, midwifery and health visiting (Mulhall 1996). Much epidemiological research informs the planning and implementation of health-related policy and has a fundamental impact on the way that the nursing profession delivers care. Unfortunately, many nurses are unaware of the impact that epidemiology has on their working practice. Nursing could be perceived as being in a better position than medicine to endorse an epidemiological approach to care. Despite epidemiology having its roots in medicine, nursing's nature is seen to be more encompassing and holistic in its outlook than the medical profession. It is this mutual holistic, less structured approach, focusing not just on individuals but on groups and communities, along with its preventive strategies instead of curative ones, that makes an epidemiological approach an ideal strategy for nursing to incorporate into its professional practice (Whitehead 2000).

An understanding of epidemiology is considered to be one of the five domains of specialist ICN knowledge (see p. 22). The domain requires the practitioner to apply epidemiological knowledge to prevent and control infections and communicable diseases (ICNA 2000).

The principal uses of epidemiology can be summarized as:

- The investigation of the causes and natural history of disease, with the aim of disease prevention and health promotion
- The measurement of healthcare needs and the evaluation of clinical management, with the aim of improving the effectiveness and efficiency of healthcare provision (Farmer et al 1996).

These aims rely upon detailed investigation of the relevant population groups in order to discover their health needs. Epidemiologists therefore require a knowledge of demographic patterns.

Demography

Demography is the study of whole populations of people. It is concerned with the major events of births and deaths and other important transitions in people's lives. Demographic data are used to make forecasts and aid decision making in both the public and private sectors. The basic data come from censuses; registrations of births, deaths and marriages; surveys and other recorded information. Epidemiologists use demographic information as a basis for their work.

In 1992, a changing age distribution of measles was noted and changes were made to the national immunization strategy. To prevent an epidemic of measles in school-age children, mass measles/rubella immunization was carried out in November 1994. This measles/rubella immunization campaign reached over 8 million children. It involved highly detailed local and national planning, with a vast number of doctors, nurses and other health personnel, particularly in the schools health service, taking part. Susceptibility to measles in this target population has dropped dramatically, and the few cases of measles since the campaign have occurred mostly in adults or infants too young to be protected by immunization. The inclusion of rubella vaccine greatly reduced the susceptibility to rubella in males, and therefore reduced the risk to susceptible pregnant women and their unborn babies. It was decided to follow-up this campaign by introducing a two-dose strategy for measles/mumps/rubella (MMR) triple vaccine to prevent further accumulations of children at risk from these diseases (DoH et al 1996). Since its introduction there have been concerns about possible links between the MMR vaccine and autism. The incidence of autism in the UK has increased noticeably over the past 10 years and it has been suggested that this rise coincides with the introduction of the MMR triple vaccine in 1988. Kaye et al (2001) undertook a time trend analysis of the data to assess the relationship of autism to the vaccine. From 1988 to 1993 there was a four-fold increase in the risk of autism in boys aged 2 to 5 years. During the same time period, the coverage of the MMR vaccine remained constant at a prevalence of 95%. Kaye et al (2001) concluded that current evidence was against a causal association between the MMR vaccine and the risk of autism. Many other experts consider there to be a lack of epidemiological evidence showing an association to either prove or disprove causality. Because of the high level of public concern about a possible link, this is an area that requires further study. However, it is thought that the benefits of immunization far outweigh any risk associated with MMR vaccination. Measles, mumps and rubella, if left unchecked, can cause considerable sickness and death.

Social epidemiology

Social epidemiology, together with the new public health, is that branch of the discipline that considers socioeconomic and cultural factors and their impact upon a population's health. A major consideration regarding the use of epidemiology, which underpins the work of health professionals today, is equity in relation to healthcare needs (Fig. 3.2). Equity is the essence of health for all by reducing the disparities in the health status between countries and between groups of people in countries. Health professionals can assist with this by helping individuals achieve their full physical, mental and social potential. The prevention of disease and promotion of health are important strategic issues to give people a positive sense of health. Many sectors of society need to collaborate to ensure health and protection from risks in the physical, economic and social environment. A harmonious health service should meet the basic needs of each community by focusing on primary healthcare with adequate referral services and affordable, high-quality care.

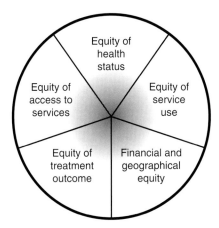

Figure 3.2 Aspects of equity.

Types of epidemiological study

Many studies are not clear-cut and cannot be fitted into just one of the categories outlined below. In fact, most health and disease investigations involve undertaking different types of study. However, the differentiation into the different categories helps to provide a framework for understanding the various methods employed in epidemiological research.

Descriptive studies

These are used to demonstrate the amount and distribution of disease in populations. A descriptive study can include a whole population or a specially selected sample from it in order to identify patterns of distribution. Who is affected, where the disease occurs and when it occurs are identified in descriptive studies. Questionnaires, home visits, physical examinations and interviews are examples of ways of obtaining data, as are the use of routinely collected mortality and morbidity statistics and hospital records.

Cohort studies

Cohort studies compare people exposed to a suspected cause and those not exposed. They are designed to define the causes or determinants of diseases more precisely than is possible using descriptive studies only. Data obtained from cohort studies can be used to calculate and compare incidence rates of a disease in individuals exposed to the suspected causal agent and those not exposed. From the results, it is often possible to identify ways of preventing, treating or controlling the disease.

People to be studied – the subjects – are selected because they are, or might be, exposed to the causative agent under scrutiny. Once identified, subjects in a cohort study are monitored and followed-up for a period of time, often many years. Characteristics of those people who develop the disease can then be reliably compared with those who do not, thus providing health planners with valuable information that can be applied to healthcare (see Box 3.3).

■ BOX 3.3   Example of a cohort study

In a study in Britain, a group of women who suffered from rubella in pregnancy were followed up for 2 years after the birth of the child. One in six of the children whose mothers developed rubella during the first 2 months of pregnancy had a congenital deformity – a far higher incidence than among children born after normal pregnancies (Barker & Rose 1990).

Probably the most well-known cohort study was that concerning smoking and mortality among British doctors (Doll & Hill 1964). The researchers sent questionnaires on smoking behaviour to all doctors on the British medical register and then followed-up the cohort (i.e. those who replied), monitoring subsequent deaths. Several causes of death were found to be associated with smoking. The most notable finding was the association between lung cancer and death, particularly in males.

A different type of cohort study – retrospective cohort study – was undertaken to identify the cause of an outbreak of cryptosporidiosis associated with an educational farm visit. In April 1995, a party of 43 school children (from 8 to 11 years of age) and four members of the school staff spent a week at an educational farm. Five days after returning home from the trip an outbreak of diarrhoea amongst the party members was reported by the school to the local environmental health department. Details of farm activities were recorded and all members of the school party were interviewed, using a questionnaire to gather information about personal history, illness and animal contact. Risk factors related to the 27 children and four staff identified as cases, showed that those who had handled calves were 3.8 times more likely to develop cryptosporidiosis, and those who habitually bit their nails or sucked their thumbs were an additional 1.5 times more at risk. The study highlighted the fact that infection occurred despite the supervision of children's handwashing practices, which was carried out. Recommendations made following the study included more publicity regarding the infection hazards of farm visits and a suggestion that further studies of the transmission of *Cryptosporidium* in the farm environment should be undertaken (Evans & Gardner 1996).

Case-control studies

Case-control studies compare two groups, one of which has the condition being investigated and the other which has not. However, the two groups must be matched on all other factors that could otherwise affect the conclusions.

An example of a case-control study is provided by an Australian study that implicated maternal rubella as a cause of congenital cataract. A comparison was made between those with the condition and those without. It was shown that the suspected cause, a history of maternal rubella, occurred more frequently among those with congenital cataract than among the control group without cataract. In 68 of the 78 children with congenital cataract, there was a history of maternal rubella (Barker & Rose 1990).

The subjects in a case-control study are therefore identified either because they have the disease (cases) or because they do not (controls).

■ **REFLECTIVE PRACTICE 3.2 Finding your control group**

Examples of groups from which control subjects can be recruited are listed below (Farmer et al 1996). What sources of control groups might be suitable for a case-control study connected with your specialty or interest?
- People working in the same factory, attending the same school or living in the same locality as cases
- Routine registers such as birth registers, electoral rolls, payrolls, school rolls or practice lists. However, each of these – potentially – has its own selective bias, which needs to be considered
- Hospital patients – usually those with conditions believed to be unrelated to the factors being studied. However, bias can occur because other diseases suffered by the patients could have affected exposure to the causal agent under investigation. Also, people who live in poor social environments are more likely to be admitted to hospital, which could introduce a social class bias
- Relatives and spouses – are often willing to cooperate and might be easily accessible. However, they are unsuitable when genetic or home environment factors are being studied because they would be too similar to the cases
- Some controls are recruited through random digit dialling using telephone exchanges in whose area cases are resident. Controls who fail to meet basic requirements are discarded.

Intervention studies

These are studies where some action is taken and the effects of that action are measured. They are usually experiments designed to assess the effectiveness of interventions in healthcare, including treatment, prevention and control measures, and the way in which healthcare is provided. They can be used to compare the results of different interventions, e.g. wound healing techniques. The most familiar study design of this kind is the clinical trial.

Randomized controlled trials (RCTs)

The basis of a clinical trial is the random allocation of individuals in a population to 'test' and 'control' groups. This is to ensure that those treated and those not treated are exactly similar in all respects before the treatment being studied is applied. This guards against the possibility that some factor other than the intervention could account for differences in outcome between the two groups. The intervention under trial is applied to the test group but not to the control group. The effect of the action taken is judged by comparing outcomes in both groups (Farmer et al 1996), e.g. in a vaccine trial the findings might be:

- incidence in vaccinated children = 5 per 1000
- incidence in unvaccinated children = 50 per 1000.

■ REFLECTIVE PRACTICE 3.3   Ethical considerations

The ethical questions that arise in the planning and conduct of randomized controlled trials are shown below (Farmer et al 1996). Consider these in relation to a possible trial related to your work (e.g. treatment for a communicable skin disease), in which you could be invited to take part:

• What are the possible risks of treatment and of failure to treat?
• Is it right to expose some people to possible harm from an untested treatment or to withhold from others a possibly beneficial treatment?
• Is it right to introduce a new treatment without first assessing its safety and benefits by means of a properly conducted trial?
• To what extent should a trial be explained to the subjects before they agree to take part?
• How can the welfare and safety of participants be safeguarded while preserving the principle of 'blind' assessment?

Many of the technical procedures undertaken and much of the equipment used during the provision of nursing care could usefully be examined for their efficiency and effectiveness using RCTs. Practitioners could try to answer such questions as 'Which bladder washout should I use when a urethral catheter is blocked?', 'Is this cheaper disinfectant as effective as the one in current use?', 'Should the insertion sites of intravenous cannulae be covered by sterile dressings?' (Mulhall 1996).

Double-blind trials

People can affect the results of a trial because they (often unwittingly) interpret the data in the light of what they expect or guess might happen. Double-blind trials prevent this happening, e.g. in clinical trials of a new medication, one group of people receives a placebo and the other group is given the drug on trial. Neither the person supplying the drug nor the patients know which one they are receiving. Double-blind preventive trials are sometimes carried out, for instance to test the effectiveness of vaccines.

SOURCES OF HEALTH INFORMATION

The question 'What is health?' is frequently asked but the answer remains elusive. People's own sense of wellbeing is closely related to their expectations of health and life, and it is not possible to measure these in an objective way. To measure and compare the health of groups and populations, indices of death and disease have to be used. Such sources have many limitations, which need to be considered when using and interpreting data.

The Office for National Statistics

The Office for National Statistics (ONS) was formed in April 1996 from a merger of the Central Statistical Office and the Office of Population Censuses and Surveys. The new organization aims to bring together all the important data about the lives of everyone in the UK, in a way that is accessible to all. It is independent of any other government department and claims to be accurate and objective in its reporting of data. It organizes the national system of registering births, deaths and marriages, which began in England and Wales in 1837. One major study it has taken over is the census.

Census data

Most developed countries undertake regular, detailed censuses of their populations to provide current information and to aid future planning. Since 1801 there has been a full census every 10 years in the UK, except in 1941 during the Second World War. Modern censuses are generally thought to be very accurate, apart from some problems of concealment or misreporting of census data, and slight under-recording because some people are not at a formal address on census night.

Between censuses

Population size and characteristics in non-census years are estimated by deducting deaths and emigrants from numbers recorded in the census, and adding births and immigrants. Errors are possible in these estimates, and these are compounded as time passes.

Mortality data

The term 'mortality' refers to the number of deaths within a population. Collection of the data is organized in England and Wales by the ONS, being gathered locally by registrars appointed in each local authority. The registration of deaths provides an accurate source of information for numbers of deaths to be recorded.

Standardized mortality rates

As crude mortality rates are of limited use, the standardized mortality rate (SMR) is often calculated instead. The SMR makes a comparison between mortality from a specific disease (or from all causes) in a designated group (e.g. a social class) and a standard, reference population. Identification of inequalities in geographical or occupational health status can be demonstrated in this way.

Infant mortality rates

Special mortality rates are defined for infants at specific time periods. On 1 October 1992, the legal definition of a stillbirth was altered from a baby born dead after 28 complete weeks of gestation or more, to one born dead after 24 complete weeks of gestation or more. Comparisons with earlier years must take this legal definition into account.

Morbidity measures

Complementary to mortality data are statistics on morbidity, which refer to the amount and types of illness affecting a population. There are a number of sources for gathering such data, including:

- notifications of infectious diseases
- hospital data
- notification of prescribed and other industrial disease and accidents
- notification of episodes of sexually transmitted diseases (STDs)
- notification of congenital malformations
- registration of handicapped persons
- registration of cancer
- registration of abortions.

Other sources include school health records, records of industrial injury and records from the armed services. There are many limitations, however, associated with morbidity data. Some collected data refer to clinic attendances (e.g. to the STD clinic) and not to individuals, so that actual numbers of people affected are not known. Under-reporting by medical practitioners varies between areas of the country and different conditions (Victor 1995). Undernotification of tuberculosis, particularly in patients with HIV infection, has been well documented. The main purpose of notification is to ensure that contact-tracing procedures are instituted. Failure to notify can result in lack of detection of associated cases or failure to manage contacts correctly (DoH 1996).

Surveys of health status

Special surveys are arranged to collect data relevant to morbidity. These are an essential part of measuring the health of the population because they can cover people who are not in contact with healthcare services. Ideally, such surveys should be national in scope, representative of the population from which they are drawn, comprehensive in coverage of topics, sufficiently large to allow comparisons across places and people and repeatable at intervals to demonstrate trends over time.

The General Household Survey (GHS) has been carried out annually since 1971 on about 10 000 households by the ONS. Data is collected concerning the prevalence of both acute and chronic health problems, although the survey excludes children and people in institutions from its sample. The Health Survey for England is a national survey that meets the criteria above and includes children in its focus.

SURVEILLANCE

Surveillance, especially for hospital-acquired infections, has long been established as a key element of all infection control programmes based on the study on the efficacy of nosocomial infection control (SENIC) project (Haley et al 1985). Surveillance provides data useful for identifying infected patients, determining the site of infection and ascertaining factors that contribute to hospital-acquired infection. This data enables the calculation of the rate of infection, which facilitates the monitoring of infection trends with respect to time, place and infection site. Surveillance also allows infection control interventions and evaluates their efficacy. Surveillance must be routine and timely, utilizing standard definitions and providing feedback to clinicians and managers. Such feedback can provide the basis for education, policy development and staffing levels. One method of feedback that is gaining approval is that of statistical process charts. These are based on engineering quality models, the basic underlying principle of which is that all processes (e.g. individual factors contributing to infection) vary and the end results (e.g. hospital-acquired infection rates) can be described in statistical terms (Sellick 1993). These charts have been used to provide feedback on infections such as methicillin-resistant *Staphylococcus aureus* (MRSA) and *Clostridium difficile* (Benneyan 1998, Curran 2001).

Surveillance of communicable diseases

In 1990, the government's Unlinked Anonymous HIV Surveys were established to supplement data already collected by voluntary confidential testing, and to provide a more accurate picture of the epidemic. The surveys take place in certain genitourinary medicine (GUM) clinics, centres for injecting drug users (IDUs) and antenatal clinics; screening of dried blood spots from neonates is also carried out. Results show that prevalence rates among IDUs were 3% for men and 4% for women in London and the south east, and less than 1% in both men and women elsewhere. This group remains vulnerable because about one-fifth of current IDUs report sharing injection equipment, with young injectors and women reporting significantly higher rates of sharing (DoH 1996).

Surveillance of hospital-acquired infection

Although there is no single or 'correct' method of surveillance, the foundation of an effective system is based on sound epidemiological principles. Surveillance is a comprehensive method of measuring outcomes and related processes of care, analysis of the data and providing information to those providing clinical care. As such, surveillance can form part of clinical audit and clinical governance, assisting in reducing the frequency of adverse events of infection or injury. To ensure the quality of surveillance, seven recommended areas should be considered (Lee et al 1998):

1. How to assess the population of interest
2. How to select the outcome or process for surveillance (outcomes = infection, process = steps taken to achieve an outcome, e.g. compliance with policy)
3. How to use valid definitions to enhance consistency, accuracy and reproducibility of surveillance information
4. How to collect and manage data – this should be done by knowledgeable professionals, qualified by training and experience
5. How to calculate and analyze surveillance rates – the methodology used to do this must be consistent over time, so that each surveillance component can be interpreted accurately

6. How to apply risk stratification methodology to enable comparison of results
7. How to incorporate reporting and using surveillance information into the development of each surveillance component.

In 1963, Alexander D. Langmuir stated that 'Good surveillance does not necessarily ensure the making of the right decisions, but it reduces the chances of wrong ones' (Langmuir 1963). A well implemented surveillance plan will have a pivotal role in supporting high-quality care initiatives by providing systems for monitoring, measuring and reporting important outcomes.

Nurses are involved in many surveillance activities in the course of their work and most of these will focus on the individual. One area where surveillance on a larger scale has a long history of nursing involvement, is the recording and control of hospital-acquired infections. Using prevalence and incidence data, most hospitals have recorded clinical evidence of all staphylococcal infections since 1959 (Mulhall 1996). In 1990 it was reported that 87% of infection control teams (ICTs) collected data concerning the rates of 'alert organisms', i.e. microorganisms such as methicillin-resistant staphylococci, which might cause potential cross-infection problems (Glenister et al 1990). Studies show that laboratory-based ward surveillance is the most sensitive and time-efficient system for detecting patients with infections. A comprehensive method of surveillance carried out by experienced, trained infection control personnel using all the sources of information available in detecting hospital infection was identified by Glenister et al (1992), who assessed the effectiveness of eight different surveillance methods in her study (see Box 3.4).

Whatever method of collection of data is decided upon by the infection control committee, it is vital that the criteria to which the infection control staff work have been fully discussed and agreed by the clinical staff concerned. Increased compliance with the aims of the ICT can be achieved if feedback of results is shared promptly.

■ **BOX 3.4   Surveillance methods** (Glenister et al 1992)

- Laboratory-based
- Laboratory-based telephone
- Risk factor
- Ward liaison
- Temperature chart
- Treatment chart
- Temperature and treatment chart
- Laboratory-based and ward liaison.

Health-associated infection surveillance scheme

In October 2000, the government announced that every NHS Trust in England must monitor levels of hospital-acquired infections, and that this would focus on infections that pose a serious threat to the health of patients.

From April 2001, universal bacteraemia surveillance, focusing initially on MRSA and with data reported on a quarterly basis, has been compulsory. It is the intention that such data, in table format, will be accessible by the general public from April 2002. This is considered to be the first step in improving surveillance of antimicrobial resistance and healthcare-associated infections. Collection of the data will be through the current public health reporting systems (DoH 2001).

Post-discharge surveillance

Over the past decade, the introduction of daycare surgery (and also increased medical costs) has resulted in a shorter hospital stay for patients. Surgical procedures are increasingly performed in outpatient departments and general practitioner (GP) surgeries. After a literature review, Holtz & Wendell (1992) found that post-discharge infections were more likely to occur in patients with a shorter length of stay in hospital. Most infections did not become apparent until after patients had been discharged.

CLINICAL AUDIT

When the government reorganized the NHS in 1990 it introduced the concept of audit as the main mechanism by which efficiency and value for money should be monitored (NHSME 1993). Audit allows for a systematic and more critical look at the effectiveness of the service by:

- scrutinizing current practices
- comparing practices against agreed standards
- assessing whether resources are used to optimum advantage.

A sound audit that identifies the strengths as well as the weaknesses of a service can make staff feel valued and provide a dynamic way of helping carers do a better job. It is also important to note that nowadays the general public expects high standards of care and that the government demands accountability at all levels.

The audit cycle shown in Figure 3.3 is the method used to carry out audit. The key stages are described by Buttery et al (1995) as:

- *Stage 1*: development and setting of standards
- *Stage 2*: measurement of compliance with standards (expected level of performance)
- *Stage 3*: making recommendations and drawing up action plans for increasing compliance with standards
- *Stage 4*: implementing recommendations and action plans
- *Stage 5*: evaluating whether recommendations and actions have been implemented and whether compliance with standards has increased.

Standards and criteria

A standard can be defined as the essential acceptable level of performance necessary for the safe and proper care of the patient to be maintained.

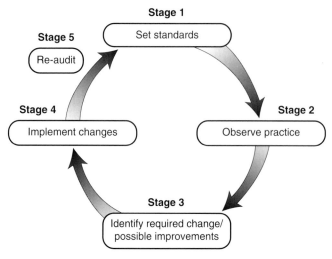

Figure 3.3 The audit cycle.

Criteria are the elements that are relevant to the achievement of that level of performance. According to the King's Fund organizational audit, 'The standard is the overall goal … The criteria are the mechanisms which have to be in place to achieve the standard'. As criteria are used as measurements of standards, these should be sufficiently distinct to be able to say whether they are present or not.

Standards can be mandatory or voluntary. Mandatory standards are produced by government agencies and professional organizations. Voluntary standards are developed locally, usually in response to complaints from patients or concerns of clinical or managerial staff. Alternatively, there might be a desire to review compliance to existing guidelines and protocols. In locally set standards, all the staff are involved and collectively agree on the level of care they consider desirable. Because the evaluation or measurement of the actual practice is against these standards, the staff are more likely to implement change because there is a sense of ownership of the standard of care thought to be both ideal and achieveable. According to Grol et al (1988) involvement of staff can be a vital factor in the success of audit.

Clinical governance is the current framework by which the NHS improves the quality of services and safeguards high standards of care (NHSE 1999). Its aim is to focus on identifying and implementing services to ensure clinical quality.

Methods of audit

The audit can be uniprofessional or multidisciplinary. Individual disciplines can examine their own practice or be part of a clinical audit that reflects the combined efforts of many professionals in caring for patients. Audits can be designed to assess the core elements of the whole service (organizational audit) or the process of care and outcome of a service (clinical audit).

Patient records chart the care administered to individual patients and failure to document clinically significant information can be interpreted as lack of care. Although the often-quoted axiom 'If it wasn't charted, it wasn't done' can be seen as an unfair criticism by nurses, who argue that they place a higher priority on the delivery of care than on its documentation, according to Coldwell & Page (1996) there are serious implications of not documenting care. A failure to maintain accurate nursing records impacts on organizations, patients and individuals. Increasingly, the managerial, financial and statistical information extracted from case notes is used for the day-to-day running of the NHS (Audit Commission 1995) and in the future there might be a financial dimension to poor record keeping. A nurse's neglect to document patients' needs and services could suggest to insurers that the patients were admitted unnecessarily or that the services given were not appropriate for the diagnosis (Edelstein 1990).

Coldwell & Page (1996) claim that poor record keeping can directly influence the quality of care given. Records act as a principal means of communication amongst all healthcare providers sharing the care of a patient. Not communicating important messages from or to the patient or family can cause distress and could result in important clinical facts being overlooked. Inadequate communications can also lead to discontinuity of care between different practitioners, professional groups or on different days, and even to the omission of significant aspects of care.

An increasing number of litigations by and complaints from patients have highlighted the poor quality of records. Individual professionals might be required to appear as witnesses and defendants in law courts and, if found to be negligent, would be investigated by their professional bodies.

Audit and infection control

The impact of audit is not always dramatic or easy to demonstrate. Surveillance of infections has been shown to reduce the infection rate, although it has its limitations. Audit, on the other hand, can establish whether the measurable elements or criteria for good practice are present.

The primary role of an infection control programme is to reduce the risk of hospital-acquired infection and so to protect patients, employees and visitors. The detection of infections, the containment of outbreaks, the introduction and implementation of appropriate policies for safe practice and the education of all staff members are central to achieving this objective.

Informed care suggests that practices are carried out from a sound knowledge-base and that practitioners are able to justify each action that they take. It is likely that the future function of the ICN will be to respond to the gaps and problems identified through audit. The West Midlands Audit Tool is now a well-established audit tool, developed by ICNs, for auditing the patient environment and the knowledge and practice of those providing the care. These are now being considered as performance indicators for monitoring the effectiveness of infection control.

Clinical guidelines

Guidelines provide statements of good practice that are evidence based and can be adapted for local use as a baseline for polices and procedures. They enable clinical effectiveness and risk management teams to focus audit on appropriate infection prevention and control interventions. The majority of guidelines in the UK have been aimed at the medical staff. There is an underlying belief that 'clinical guidelines based on the systematically analysed results of the research and carefully introduced to doctors can improve clinical practice and outcome' (Grimshaw & Russell 1993).

CONCLUSION

The focus of healthcare is changing to that of prevention, resulting in a need to understand the issues surrounding public health. The major purposes of epidemiology in relation to nursing are to help in the understanding of: (i) disease causation; (ii) its distribution; (iii) its determinants in relation to person, place and time; and (iv) its natural history. Nurses who understand the epidemiology of a disease or condition will know who in a group is most likely to be at risk, e.g. if they are in a particular age-group or health category. Nurses are therefore key professionals in limiting disease and promoting health.

REFERENCES

Ashton J, Seymour H 1991 The new public health, 3rd edn. Open University Press, Buckingham

Audit commission 1995 Setting the records straight. A study of hospital medical records. HMSO, London

Baggott R 1994 Health and health care in Britain. Macmillan, London

Barker DJP, Rose G 1990 Epidemiology in medical practice, 4th edn. Churchill Livingstone, Edinburgh

Benneyan JC 1998 Statistical quality control methods in infection control and hospital epidemiology. Part I: Introduction and basic theory. Infection Control and Hospital Epidemiology 19:194–214

Billingham K 1994 Beyond the individual. Health Visitor 67(9):295

Buttery Y et al 1995 How is audit different from research? Network 21:7

Coldwell G, Page S 1996 Just for the record. Nursing Management 2(9):12–13

Curran ET 2001 Monitoring quality. British Journal of Infection Control 2(1):20–23

Department of Health (DoH) 1992 The health of the nation: a strategy for health in England (Cm 1986). HMSO, London

Department of Health (DoH) 1996 On the state of the public health 1995. HMSO, London

Department of Health, Welsh Office, Scottish Office Department of Health, DHSS (Northern Ireland) 1996 Immunisation against infectious disease. HMSO, London

Department of Health (DoH) 1999 Corporate governance in the new NHS: controls assurance standards 1999/2000: Risk management and organisational controls.

HSC 1999/23. HMSO, London. Available: http://tap.ccta.gov.uk/doh/rm5.nsf/Publications?Open View

Department of Health (DoH) 2001 Healthcare acquired bacteraemia surveillance: statement. Available: www.doh.gov.uk/hai/habs.htm

Department of Health (DoH) 2002a Shifting the balance of power: the next steps. HMSO, London. Available: www.doh.gov.uk/shiftingthebalance/index.htm

Department of Health (DoH) 2002b Getting ahead of the curve. HMSO, London. Available: www.doh.gov.uk/cmo/publications.htm

Department of Health and Social Security (DHSS) 1988 Public health in England: report of the Acheson committee of inquiry into the future development of the public health function (Cm 289). HMSO, London

Doll R, Hill AB 1964 Mortality in relation to smoking: ten years' observation of British doctors. British Medical Journal i:1399–1410

Edelstein J 1990 A study of nursing documentation. Nursing Management 21(11):40–46

Evans MR, Gardner D 1996 Cryptosporidiosis outbreak associated with an educational farm holiday. Communicable Disease Report 5(6):81–86

Farmer R, Miller D, Lawrenson R 1996 Lecture notes on epidemiology and public health medicine, 4th edn. Blackwell Science, Oxford

Glenister HM et al 1990 Surveillance of hospital infections in the United Kingdom. Infection Control and Hospital Epidemiology 11:622–623

Glenister HM et al 1992 An 11 month incidence study of infection in wards of a district general hospital. Journal of Hospital Infection 21:261–263

Griffiths-Jones A 1997 Tuberculosis in homeless people. Nursing Times 93(9):60–61

Grimshaw JM, Russell IT 1993 Achieving health gain through clinical guidelines. Developing scientifically valid guidelines. Quality in Health Care 2:243–248

Grol R et al 1988 The effects of peer review in general practice. Journal of Royal College of General Practitioners 38:10–13

Haley RW, Culver DH, White JW 1985 The efficacy of infection surveillance and control programs in preventing nosocomial infections in US hospitals. American Journal of Epidemiology 121:182–205

Health and Safety Commission (HSC) 1992 Management of health and safety at work: management of health and safety at work regulations 1992: approved code of practice. HMSO, London

Holtz TH, Wendell RP 1992 Post discharge surveillance for nosocomial ward infection: a brief review and commentary. American Journal of Infection Control 20(4):206–213

Infection Control Nurses Association (ICNA) 2000 Professional core competencies for infection control nurses. ICNA, Bathgate, Scotland

Kaye JA, Melero-Montes M, Jick H 2001 Mumps, measles, and rubella vaccine and the incidence of autism recorded by general practitioners: a time trend analysis. British Medical Journal 322:460–463

Lalonde M 1974 A new perspective on the health of Canadians. Government of Canada, Ottawa

Langmuir AD 1963 The surveillance of communicable diseases of national importance. New England Journal of Medicine 268:182–191

Lee TB et al 1998 Recommended practices for surveillance. American Journal of Infection Control 26(3):277–288

Mulhall AB 1996 Epidemiology, nursing and healthcare: a new perspective. Macmillan, Basingstoke

National Health Service Executive (NHSE) 1994 Effective health care, implementing clinical practice guidelines. NHSE, Leeds

National Health Service Management Executive (NHSME) 1993 Improving clinical effectiveness (EL(93)115). DoH/NHSME, Leeds

Pearson AD, Hamilton GR, Healing TD 1996 Summary of a report of the working party on tuberculosis of the London group of consultants in communicable disease control. Journal of Hospital Infection 33:165–179

Sellick JA 1993 The use of statistical process control charts in hospital epidemiology. Infection Control and Hospital Epidemiology 14(11): 649–656

Stanford J 1990 Professional care for people with HIV/AIDS. Professional nurse: patient education plus. Austen Cornish, London, pp 32–35

Victor C 1995 Information and health promotion. In: Pike S, Forster D (eds) Health promotion for all. Churchill Livingstone, Edinburgh, pp 69–80

Whitehead D 2000 Is there a place for epidemiology in nursing? Nursing standard 14(42):35–39

World Health Organization (WHO) 1978 Alma Ata declaration. WHO, Geneva

World Health Organization (WHO) 1993 Health for all targets: the health policy for Europe. WHO Regional Office for Europe, Copenhagen

World Health Organization (WHO) 1994 International classification of diseases. WHO, Geneva

World Health Organization (WHO) 1995 Tuberculosis trends in Central and Eastern Europe. Weekly Epidemiology Review 70:21–24

Knowledge management

4

■ CONTENTS

SUMMARY

This chapter considers the context of health information and offers some guidance on accessing the evidence. Also included is a list of useful resources.

INTRODUCTION

In 1998 the NHS Executive (NHSE) published *Information for Health*. This was followed in 2001 by *Building the Information Core: Implementing the NHS Plan*. These two documents created a 7-year plan to ensure information is used to help patients receive the best possible care. Their emphasis is on the 'I' rather than the 'T' of information technology and a key aim of the strategy is to enable clinicians to access the healthcare knowledge-base. The strategy also includes the commitment that patients, the public and carers will be able to access the information they need to make informed decisions about their healthcare. Its aim is to promote health through increased efficiency, accuracy and the provision of up-to-date information across the NHS. This includes acute and non-acute hospital care, community care, primary care, commissioners and support services.

   Government policy is one of the major imperatives driving the current healthcare agenda forwards, the other is the emerging importance of electronic resources. At the centre of the government's health policy is the objective of ensuring that patients receive the best possible healthcare.

Three factors – clinical governance, evidence-based practice and lifelong learning – are having an impact on health information providers and services. The concept of clinical governance was first introduced in *The New NHS: Modern and Dependable* (DoH 1998), which placed quality of care directly on the Chief Executives of NHS Trusts. In *A First Class Service: Quality in the New NHS* (NHSE 1998a) it was stated that 'evidence-based practice must be in everyday use'; the need for a culture of lifelong learning by all healthcare professionals was also emphasized. *Clinical Governance: Quality in the NHS* (DoH 1999) acknowledges that health professionals need knowledge from research to support their clinical decisions and that new skills are required by providers of health information services and their users to access this. Infection control practitioners need to maintain their own knowledge and skills and to be an educational resource for other healthcare workers. To achieve this, they need to be fully conversant with how to access the evidence base.

FINDING THE EVIDENCE

Evidence-based nursing, according to the Centre for Evidence Based Nursing website, is 'the process by which nurses make clinical decisions using the best available research evidence, their clinical expertise and patient preferences, in the context of available resources'.

Making clinical practice more effective requires easy access to the best current knowledge. The range of resources required for the practice of evidenced-based healthcare is growing, and it changes all the time. Many resources are available to support evidence-based practice: databases such as Medline and the Cochrane Library, evidence-based journals, the National Electronic Library for Health, the Internet, guidance from the National Institute for Clinical Effectiveness (NICE) and health libraries are some that are available.

These resources are available 24 hours a day, 7 days a week in the workplace or from home for those with Internet or NHSnet access. Targets were set in *Information for Health* (NHSE 1998b) to provide all staff with access to NHSnet and, as more wards and clinics are connected to NHSnet, it should become more convenient to access the evidence from the workplace, instead of visiting the library to use CD ROMs.

WHO CAN HELP?

Library and information services have a key role in developing an evidence-based NHS by acting as a gateway to the knowledge-base of healthcare. Libraries are at the heart of creating the learning environment and offer life-long learning facilities for professional development for all NHS practitioners. In *Working Together with Health Information: a Partnership Strategy for Education, Training and Development* (NHSE 2000) it was noted that 'library and information services are the bedrock of education and training and are critical to the development of evidence-based practice and clinical effectiveness'.

The importance of librarians is becoming more apparent as a consequence of a series of initiatives, including evidence-based practice, clinical governance and a statutory duty for quality (NHSE 2001). Although direct access to knowledge databases will grow, librarians will continue to support healthcare staff in finding the best evidence in the fastest possible time. Librarians are able to support clinical governance by teaching users how to find material, filter out the best evidence and navigate the Internet. They can support knowledge management services by facilitating information flows and by providing access to electronic information.

There are over 600 libraries in NHS Trusts and health authorities, providing access to the knowledge-base for staff involved in patient care, research, management and education, and training. The majority are multiprofessional facilities providing users with access to information via intranets and the Internet, enquiry services, literature searching, current awareness, loans and the supply of documents not held locally.

Your local librarian/knowledge manager can provide:

- Access to a range of global electronic 'evidence-based' information sources, either in the library or at your desk or from home
- Training in information and knowledge management skills
- Training in evidence-based practice skills and how to use databases
- A current awareness service and alert you to new sources of information
- Up-to-date latest research evidence
- Information on 'who is doing what' locally in evidence-based practice
- Advice on the most effective ways to search and the sources to use
- Advice on evaluating sources/articles
- Documents and other resources rapidly and cost-effectively.

A ROUGH GUIDE TO A LITERATURE SEARCH

- Identify the key subject of your search
- Select the sources, e.g. the Cochrane Library, Medline or the National Research Register (to discover if anyone else has already covered your topic)
- Carry out your search, narrowing your search terms or broadening them as appropriate
- Assess the relevance of the material retrieved
- If full text is available, download it immediately. If it is not, ask for the relevant articles from your library.

The most effective way to learn is to book a training session with your library service.

THE INTERNET OR WORLDWIDE WEB

The Internet is an electronically connected network of computers around the world that share information. The worldwide web is the information published on web pages using text, images, sound and video. When you 'search the Internet' you are actually searching the worldwide web *using* the Internet.

What information can be found on the web?

The worldwide web contains information on just about any topic. This information might be accurate and of high quality, but it could also be inaccurate and unauthoritative. Anyone can publish on the web – organizations, private companies, governments, individuals. Some sites are offensive and most organizations have an Internet policy that all users must sign up to before access is granted. It is important to remember that, despite the claims of Internet service providers (ISPs) the Internet will never be able to provide the answers to all questions. Traditional sources are still important for obtaining access to older information.

Browsers and home pages

A browser is a piece of software that allows you to see and read the information on the web.

A home page is the introductory or first page of an organization's or individual's website. A home page can be more than one screen long – to see everything on one page click on the bar on the right to scroll up and down. You can also use the arrow keys and the Page Up and Page Down keys to move up and down.

Navigation tools

The buttons along the toolbar at the top of your screen have the following functions:

- Back – takes you back one page at a time
- Forward – takes you forward one page at a time
- Home – takes you back to the home page used by your machine as the default when first switched on. You can choose your own or it might have been chosen for you by your Information Technology department
- Stop – stops a search in progress or a download
- Print – prints the web page you are looking at (remember to click the cursor within the page first or you may end up with a blank sheet of paper)
- Refresh – reloads a page. This is useful when information is changing rapidly (e.g. share prices), if the link has broken or if the page has frozen. If this does not work after three attempts there is a problem with access to the Internet or the web page itself has a problem (usually maintenance or congestion on the web)
- Favourites – you can add sites you visit frequently to your Favourites folder to enable quick access and reduce the amount of typing (and also the chance of typing errors)
- History – this can be the most useful button of all, it contains a list of the sites you have visited recently. This is helpful if you forgot to add a site to your favourites and need to look at it again.

One of the useful things about the Internet is that you can follow links using the mouse. Links are usually shown in blue text and underlined. Clicking with the left mouse button on a link will take you to a different page or to a different website. The majority of sites change the colour of the link to purple when you click on it, so you know you have already been there. It is easy to get lost when following links and be unable to get back to the page where you began, therefore care is needed, especially if you are a novice searcher.

Surfing tips

If you know the site you can type the address (or Uniform Resource Locator (URL)) directly into the address box at the top of your screen (e.g. http://www.doh.gov.uk).

If you do not know the address of the site, then you will need to use subject indexes and search engines. Use subject indexes like Yahoo to browse for information and sites on particular topics. Use keyword search engines like Alta Vista or evaluated subject catalogues like OMNI and the Our Healthier Nation Gateway to search for specific information.

One of the problems of searching the web is that it can be very slow. There are several ways of getting around this.

- Try to avoid peak times, e.g. if you want access to servers in North America, the early morning (when it is still night in the US) is usually better than the afternoon.
- If you are using a graphical browser like Netscape, try turning off the graphics. (On Netscape click on Options right at the top of the screen, above the tool bar, and then click on Auto Load Images.) This should make the loading of pages with images faster but is no use if you want images, and it can make the layout of some pages look quite poor. So, when you come across images you want to see, you will have to click on Auto Load Images again to turn the facility back on, and then reload the page (this should be reasonably quick as it will have been cached, i.e. saved into your machine's hard drive).

USEFUL RESOURCES

Increasingly, regional library services are banding together to subscribe to services, such as OVID and Biomed, that provide full-text versions of articles in journals and other publications. These can be used from work or home. Ask your librarian what is available in your organization. The majority of library and information services also belong to regional and national schemes with cooperative photocopying agreements, so those articles not available electronically can usually be obtained within a few days from elsewhere.

The majority of journals available via the Internet now offer a table of contents service, which sends you an e-mail whenever a new issue is published. This is a very easy way of keeping up-to-date with the literature. This service is usually free, although accessing the full text usually requires a full subscription. Again, ask your librarian whether the organization has one.

There are also news services that e-mail daily listings of health-related items direct to your computer.

Associations

Most professional organizations now have their own websites, where you can access guidelines, press releases, etc. There is often a password-protected area for members only, where more sensitive material is available.

The Royal College of Nursing (RCN) provides members with free personal Internet access to the British Nursing Index (BNI Plus) – a database indexing over 220 core nursing journals – together with World Information Nursing, including references to additional English language journals selected from Medline. The *Journal of Advanced Nursing, Journal of Clinical Nursing, International Journal of Nursing Practice* and the *Journal of Nursing Management* are among some of the journals available.

Initially the service is being piloted for 1 year. RCN members must register for the service by visiting the RCN website at www.rcn.org.uk, by e-mailing eservices@rcn.org.uk or by telephoning the RCN.
http://www.rcn.org.uk

UK Infection Control Nurses Association
http://www.icna.co.uk/

Electronic journals

American Journal of Infection Control
http://www.harcourthealth.com/scripts/om.dll/serve?action=searchDB
&searchdbfor=home&id=ic

Internet Journal of Advanced Nursing Practice
1997 vol 1(1) onwards.
http://www.ispub.com/journals/ijanp.htm

Journal of Hospital Infection
http://www.harcourt-international.com/journals/jhin/

Nursing Standard Online
http://www.nursing-standard.co.uk/

Nursing Times
http://www.nursingtimes.net/

Government sites

Clinical Governance Support Team
The NHS Clinical Governance Support Team has been created to help deliver the successful implementation of clinical governance 'on the ground'. This pilot website has been set up as a means of exchanging information and the best ideas and practice in clinical governance.
http://www.cgsupport.org/

Clinical Governance Development Network
This provides access to information on the development and implementation of clinical governance in the NHS in England. There are pages

describing local, regional and national activity, together with opportunities for requesting assistance with projects, and a discussion forum.
http://www.doh.nhsweb.nhs.uk/nhs/clingov.htm

Commission for Health Improvement
http://www.chi.nhs.uk/

Department of Health
This site gives access to the latest news and information about the department and its work. It also offers easy access to a wide range of publications, policy and guidance. It also includes links to several other key sites.
http://www.doh.gov.uk/

Department of Health Circulars on the Internet (COIN)
Includes full text access to the contents of the COIN database, Current local authority circulars (LACs) and Local Authority Social Services Letters (LASSLs).
http://www.doh.gov.uk/publications/coinh.html

Department of Health Hospital Acquired Infection site
http://www.doh.gov.uk/hai/index.htm

Department of Health Publications on the Internet (POINT)
The Department of Health's Internet service providing access to bibliographic details of Departmental publications from 1996, with full text of publications where available electronically.
http://www.doh.gov.uk/publications/pointh.html

National Institute for Clinical Excellence (NICE)
http://www.nice.org.uk/

NHS A–Z HelpDirect
Used by health and social care professionals, the voluntary sector, helplines and health information services, human resource managers and the public. It is available on the Internet as part of NHS Direct Online and also as a stand-alone site.
http://www.nhsatoz.org/nhsd/

NHS Learning Zone (Benchmarking)
Includes links to the NHS Trust Benchmarking Database, as well as to reports of other benchmarking activity in the NHS, including: effective prescribing; HA public health functions; secondary care services; thrombolysis project; primary care; mental health services.
http://www.doh.nhsweb.nhs.uk/learningzone/benchmrk.htm

NHS Modernisation Agency
http://www.modernnhs.nhs.uk/

NHS UK
This is the official gateway to National Health Service organizations on the Internet. It connects to local NHS services and also provides national information about the NHS – what it does, how it works, and how to use it.
http://www.nhs.uk/

Our Healthier Nation website
http://www.ohn.gov.uk/

Public Health Laboratory Service (includes the Communicable Disease
Surveillance Centre)
http://www.phls.co.uk/

Government policy documents

The New NHS. Modern, Dependable (Cm 3807). 1997
http://www.official-documents.co.uk/document/doh/newnhs/
newnhs.htm

NHS Plan
http://www.nhs.uk/nationalplan/

The NHS Plan: priorities
http://www.nhs.uk/thenhsexplained/priorities.asp

Clinical Governance (HSC 1999/065).
http://tap.ccta.gov.uk/doh/coin4.nsf/Circulars?ReadForm

Help with using the Internet

Internet Medic
A free online tutorial teaching medical Internet information skills.
http://omni.ac.uk/vts/medic/

BIOME resource evaluation guidelines for general and internet-based information sources.
http://biome.ac.uk/guidelines/eval/

Library websites

The British Library
Digital access to the collections of the National Library. Free access to over
8.5 million records available from the Online Public Access Catalogue.
www.blpc.co.uk

The British Library Health Care Information Service
Comprehensive coverage of medicine and healthcare across several British
Library services. Subjects covered by the Healthcare Information Service
include: medicine; complementary and alternative medicine; allied health
professions – including physiotherapy, occupational therapy, speech and
language therapies; podiatry; nursing; healthcare management; pharmaceuticals; healthcare services and products; history of medicine; telemedi-
cine information service. Also includes tutorials on searching for healthcare
information on the Internet.
http://www.bl.uk/services/stb/hcis.html

National Electronic Library for Health
http://www.nelh.nhs.uk/

Nursing resources

BUBL LINK

BUBL LINK is the name of a catalogue of selected Internet resources covering all academic subject areas and catalogued according to DDC (Dewey Decimal Classification). All items are selected, evaluated, catalogued and described. Links are checked and fixed each month. LINK stands for Libraries of Networked Knowledge.
http://bubl.ac.uk/link/

Centre for Evidence Based Nursing (CEBN)
http://www.york.ac.uk/depts/hstd/centres/evidence/cebn.htm

Cochrane Library
http://www.nelh.nhs.uk/cochrane.asp

Medline
http://www.ncbi.nlm.nih.gov/entrez/query.fcgi

Nursing, Midwifery and Allied Health Professions (NMAP)
A gateway to evaluated, quality Internet resources, aimed at students, researchers, academics and practitioners in the health and medical sciences. Content providers from relevant professional organizations help to ensure that NMAP meets the needs of the professions. It is closely integrated with the OMNI gateway (This site has replaced 'Nursing and Health Resources on the Internet').
http://nmap.ac.uk/

OMNI
Free access to a searchable catalogue of Internet sites covering health and medicine.
http://omni.ac.uk/

Netting the Evidence
Netting the Evidence is intended to facilitate evidence-based healthcare by providing support and access to helpful organizations and useful learning resources, such as an evidence-based virtual library, software and journals.
http://www.shef.ac.uk/~scharr/ir/netting/

Public health sites

Public Health Laboratory Service (includes the Communicable Disease Surveillance Centre)
http://www.phls.co.uk/

Public Health Observatories
http://www.pho.org.uk/index.htm

Research

RCN Research
This site has been developed to provide an easy-to-access means of sharing information on research and practice development in nursing, and is designed to be fully interactive. The site will be permanently 'under construction' so

that it develops in line with the needs of professional nurses endeavouring to conduct relevant research and keep abreast of current activities in research and practice development. The site provides a framework for sharing information about research networks, policy issues, ethics, funding, training and support units, dissemination and utilization and practice development.

http://www.man.ac.uk/rcn/

Search engines

Alta Vista
http://uk.altavista.com/

Ask Jeeves
http://www.ask.co.uk/

Google
http://www.google.co.uk/

Yahoo
http://www.yahoo.co.uk

REFERENCES

Department of Health (DoH) 1998 The new NHS: modern, dependable. HMSO, London

Department of Health (DoH) 1999 Clinical governance: quality in the NHS (HSC(99)065). DoH, London. Available: http://tap.ccta.gov.uk/doh/coin4.nsf/Circulars?ReadForm

NHS Executive (NHSE) 1997 Education and training planning guidance (EL(97)58). NHSE, Leeds

NHS Executive (NHSE) 1998a A first class service: quality in the new NHS (HSC 1998/113). NHSE, Leeds

NHS Executive (NHSE) 1998b Information for health: an information strategy for the new NHS (HSC 1998/168). NHSE, London, 24 September

NHS Executive (NHSE) 2000 Working together with health information. A partnership strategy for education, training and development. NHSE, London

NHS Executive (NHSE) 2001 Building the information core: implementing the NHS plan. NHSE, London

Infection control and developing countries

5

■ CONTENTS

SUMMARY

Many simple but effective measures can be applied to control infections and infectious diseases. However, the resources necessary for even the simplest of these actions is often lacking, or is not applied, in many developing parts of the world. This chapter examines the problems faced by poorly resourced countries and how they can be helped by the more developed, wealthier nations.

INTRODUCTION

Approximately 4 billion people, or 80% of the total global population, live in developing areas of the world (Isturiz & Carbon 2000). Poverty and overcrowding, the two main features of developing countries, impact on health, creating a continual burden on resources for health. Food, water and adequate sanitation, universally accepted as foundations for good health, are often lacking. The situation is often compounded by population increase. In many instances, a country's already limited resources are stretched further by the burden of displaced people from neighbouring warring or politically unstable countries. These refugees tend to be put into crowded settlements without even the very basic amenities, such as water and sanitation, and often do not receive an adequate supply of food. Inevitably, this creates an environment ripe for the spread of infectious disease.

Vulnerability to infection is increased by malnutrition resulting from disease, inadequate food or lack of proper food supply. According to the World Health Organization (WHO), infectious diseases are the leading killers of young people in developing countries (WHO 2000a). Among the global poor, communicable diseases are responsible for 58.6% of deaths (Gwatkin & Guillot 2000).

PROBLEMS FACED BY DEVELOPING COUNTRIES

Sanitation and water supply

Water is needed for drinking, cooking and personal hygiene and general household and community cleanliness. Lack of water leads to poor sanitation, and poor household and community sanitation is a major risk to health. According to the World Health Organization (WHO 1997), nearly two-thirds of all people in developing countries do not have sanitary excreta disposal and 25% of the world's population does not have a safe water supply. Figure 5.1 identifies the population in developing countries who remain unserved by a water supply and sanitation.

The WHO (1997) report states that: 'The poorest 1000 million people on Earth are seven times more likely to die from infectious diseases and maternal and perinatal conditions – most of which are directly related to poor sanitation – than are the least poor 1000 million'. The diseases listed include:

- schistosomiasis: estimated current global prevalence of 200 million cases
- typhoid fever: 16–17 million cases
- intestinal helminthic infections: 1500 million people infested
- various diarrhoeal diseases – over 2 million infant and child deaths annually.

These diseases result in anaemia and malnutrition, especially in children and in women of childbearing age. The infant and child mortality rate would appear to relate directly to the access of safe water and adequate sanitation. As Table 5.1 shows, there is a marked contrast in the infant and child mortality rates between countries with poor and good access to water and sanitation.

A lack of awareness of the risks associated with sanitation is currently apparent in the rural villages in North Pakistan, where human excreta are used as manure. Women carry out the task of spreading the excreta onto the

Sanitation

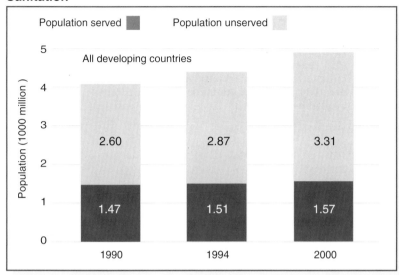

Water supply

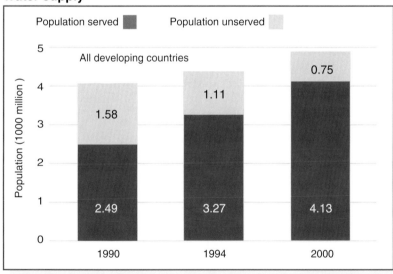

Source: WHO

Figure 5.1 The proportion of the population in developing countries who do not have sanitation and a water supply. (After Environmental Matters EB101/19 1997, with permission of WHO.)

fields. The importance of washing hands, especially before breast-feeding and cooking, is not appreciated. Children play on these fields, increasing the risk of transmission of infectious diseases. The situation is compounded by the fact that water is in short supply or frozen during many months of harsh winter.

Table 5.1 Infant mortality, child mortality, water supply and sanitation coverage, and GNP per capita in six countries, 1994 and 1995

Country	Infant mortality rate (1995) (0–1 year) per 1000 live births	Child mortality rate (1995) (0–5 years, cumulative) per 1000 live births	Access to safe water (1994) (percentage of population)	Access to adequate sanitation (1994) (percentage of population)	GNP per capita (1995) (US$)
Afghanistan	159	251	10	8	<765
Chile	15	17	96	71	4160
Ghana	77	113	56	42	390
Guinea-Bissau	135	207	57	20	250
Philippines	39	48	84	75	1050
Sweden	5	6	100	100	23750

Source: WHO, 1996.

Food hygiene

WHO estimates that, worldwide, almost 2 million children die every year from diarrhoea, most of this caused by microbiologically contaminated food and water (WHO 2001).

Major infectious diseases

Human immunodeficiency virus (HIV), tuberculosis (TB) and malaria cause over 300 million illnesses and more than 5 million deaths each year. Approximately half of infectious disease mortality can be attributed to these three diseases (WHO 2000b). In addition to suffering and death, they are associated with economic and social burdens.

Maternal and child deaths

Rosenfield (1989) describes maternal mortality as one of the great neglected problems of healthcare in developing countries. According to Rosenfield (1989), approximately 500 000 women die each year from pregnancy-related causes; more than 98% of these deaths occur in the developing world. In 1995, the estimated number of maternal deaths for the world was 515 000. Half of these deaths occurred in Africa, about 42% in Asia, 4% in Latin America and the Caribbean, and less than 1% in the more developed regions of the world (WHO 1995).

Antibiotic resistance

Infections caused by antibiotic-resistant bacteria are a global problem. Increased morbidity and mortality, as well as the use of more expensive and sometimes very toxic antimicrobials, are associated with resistant microbes. Anti-infective drugs are amongst the most widely used class of drugs in the world, accounting for over 25% of drug costs in many hospitals and a very high proportion of prescriptions in the community, especially in the developing world (Smith et al 1991). This is because the greatest contributor to disease is infectious in aetiology, requiring antibiotics (Duse & Smego 1999).

Poverty and inadequate access to drugs lead to antimicrobial resistance. Poor patients resort to poor quality or counterfeit drugs, or to truncated courses of treatment that result in a selection of resistant organisms (WHO 2000a). Prolonged illness, often resulting in death, and prolonged hospital stays result in lost wages, lost productivity and family hardship.

Diarrhoeal diseases caused by multi-drug-resistant microbes are believed to have claimed the lives of more than 2.2 million people in 1998 (WHO 2000a).

Several factors have been identified as contributing to the development of resistance in developing countries (Duse & Smego 1999, Folb & Dukes 1994, Forder 1995, Isuturiz & Carbon 2000, Kunin 1990). These include:

- the fact that empirical treatment costs less than diagnostic investigations
- the high cost, inadequacy or total absence of diagnostic services
- general practitioners (GPs) who are inadequately educated regarding the treatment of infectious diseases
- inappropriate or over-prescribing by unskilled, less well trained and un-updated practitioners in places where professional healthcare is absent
- prescription by practitioners whose only source of learning is promotional activities by pharmaceutical companies
- a tendency for dispensing doctors to overprescribe; these people not only prescribe but often also sell the drugs
- a desire to prevent infection before it occurs and the fear of therapeutic failure
- patient pressure
- patients in the community being erratic when taking their medication, e.g. taking antibiotics at a self-determined dose or only until they feel better
- unused antibiotics being saved and used for future self-diagnosed illnesses
- saved antibiotics being offered to other members of the family and to friends
- antibiotics that are freely available over the counter and in the street markets
- unrestricted availability of poor-quality, ineffective and potentially dangerous counterfeit medicines. It is estimated that nearly one-fifth of the world's trade in pharmaceuticals involves counterfeit medicines. Aggressive marketing by the pharmaceutical industry and the promotion of inappropriate and expensive broad-spectrum agents lead to improper use of antibiotic agents
- poor microbiological support in hospitals, which leads to extended hospitalization and the increased use of antimicrobials
- the ease of international travel, which provides an easy means of dissemination of antibiotic-resistant genes, both globally and locally.

HOSPITAL INFECTIONS IN DEVELOPING COUNTRIES

Hospital infection is one of the most adverse outcomes of hospitalization, both nationally and internationally (Daniel 1977, Lima et al 1993, Mayon-White et al 1988, Sithikesorn et al 1989, Sramova et al 1988, Srisuspan et al 1989, Wagner et al 1990). Yet the amount of attention paid to the control of hospital-acquired infection is related broadly to the level of provision of general healthcare (Meers 1988).

Information on the magnitude of hospital-acquired infections in developing countries is difficult to obtain. Studies with published data are limited; they are often from a single hospital or specialty, and cover few countries (Mortensen 1991). Other sporadic reports showing very low incidence rates are thought to be based on inadequate surveillance (Ponce-de-León & Rangel-Frausto 1993).

In a WHO-initiated survey of hospital-associated infection in 1983–85 in four WHO regions – European, Mediterranean, South East Asia and Western Pacific – data from 55 hospitals in 14 countries showed an average prevalence rate of 8.7% (range of 7.7–11.8%) (Mayon-White et al 1988). A 9-month study in Tikur Anbessa Hospital in Addis Ababa in Ethiopia (Habte-Gabr et al 1988) detected a 16.4% prevalence of hospital-acquired infections in surgical patients. Studies quoted by Orrett et al (1998), report infection rates of 27%, 15.5% and 24.6% among surgical patients in regional hospitals in Jamaica. Their own study in San Fernando General Hospital, Trinidad, identified 10 per 100 admissions. Equally high rates, often reaching 25%, have been identified in other studies (Haley 1991, Nettleman 1993a, Western et al 1982). Ponce-de-León (1991) reported that the average hospital-wide rate of hospital-acquired infections in Mexico was around 15%, and that this rate approached 26% in hospitals with fewer resources.

Berg et al (1995), identified rates of nosocomial infection of between 7 and 64% in intensive care units (ICUs) in Guatemala. The absence of other comparative ICU infection rates from developing countries is attributed to the lack of an infection control infrastructure and the paucity of resources and facilities for performing regular surveillance (Ponce-de-León 1991, Rhinehart et al 1991). In a country hard-pressed to manage and control ordinary infections, the issue of hospital-acquired infections does not always receive attention or priority (Meers 1988). Other factors, such as control of overpopulation, malnutrition and childhood diseases, take priority over hospital-acquired infections (Forder 1995).

Mortality related to hospital-acquired infections

Hospital-acquired (or nosocomial) infections are, directly or indirectly, among the most important causes of death in the developing world (Duse 1998). This is based, according to Duse and Smego (1999), on the assumption that there is a hospital-acquired infection rate of 15%, with an associated attributable mortality of 5% in all hospital-acquired infections. In Mexico, hospital-acquired infections are thought to be the third most common cause of mortality, behind enteric infections and pneumonia (Ponce-de-Léon 1991). Berg et al (1995) found a 24% mortality associated with hospital-acquired infections in ICUs in Guatemala.

Many hospital infection outbreaks in developing countries have been associated with substantial mortality (Adeyemo et al 1993, Banerjee et al 1993, Hammami et al 1991, Murphy et al 1994, Sirinavin et al 1991, Stephen & Lalitha 1993). A bacteraemia and meningitis epidemic due to *Serratia marcescens* caused 69% mortality in a general hospital in Mexico (Zaidi et al 1989).

Cost of hospital-acquired infections

There are very few studies focusing on the economic aspects of healthcare, especially infection control, in developing countries (Pannuti 1991). Ponce-de-Léon (1991) estimated that the annual cost of hospital infections in Mexico approached US $450 million in 1991. This estimate did not include the cost of antimicrobial therapy, thought to exceed US $50 a day. Orrett et al (1998), have estimated the cost of extra days stayed for hospital-acquired infection in a hospital in Trinidad to be around US $697 000 per year, which is approximately 5% of the annual hospital budget.

HOSPITAL INFECTION CONTROL – A LOW PRIORITY

Developing countries face two problems: limited resources for healthcare and lack of awareness of the importance of preventing hospital-acquired infections (Ponce-de-Léon & Rangel-Frausto 1998). Many countries are afflicted by a serious economic crisis and available resources for healthcare are severely limited (Pannuti 1991). Interest in hospital-acquired infections is therefore, not always a priority.

There is often a two-tier system of healthcare – private (or semi-private) and government-run hospitals. The interest in the economic advantage of infection control, often apparent to the administrators running private hospitals, is not always present in government healthcare facilities and infection control is seen as an easily dispensable discipline and often the first-line target for budget cuts (Duse 1998).

According to Ponce-de-Léon (1991), governments throughout the world, with few exceptions, consider investment in health to be non-productive. Health sectors are said to have 'survival budgets' (Duse 1998). In South Africa, the budget allocated to healthcare accounted for 9.9% of the total estimated government expenditure in 1996–97. In Pakistan, a total of 3.23% of the total government expenditure is allocated to healthcare (Zeenat Kanji, personal communication, 2001). Other problems include:

- inadequate or limited training of staff
- lack of good staff morale
- overcrowded and understaffed wards
- lack of potable water for drinking and washing, or contaminated water

- contaminated blood products
- scarcity of and the high cost of soap
- a lack of ability to perform microbiological tests
- limitations imposed on administration to deal with problems of hospital-acquired infections (Cavalcante et al 1991, Nettleman 1993b, Schlabach 1988, Wey 1995).

LACK OF KNOWLEDGE AMONG HEALTHCARE PERSONNEL

Cross-transmission of infection from healthcare personnel to patients is often associated with lack of knowledge and awareness. This ignorance can also lead to unnecessary practices, which consume scarce hospital resources. The hospital environment is often considered to be the main source of hospital-acquired infection. Issack (1999) cited the following instances of unnecessary practices, presumably performed in the belief that they would reduce the incidence of infection: routine environmental sampling from the walls, floor and, even the toilets, of operating theatres, intensive care units and surgical wards. Another example is the routine use of disposable overshoe covers when entering neonatal and intensive care units.

Issack (1999) describes a similar lack of knowledge among clinicians about causes and prevention of hospital-acquired infections. Examples include:

- not being aware that the origin of *Escherichia coli*, with different antibiograms, could be patients themselves
- being surprised at the occurrence of a multi-resistant *Klebsiella* septicaemia in a neonatal unit because the unit had been fumigated less than a month previously
- fumigation of an operating room with formaldehyde at the request of the surgeon because surgery had been performed on a case of gas gangrene
- environmental sampling from the operating room instead of from wound swabs from patients who had developed wound infections.

Unnecessary practices attributed to lack of knowledge

Unnecessary practices identified in a nationwide survey of hospitals in Thailand by Kunaratanapruk and Silpapojakul (1998) reflect many similar practices observed by the author in healthcare establishments in Pakistan. These include:

- Ward floors being washed with disinfectants. Studies have shown that bacteria on floors are not associated with hospital-acquired infections and that infections are not significantly different whether floors are cleaned with disinfectant or with ordinary household detergent (Danforth et al 1987, Daschner 1984, Maki et al 1982).

- Aerosol disinfection using disinfectant spray. Benzalkonium chloride is often used for this purpose, especially in operating rooms and intensive care units (Kunaratanapruk & Silpapojakul 1998). Studies indicate that bacteria sampled from the air, unlike those from the hands of healthcare personnel, do not cause surgical wound infections (Ayliffe 1991, Donowitz 1991).

• Fogging: operating rooms and isolation rooms are often disinfected using formaldehyde and a fogging machine. This form of disinfection is said to have little merit (Beeby et al 1967, CDC 1972). Apart from the human resource needed to perform the procedure, fumigated rooms have to be taken out of commission to allow the vapours to evaporate, adding to the cost of care.

• Ultraviolet lights: these are used in the operating rooms in the belief that they would protect surgical wounds from airborne infection. Apart from a slight benefit in 'ultra clean' operations, ultraviolet light has been found to have little effect on the incidence of postoperative wound infections (NRC 1964). Hot temperatures and high humidity, often encountered in developing countries, can compromise the bactericidal effect of ultraviolet irradiation (Riley & Kaufman 1972).

• Wearing gowns when entering critical care units is often a routine infection control measure. Gowns, masks, hats and overshoes were worn in neonatal phototherapy rooms in Pakistan. However, studies have failed to demonstrate that gowns prevent hospital-acquired infection in critical care situations (Donowitz 1986, Thakaran et al 1989).

PRACTICAL ISSUES AFFECTING HOSPITALS

Water supply

Lack of piped water is often a feature in hospitals and healthcentres in rural areas. The water is collected from wells and stored. The use of water in these circumstances is frugal, especially during dry periods of the season or drought.

The water supply in big city hospitals is often turned off for long periods each day (private and semi-private hospitals tend to be better catered for). This lack of water creates a major difficulty for hand hygiene or routine cleaning of the hospital.

Reuse of syringes and needles

According to WHO Fact Sheet no. 253 (WHO 2000c), worldwide, 8–16 million hepatitis B, 2.3–4.7 million hepatitis C and 80 000–160 000 HIV infections are estimated to occur yearly from the reuse of syringe needles without sterilization. The reuse of disposable syringes and needles for injection is common in certain African, Asian and Central and Eastern European countries.

The practice of scavenging on waste disposal sites is common in many developing countries. The scavengers expose themselves to infectious material and disposed, used needles and syringes.

Clinical waste

Almost 80% of wastes generated by healthcare activities are general household type wastes and 20% is hazardous material that could be infectious, toxic or radioactive. Infectious and anatomic wastes represent up to 15% of the total waste from healthcare activities (WHO 2000c).

Many hospitals and healthcare facilities do not have a system of safe disposal, and their waste is disposed of on sites that are easily accessible to the public. Landfill is an alternative to waste sites but can result in contamination of drinking water. WHO Fact Sheet no. 11 (WHO 2000d) recommends placing solid waste contaminated with blood, body fluids, laboratory specimens or body tissue into leak-proof containers and burying it in a pit 7 feet deep and at least 30 feet away from a water source. It suggests that blood and body fluids, as liquid waste, should be poured down a drain connected to an adequately treated sewer or pit latrine.

Disposal of sharps

Puncture-proof commercial containers are expensive and not readily available. Alternatives such as tins with lids, thick plastic bottles, heavy plastic or cardboard boxes are considered suitable (WHO 2000d). It is recommended that the sharps containers are buried in a deep pit if they cannot be incinerated.

Decontamination

Inadequate training, monitoring and education on basic hygiene are as much a factor in the inappropriate decontamination of used equipment as inadequate facilities such as lack of running water, disinfectants and sterilizers. In a survey of health clinics in the United Republic of Tanzania, 40% of presumed sterile reusable needles and syringes were contaminated with bacteria (WHO 2000d). A method of risk assessment is recommended for safe decontamination of used patient-care items.

INFECTION CONTROL STRUCTURE IN DEVELOPING COUNTRIES

An infection control programme that includes organized surveillance, control activities, an infection control doctor, one infection control nurse per 250 beds, and a system for reporting infection rates to surgeons has been found to help reduce the rates of hospital-acquired infection by 32% (Haley et al 1985).

Similarly, infection control programmes have been shown to have an impact on hospital-acquired infection rates in Ibadan (CISC 1979, Scott-Emuakpor 1970), Lagos (Anyiwo et al 1980, Daniel 1977), Iran (Kimberlin & Hariri 1981) and Kuwait (Larson 1987). The effectiveness of an infection control programme has been verified in a 600-bed federal hospital in Sao Paulo, where hospital-acquired infection rates were lowered from 11.8% to 7.4% (Wey 1995). The introduction of infection control and drug use evaluation led to a decrease in wound infection rates from 24.4% to 3.45%, and a 71% decline in the global incidence of infection in the intensive care unit in one Brazilian hospital (Cavalcante et al 1991). In the same hospital, the urinary infection rate was reduced from 100% in 1986 to 15% in 1989 by changing from open drainage bags to a closed drainage bag system and by establishing catheterization policies: the cost of treating each urinary tract infection was placed at US $500. The hospital also recorded a 74% reduction in the surgical prophylactic use of antibiotics. The total estimated saving resulting from these measures was US $2 million.

In another hospital in Brazil, the rate of hospital-acquired infection fell from 12% of hospital admissions to 7.3% following the institution of an effective infection control programme (Nettleman 1993b). According to Nettleman (1993b), US $300 million to $1.4 billion could be saved annually in South America, and US $230 million to $2.3 billion could be saved annually in Asia, if effective infection control programmes were established.

However, with the exception of private hospitals and some academic teaching institutions, a formal structure with an infection control team (ICT) and infection control committee is not widely applied.

Infection control doctors (ICDs)

ICDs are often in short supply in developing countries. This is mainly due to lack of interest in the discipline of infection control (Duse 1998). If available, they carry the infection control responsibility for a number of hospitals in the region.

Infection control nurses (ICNs)

ICNs, if present, often take lead responsibilities for the service in developing countries. This is seen as appropriate by Meers (1988), who considers nurses to be particularly suited to taking the lead in the prevention of infection and has suggested that a special initiative towards their education is the most effective and appropriate initial approach in tackling infection. This approach is strongly supported by experiences from Iran (Kimberlin & Hariri 1981) and Chile (Goldmann et al 1988).

The training of ICNs is often 'on the job' with limited support from the microbiologist, infectious diseases doctor or epidemiologist (if they exist). However, formal certificated courses are available in some countries (Duse 1998).

Link nurses

According to Duse (1998), the link nurse system (Horton 1988) is unlikely to succeed in South Africa because professional nurses are in short supply due to severe cuts in health budgets. They are heavily overworked, generally underpaid and often demoralized, leaving them with little incentive to take on additional responsibilities. However, link nurses were recently introduced by the author into healthcare centres and hospitals in North Pakistan and Aga Khan hospitals in Kenya. This system of creating infection control awareness at local level remains to be evaluated.

Surveillance

Surveillance is considered to be the logical initial step of any infection control programme in developing countries (Ponce-de-León & Rangel-Frausto 1998). The value of surveillance to generate funding for infection control programmes and to direct the priorities of that programming is well established. In Kuwait, government support for an infection control programme was obtained when healthcare policymakers were able to demonstrate that hospital-acquired infections were adding US $267 000 per day to hospital costs (Larson 1987). The Ministry of Health of Thailand has estimated that the annual US $40 million cost of hospital-acquired infections can be reduced by 30% in 5 years with a yearly investment of US $90 000 (Sudsukh 1989).

Surveillance of hospital infection and feedback of infection rates are seen as the backbone of hospital infection prevention and control efforts. The data can help gauge performance, influence changes in practice and measure the effect of change (Huskins et al 1998).

Duse (1998) maintains that the profile of infection control can be raised by the dissemination of locally derived or published information related to the morbidity and mortality rates associated with hospital-acquired infection. Limsuwan and Danchaivijitr (1988) suggest that information based on local studies is likely to be more helpful in developing better and more economical approaches than results from the developed, wealthier countries. Countries with few resources differ from industrialized nations with regard to the prevalence of diseases, population profiles and types of healthcare system (McInnerney 1990, Nundy 1984).

The surveillance programme should reflect the special characteristics of the hospital, the expected goals and the available resources (Ponce-de-Léon & Rangel-Frausto 1998). The magnitude of the problem identified by the surveillance programme can be overwhelming and Mortensen (1991) considers a programme of specific targets, based on the local problems (Haley 1985), to be more acceptable. Ponce-de-Léon and Rangel-Frausto (1998) recommend that hospitals with limited resources begin with the surveillance of critical areas such as emergency room/intensive care units, because these areas are the loci of >40% of bloodstream and pulmonary infections.

EDUCATION IN INFECTION CONTROL

Ponce-de-Léon (1991), suggests that both medical and nursing training programmes need to include more information on the risks associated with hospital treatment as far as it relates to hospital-acquired infections in particular and iatrogenic disease in general. Ponce-de-Léon and Rangel-Frausto (1998) also maintain that nurses need to be the first group of healthcare personnel to receive the continuing education programme directed at controlling and preventing hospital-acquired infections. The reasons cited for this are:

- nurses have the greatest contact with patients and are therefore the personnel who carry the greatest risk of transmitting organisms
- nurses are therefore a very important link in the pathway for interrupting infection transmission
- nurses are one of the most receptive and enthusiastic groups of professionals

- nurses are willing to follow control practices
- nurses are present everywhere and are associated with practically every procedure within the hospital.

The authors believe that if nurses are aware of the importance of their participation in infection control, then the procedures will be followed correctly and the success of the programme will be guaranteed. This will also help create an environment of ownership and collaboration.

Infection control policies and guidelines

Many unnecessary practices exist and proliferate out of ignorance. Often, guidance from developed countries is used to introduce infection control measures. However, these will need to be modified to suit local facilities and should be based on the actual capabilities of the hospital and its personnel. Ponce-de-Léon and Rangel-Frausto (1998) maintain that failure to meet even a few regulations will result in all the proposed regulations being viewed as unrealistic, and therefore impractical, by the hospital's administrative team.

A well-organized and supported infection control structure is essential to even the most tested and tried guidelines. Ponce-de-Léon and Rangel-Frausto (1998) suggest enlisting the support of people who are politically prominent in the hospital by encouraging their participation in the infection control programme as advisers or members of the infection control committee. Once involved, they will become natural allies and will appreciate the need for their collaboration to ensure its success.

This would undoubtedly help to raise the profile of a service where the primary worker is the ICN. This is because the ICN is often a female in a male-dominated society, and there is frequently a bias based on gender in those less developed countries where the emancipation of women is slow (Meers 1988).

PERFORMANCE EVALUATION

Continuous quality improvement (CQI) is considered a suitable method for evaluating the effectiveness of infection control programmes in low- and middle-income countries (LMI) because it emphasizes the analysis and optimization of systems of care in the context of existing resources (Huskins et al 1998). The bulk of the public healthcare money in LMI countries is consumed by hospitals (Barnum & Kutzin 1993, World Bank 1993) and an efficient follow-up of infection control programmes would permit the early detection of resource waste within the programme (Pannuti 1991).

INFECTION PREVENTION MEASURES

Many infection prevention measures are low cost but highly effective. The use of closed sterile drainage or indwelling urinary catheters, proper cleaning and disinfection of respiratory therapy equipment, use of boiled water in humidifiers are all measures with proven efficacy (Huskins et al 1995, Rhinehart et al 1991).

Many alternatives are possible if supplies are not available. For example (WHO 2000d):

- using plastic bags or condoms as gloves
- using cooking utensils to boil equipment
- exploring herbal or traditional alternatives to detergents and soaps
- using leaves, thimbles or plastic wraps instead of bandaids to protect cuts.

Schlabach (1988) recommends other similar practical alternatives:

- dressings made from shredded paper, mechanical waste or trimmings from local textile plants covered with a layer of gauze and sterilized
- clean cloths, torn into strips and sewn together to make bandages
- scotch tape or masking tape as an alternative to adhesive plaster tape.

Other infection control measures recommended are:

- drying used floor mops in the sun after cleaning
- sun-drying of linen used on patients with wounds
- leaving clean, non-draining wounds exposed in tropical climates where the atmosphere is warm and humid. Several hours after surgery, the non-draining incision of non-draining wounds have been found to be sealed with a dried serum coagulum.

All the above practices can be introduced at very little cost. However, the introduction and maintenance of such practices require knowledge and training on risk identification and management in infection control. The resource to train healthcare personnel is often lacking.

The information provided in Section 2 of this book, entitled Infection control knowledge and practice, can be used to form the basis of an educational input in both the basic and continuing nurse education programmes in all healthcare establishments in any country. The principles indicated can be adapted to local facilities.

How can we help?

The industrialized nations have resources, peoplepower and expertise in infection control, and these could be shared with colleagues in developing countries. Mortensen (1991) suggests a sponsored exchange and/or the production of education material, such as audiovisual aids and other useful materials. Also suggested is the sharing of resources in the form of financial support to enable the participation of experts in training courses based on local surveys of hospital-associated infections. The guidelines thus developed would be based on local needs and available resources.

The current proposal by the Infection Control Nurses Association (ICNA) to adopt a (developing) country in order to share knowledge and expertise (personal communication) is highly commendable. ICNs and ICDs, Public Health Physicians and health service managers and executives should all support this venture.

The commercial companies associated with healthcare products can also help. South Africa has introduced pharmaceutical-sponsored regional infection control programmes. The companies adopt a province/region and provide financial support for the development of infection control programmes, including follow-up audits. These consist of formal lectures on the basics of infection control and road shows, where trained practitioners do on-site visits, develop policies and solve problems in hospitals with limited resources (Duse 1998). Such commercial-assisted infection control programmes could be duplicated in other developing countries.

CONCLUSION

Health improvements often occur with social pressure but this demands a higher level of education than is available to the majority of people in developing countries. Their schooling level is low and their health expectations are determined by socioeconomic conditions. Hospitalized patients, many of whom think themselves fortunate to have reached hospital at all, have very limited expectations from the service. They accept discomfort as a necessary part of their treatment (Meers 1988).

Colleagues in the developing world need help from the more advanced nations to enable them to improve conditions for those using the healthcare service and those who deliver care.

REFERENCES

Adeyemo AA, Akindele JA, Omokhodion SI 1993 *Klebsiella septicaemia* osteomyelitis and septic arthritis in neonates in Ibadan, Nigeria. Annals of Tropical Paediatrics 13:285–289

Anyiwo CE, Daniel SO, Ogunbi OO, Aromolaran GO 1980 Nosocomial infections – a continuing danger to patients at Lagos University Teaching Hospital. Public Health 94:229–234

Ayliffe GAJ 1991 Role of the environment of the operating suite in surgical wound infection. Review of Infectious Diseases 13(suppl 10):800–804

Banerjee M, Sahu K, Bhattacharya S et al 1993 Outbreak of neonatal septicaemia with multidrug resistant *Klebsiella pneumoniae*. Indian Journal of Paediatrics 60:25–27

Barnum H, Kutzin J 1993 Public hospitals in developing countries: resource, use, cost, financing. The Johns Hopkins University Press, Baltimore, MD

Beeby MM, Kingston D, Whitehouse CE 1967 Experiments on terminal disinfection of cubicles with formaldehyde. Journal of Hygiene (Cambridge) 65:115–130

Berg DE, Hershow RC, Ramirez CA 1995 Control of nosocomial infections in an intensive care unit in Guatemala City. Clinical Infectious Diseases 21:588–593

Calvalcante MD, Barga OB, Teofilo CH et al 1991 Cost improvements through the establishment of prudent infection control practices in a Brazillian general hospital, 1986–1989. Infection Control and Hospital Epidemiology 12:649–653

Centre for Disease Control (CDC) 1972 Disinfectant fogging, an ineffective measure. NNIS Report 1971 (third quarter) (DHEW pub. no. CDC 72-8149). United States Government Printing Office, Washington DC

Control of Infection Sub-Committee (CISC) 1979 University College Hospital, Ibadan. Epidemiological surveillance of hospital-acquired wound infections. Niger Medical Journal 9:289–293

Danforth D, Nicolle LE, Hume K et al 1987 Nosocomial infections on nursing units with floors cleaned with a disinfectant compared with detergent. Journal of Hospital Infection 10:229–235

Daniel SO 1977 An epidemiological study of nosocomial infections at the Lagos University Teaching Hospital. Public Health 91:13–18

Daschner FD 1984 The cost of hospital acquired infections. Journal of Hospital Infection 5(suppl A):27–33

Donowitz LG 1986 Failure of the covergown to prevent nosocomial infection in a pediatric intensive care unit. Paediatrics 77:35–38

Donowitz LG 1991 Benzalkonium chloride is still in use. Infection Control and Hospital Epidemiology 12:229–235

Duse AG 1998 Infection control in developing countries with limited resources. Infection Control Practices – proceedings of the 2nd Conference on Infection Control organised by 3M Healthcare, Borken, Germany. 3M Medical Markets Laboratory

Duse AG, Smego RA 1999 Challenges posed by antimicrobial resistance in developing countries. Baillière's Clinical Infectious Diseases 5(2):193–201

Folb PI, Dukes MNG 1994 Pharmaceuticals policy in sub-Saharan Africa: what more can be done (report to the World Bank)? The World Bank, Africa Technical Department, Population, Health, and Nutrition Division. The World Bank Report

Forder AA 1995 How best to utilise limited resources. Journal of Hospital Infection 30:15–25

Goldmann DA, Otaiza F, Ponce-de-Léon SR, Gutman IF 1988 Infection control in Latin America. Infection Control and Hospital Epidemiology 9:291–301

Gwatkin DR, Guillot M 2000 The burden of disease on the global poor. Current situation, future trends, and implications for strategy. Health, Nutrition and Population Series, The World Bank, Washington DC

Habte-Gabr E, Gedebou M, Kronvall G 1988 Hospital acquired infections among surgical patients in Tikur Anbessa Hospital, Addis Ababa, Ethiopia. American Journal of Infection Control 16:7–13

Haley RW 1985 Surveillance by objective: a new priority-directed approach to the control of nosocomial infections. American Journal of Infection Control 13:78–89

Haley RW 1991 Measuring the costs of nosocomial infections: methods for estimating economic burden on the hospital. American Journal of Medicine 91(suppl 3B):S32–S38

Haley RW, Culver DH, White JW et al 1985 The nationwide nosocomial infection rate. American Journal of Epidemiology 2:59–67

Hammami A, Alert G, Ben Radjeb S et al 1991 Nosocomial outbreak of acute gastroenteritis in neonatal intensive care unit in Tunisia caused by multiply drug resistant *Salmonella wien* producing SHV-2 beta-lactamase. European Journal of Clinical Microbiology and Infectious Diseases 10:641–646

Horton R 1988 Linking the chain. Nursing Times 84:44–46

Huskins WC, Soule BM, O'Boyle C, Gulacsi L 1998 Hospital infection control: a model for improving the quality of hospital care in low- and middle-income countries. Infection Control and Hospital Epidemiology 19(2):125–135

Huskins WC, O'Rourke EJ, Rhinehart E, Goldmann DA 1995 Infection control in countries with limited resources. In: Mayhall CG (ed) Hospital epidemiology and infection control. Williams & Wilkins, Baltimore, MD, pp 1176–1200

Issack M 1999 Letters to the Editor. Unnecessary hospital infection control practices in developing countries. Journal of Hospital Infection 42:339–341

Isturiz RE, Carbon C 2000 Antibiotic use in developing countries. Infection Control and Hospital Epidemiology 21:394–397

Kimberlin CL, Hariri AR 1981 Nosocomial infections – problems in a developing country. Nosocomial infections in southern Iran. Royal Society Health Journal 101:74–77

Kunaratanapruk S, Silpapojakul K 1998 Unnecessary hospital infection control practices in Thailand: a survey. Journal of Hospital Infection 40:55–59

Kunin CM 1990 Problems in antibiotic usage. In: Mandell GL, Douglas RG, Bennett JE (eds) Principles and practice of infectious diseases, 3rd edn. Churchill Livingstone, Edinburgh, pp 427–433

Larson E 1987 Development of an infection control program in Kuwait. American Journal of Infection Control 5:163–167

Lima NL, Pereira CR, Souza IC et al 1993 Selective surveillance for nosocomial infections in a Brazilian hospital. Infection Control and Hospital Epidemiology 14:197–202

Limsuwan A, Danchaivijitr S 1988 Nosocomial infection control in Thailand. Journal of the Medical Association of Thailand 71(suppl 3):1–80

Maki DG, Alvarado CJ, Hassemer CA, Zilz MA 1982 Relation of the inanimate hospital environment to endemic nosocomial infection. New England Journal of Medicine 307:1562–1566

Mayon-White RT, Ducel G, Kereselidze T, Tikomirov E 1988 An international survey of the prevalence of hospital-acquired infection. Journal of Hospital Infection 11:43–48

McInerney TG 1990 OR nursing in developing countries. Present conditions, future hopes. American Operating Room Nursing Journal 51:554–570

Meers PD 1988 Infection control in developing countries. Journal of Hospital Infection 11(suppl A):406–410

Mortensen N 1991 How countries with more resources can help. Journal of Hospital Infection 18(suppl A):382–387

Murphy SA, Lowe B, Maghenda JK, Apollo JG 1994 An outbreak of intravenous cannulae associated nosocomial septicaemia due to multidrug-resistant Klebsiella pneumoniae. East African Medical Journal 71:271–272

National Research Council (NRC) 1964 Post-operative wound infections – the influence of ultraviolet irradiation of operating room and of various factors. Annals of Surgery 160(suppl 2):1–132

Nettleman MD 1993a Global impact of infection control. In: Wenzel RP (ed) Prevention and control of nosocomial infections, 2nd edn. Williams & Wilkins, Baltimore, MD, pp 13–20

Nettleman MD 1993b Global aspects of infection control. Infection Control and Hospital Epidemiology 14:646–648

Nundy S 1984 How might we improve surgical services for rural populations in developing countries? British Medical Journal 289:71–72

Orrett FA, Brooks PJ, Richardson EG 1998 Nosocomial infections in a rural regional hospital in a developing country: infection rates by site, service, cost, and infection control practice. Infection Control and Hospital Epidemiology 19:136–140

Pannuti CS 1991 Editorial. The costs of hospital infection control in a developing country. Infection Control and Hospital Epidemiology 12(11):647–648

Ponce-de-Léon S 1991 The needs of developing countries and the resources required. Journal of Hospital Infection 18(A):376–381

Ponce-de-Léon S, Rangel-Frausto MS 1993 Organising infection control with limited resources. In: Wenzel RP (ed) Prevention and control of nosocomial infections. Williams & Wilkins, Baltimore, MD, pp 82–88

Ponce-de-Léon S, Rangel-Frausto MS 1998 Infection control in developing countries. In: Bennett JV, Brachman PS (eds) Hospital infection. Lippincott–Raven Publishers, Philadelphia, pp 291–296

Rhinehart E, Goldmann DA, O'Rourke EJ 1991 Adaptation of Centres for Disease Control guidelines for the prevention of nosocomial infections in a pediatric intensive care unit in Jakarta, Indonesia. American Journal of Medicine 91(suppl 3B):213S–220S

Riley RL, Kaufman JE 1972 Effect of relative humidity on the inactivation of airborne *Serratia marcescens*. Applied Microbiology 23:1113–1120

Rosenfield A 1989 Maternal mortality in developing countries. Journal of the American Medical Association 262(3):376–379

Schlabach WE 1988 Dealing with hospital infections in developing countries. Tropical Doctor 18:161–162

Scott-Emuakpor MB 1970 The problem of post-operative wound sepsis in a city hospital. 1. Bacteriology of post-operative infections. Journal of Tropical Medicine and Hygiene 73:39–44

Sirinavin S, Hotrakitya S, Suprasongsin C et al 1991 An outbreak of *Salmonella urbana* infection in neonatal nurseries. Journal of Hospital Infection 18:231–238

Sithikesorn J, Lumpikanon P, Bunma P, Patjanasuntorn B 1989 Nosocomial infections in Srinagarind Hospital. Journal of the Medical Association of Thailand 72(suppl 2):12–14

Smith AJ, Aronson JK, Thomas M 1991 Antibiotic policies in the developing world. European Journal of Clinical Pharmacology 41:85–87

Sramova H, Batonova A, Bolek S et al 1988 National prevalence survey of hospital acquired infections in Czechoslavakia. Journal of Hospital Infection 11:328–334

Srisupan V, Senaratana W, Pichiansathien W, Tongsawas T 1989 Nosocomial infections in Maharaj Nakhon Chiang Mai Hospital. Journal of the Medical Association of Thailand 72(suppl 2):7–11

Stephen M, Lalitha MK 1993 An outbreak of *Serratia marcescens* infection among obstetric patients. Indian Journal of Medical Research 97:202–205

Sudsukh U 1989 The control of nosocomial infections in Thailand in the future. Journal of the Medical Association of Thailand 72(suppl 2):44–45

Thakaran V, Indararuska P, Onubol A 1989 Discontinuation of wearing covergowns in ICU did not increase the nosocomial infection rate. Journal of Infectious Diseases and Antimicrobial Chemotherapy (in Thailand) 6:183–188

Wagner MB, Petrillo V, Gay V, Fagundes GR 1990 A prevalence survey of nosocomial infection in a Brazilian hospital. Journal of Hospital Infection 15:379–381

Western KA, St John R, Shearer LA 1982 Hospital infection control – an international perspective. Infection Control 3:453–455

Wey S 1995 Infection control in a country with annual inflation of 3,600%. Infection Control and Hospital Epidemiology 16(part 2):45

World Bank 1993 World development report 1993: investing in health. Oxford University Press, New York

World Health Organization 1995 Global estimates of maternal mortality for 1995: results of an in-depth review, analysis and estimation strategy. WHO, Geneva. Available: http://www.who.int/reproductive-hea.../ statement_on_maternal_mortality_estimates.en.htm

World Health Organization 1997 Environmetal matters. Report by the Director-General EB101/19. WHO, Geneva. Available: http://www.who.int/ water_sanitation_health/Environmental_sanit/envindex.htm

World Health Organization 2000a Overcoming antimicrobial resistance. World health report on infectious diseases 2000. WHO, Geneva. Available: http://www.who.int/infectious-disease-report/2000/other_versions/ index-rpt2000_text.html

World Health Organization 2000b Fact sheets. HIV, TB and malaria – three major infectious diseases threats. WHO, Geneva. Available: http://www.who.int/ inf-fs/en/back001.html

World Health Organization 2000c Waste from health-care activities. Fact sheet no 253. WHO, Geneva. Available: http://www.who.int/inf-fs/en/fact253.html

World Health Organization 2000d HIV and the workplace and universal precautions. Fact sheet no. 11. WHO, Geneva. Available: http://www.who.int/ HIV_AIDS/Nursesmidwivesfs/fact-sheet-11/index.html

World Health Organization 2001 Food safety a world-wide challenge. WHO, Geneva. Available: http://www.int/director-general/speeches/2.../ 20010314_foodchain2001uppsala.en.htm

Zaidi M, Sifuentes J, Bobadilla M 1989 Epidemic of *Serratia marcescens* bacteraemia and meningitis in a neonatal unit in Mexico City. Infection Control and Hospital Epidemiology 10:14–20

Section 2
Infection control knowledge and practice

2

SUMMARY

Safe infection control practice suggests that the most effective set of actions has been taken to protect patients from developing infections; this effective set of actions must come from an informed understanding of infection control practice. Kitson's (1995) description of clinical effectiveness as 'doing the right thing' and 'doing the thing right', sits well with the ethos of 'informed' infection control practice. To do the right thing suggests a level of knowledge that enables healthcare practitioners to 'do it right' and evaluate the outcome, which may or may not be favourable. Some patients develop infections despite 'doing the right thing' because the practitioners do not have any control over a patient's own inherent susceptibility to infection. Some patients become infected because care practices contributed to this outcome. Whatever the outcome, practitioners need to possess an adequate and appropriate knowledge-base to understand their own role in patient outcome. The practice of infection control is complex, with contributions from many components, and practitioners need to be aware of:

- inherent and changing risk factors in and for patients
- actions/planning to reflect these ever-changing risks
- the potential risks associated with each treatment/procedure/ practice
- the theory that informs each practice
- the importance of evaluating practices in relation to patient outcome.

This section examines how infections impact on patients, staff and the organization, and investigates some of the components that help promote safe practice to protect patients as well as staff.

INTRODUCTION

An infection that is present on admission or becomes evident within 48 h of admission is considered to be community acquired. If an infection occurs 48 h after admission, or follows an invasive or manipulative procedure, the term 'hospital-acquired' or 'nosocomial' infection is used (Emmerson et al 1993). A hospital-acquired infection does not mean that it occurred as a direct result of staff practices or procedures, only that it occurred during hospitalization. Hospital-acquired infections (HAIs) are recognized according to the body system that they affect. Examples of common hospital-acquired infections are surgical wound infections, infections of the urinary tract, lower respiratory tract infections (especially pneumonia) and blood infections (bacteraemia or septicaemia). The last two are the main cause of infection-related morbidity. The 1994 Prevalence Survey, which included 37 111 patients from 157 hospitals, identified the distribution of hospital and community-acquired infections by the systems shown in Table 21.1.

Table 21.1 Infections in hospital patients according to the system affected as a percentage of all infections

Infection site	Hospital-acquired infection		Community-acquired infection	
	Count	%	Count	%
Skin	370	9.6	909	15.4
Surgical wound	413	10.7	42	0.7
Lower respiratory tract	882	22.9	2282	38.7
Intra-abdominal	93	2.4	244	4.1
Burns	22	0.6	4	1.1
Continuous ambulatory peritoneal dialysis	13	0.3	19	0.3
Central nervous system	23	0.6	94	1.6
Ear	11	0.3	48	0.8
Eye	116	3.0	111	1.9
Gastrointestinal	189	4.9	287	4.9
Peripheral device	75	1.9	4	1.1
Central line	77	2.0	32	0.5
Other vascular device	15	0.4	10	0.2
Bone	54	1.4	135	2.3
Undiagnosed fever	186	4.8	183	3.1
Implant	46	1.2	32	0.5
Urinary tract	894	23.2	839	14.2
Wound drain site	20	0.5	2	0.0
Reproductive tract	34	0.9	112	1.9
Septicaemia	239	6.2	236	4.0
Upper respiratory tract	76	2.0	269	4.6
Total	3848	100.0	5894	100.0

Reproduced by kind permission of Professor A.M. Emmerson from Emmerson et al (1996).

The main hospital-acquired infections are urinary tract, surgical wound, lower respiratory tract and skin (Emmerson et al 1996). Each system is affected by a multitude of factors. The literature pertaining to each body system is vast and beyond the scope of this book; only the relevant factors will be considered here. The discussions include the application of relevant knowledge to individual practices.

The practice of infection control is complex. Each healthcare-related action requires the application of relevant knowledge from a range of specialist topics such as microbiology, immunology, epidemiology, engineering and environmental hygiene. An understanding of how infections develop and factors that influence this outcome is also crucial to safe and informed care.

The knowledge-base that defines the principles appropriate to each practice is embedded in factors that come together to form a chain of infection, illustrated in Figure 2I.1. For an infection to occur, the links in this chain have to remain intact. The links can be broken at any stage in the chain by actions appropriate to each link.

The following chapters discuss the components of each link and the practices that will break the chain.

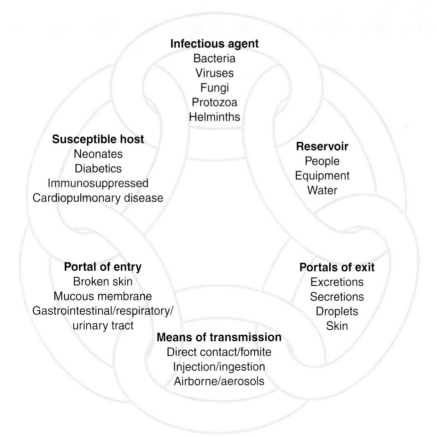

Figure 2I.1 The chain of infection.

Chapter 6 – Infectious agents

Chapter 7 – Reservoirs

Chapter 8 – Portals of exit

Chapter 9 – Means of transmission

Chapter 10 – Portals of entry

Chapter 11 – Susceptible hosts

Chapter 12 – Safe care: reflective practice

REFERENCES

Emmerson AM, Ayliffe GAJ, Casewell MW et al 1993 National prevalence survey of hospital acquired infections: definitions. A preliminary report of the Steering Group of the Second National Prevalence Survey. Journal of Hospital Infection 24(1):69–76

Emmerson AM, Enstone JE, Griffin M et al 1996 The second prevalence survey of infection in hospitals – overview of the results. Journal of Hospital Infection 32:175–190

Kitson A 1995 The multi-professional agenda and clinical effectiveness. In: Dieghan M, Hitch S (eds) Clinical effectiveness from guidelines to cost-effective practice. Health Service Management Unit, Manchester

Infectious agents

6

SUMMARY

Microorganisms are integral to infections and a basic insight into the characteristics of some commonly encountered microorganisms is essential for good infection control practice. Acting upon this knowledge will prevent the entry of disease-producing pathogens into susceptible sites on patients, ensuring a safe and informed element of practice. Figure 6.1 shows the first

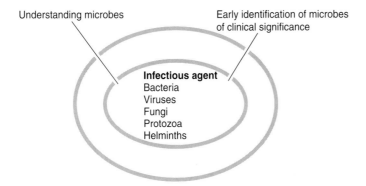

Figure 6.1 Breaking the chain of infection: infectious agents.

link in the chain of infection and the lines that break this chain. This chapter discusses the aspects of knowledge required to make these break lines.

An overview of some commonly encountered disease-producing microorganisms and their methods of transmission can be found in the Appendix at the end of this chapter. For further study, a list of recommended reading is included at the end of this chapter.

INTRODUCTION

Microorganisms are thought to have been the first living organisms on earth and can be found from the frozen wastes of Antarctica to the hottest areas in the magma core of the earth. They inhabit many parts of the world where no other organisms can survive, living in the soil, dust, water, air, food and on clothes, as well as on and in our bodies. Largely invisible to the naked eye, many microorganisms can be seen with an ordinary microscope, but viruses require an electron microscope because of their size.

The majority of microorganisms are beneficial to humans. Many are used by the biotechnology industry and they perform many useful functions in the ecological chain, being responsible for the breakdown of dead matter from plants and animals. They are also used in the production of cheese, yoghurt, beer, wine and bread.

Microorganisms that cause disease are referred to as pathogenic organisms. These include viruses, bacteria, chlamydia, rickettsiae, mycoplasma, fungi and protozoa.

Over the years, a system has evolved for identifying individual organisms by placing them into groups according to their similarities in structure. As scientific knowledge advances and more is discovered about microorganisms, they are reclassified and moved into other groupings.

BACTERIA

Bacteria are usually unicellular organisms, with a typical cell being able to carry out many different metabolic activities to increase in size and reproduce. Bacterial cells come in various shapes and sizes (Fig. 6.2).

Some bacteria form spores when environmental conditions are not suitable and can survive for a long time in the environment. One example is *Clostridium difficile*, which is responsible for antibiotic-associated diarrhoeal infections.

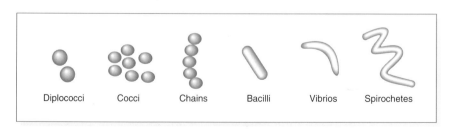

Figure 6.2 The different types of bacteria.

Classification

Bacteria are classified according to a variety of characteristics, the most important being shape and reaction to staining. Gram-staining is a method of colouring cells with dyes using a technique devised in 1884 by Christian Gram. Gram-positive bacteria stain blue after application of a methyl violet dye. Gram-negative bacteria do not retain the blue stain but, after decolourizing (e.g. with alcohol) and treatment with a red counterstain, take up a pink colour. Gram-staining and examining cells under the microscope for their shape and structure are methods used to provide a provisional identification. After the initial identification, specimens are grown on special culture medium to identify the organism. Mycobacterial species are not easily seen by Gram-staining and, for identification purposes, acid-fast stains such as Ziehl–Neelsen are used. Similarly, spirochetes are also not seen by Gram-staining so either dark-ground illumination microscopy or in a silver stain under the light microscope are used (Shanson 1999).

Replication

The main activity of bacteria is to reproduce and, under ideal conditions, some species divide by binary fission every 20 min. A single bacterium can convert itself overnight into a colony with a population of millions. The majority of microorganisms, including those important in medicine, are chemotrophs and get their energy from the oxidation of chemical compounds.

Generally, microorganisms reproduce themselves either by the simple fission of dividing one cell into two or by some form of sexual process, where genetic material from two or more cells is pooled and subsequently redistributed. A bacterium that replicates by simple binary fission produces two identical organisms, and constant repetition of this process produces a population of identical organisms. Changing the genetic composition can occur through mutation, transformation, transduction and conjugation. It is through these mechanisms that drug resistance occurs.

Toxins

Bacteria produce powerful poisons during their growth in the tissues of their hosts. Those toxins liberated by living bacteria are produced mainly by Gram-positive bacteria and are called exotoxins. These are proteins and are relatively easy to inactivate by heat. Endotoxins are released into the body when bacteria die. These are associated mainly with Gram-negative organisms and are relatively heat-stable. Endotoxins are considered less potent than the more active exotoxins.

CHLAMYDIA AND RICKETTSIAE

Chlamydia and rickettsiae are both obligate intracellular organisms, resemble bacteria and contain both deoxyribonucleic acid (DNA) and ribonucleic acid (RNA). They reproduce by binary fission and are susceptible to antimicrobial drugs that have no effect on viruses. However, they are nearer to viruses in size than bacteria and – virus-like – are unable to reproduce except inside the cells of host organisms.

Rickettsiae can survive for long periods outside their hosts at normal atmospheric temperatures. They are pathogenic to humans and diagnosis is usually from serological test. Chlamydia cannot live outside the host.

VIRUSES

Viruses are different from other organisms in that they consist of a core of one type of nucleic acid (either DNA or RNA) surrounded by a protein shell called a capsid. The purpose of the capsid is to protect the virus and to assist it to attach to the targeted host cell. When inside the human cell, the virus takes over the nuclear control of the cell and alters the cellular metabolism so that it makes new virons (Shanson 1999). Viruses attack a wide range of living organisms in the microbial, plant and animal kingdoms.

Structure

Viruses are identified by being grown in tissue culture, by special staining techniques or by electron microscope of the structure (i.e. central nucleic acid core of RNA or DNA surrounded by the capsid). Some viruses, such as the herpes viruses, have another covering called an envelope. These viruses are known as enveloped viruses; those without an envelope are called naked viruses.

Survival

Viruses are usually fragile and do not survive long outside a living cell; some, like rhinoviruses, that can survive for short periods, are responsible for colds and are spread more commonly on the hands and by direct contact than through the air by sneezing.

Viruses are prolific and can be found everywhere; many do humans no harm but some cause infections and diseases.

FUNGI

Fungi are considered to be plants that lack the green pigment, chlorophyll, that is used by plants for photosynthesis. Depending upon how they grow, fungi are described as moulds or yeasts, and some species can grow as either, depending upon the temperature and the availability of oxygen and nutrients. Fungi are eukaryotic cells. They are more complex than bacteria and reproduce sexually or by formation of spores. Those that are of medical significance do not have a sexual phase but form asexual reproductive spores. Fungal diseases are referred to as mycoses and are divided into those that affect only the skin, causing superficial infections like ringworm, and those deep infections that affect the whole body causing systemic infections, such as aspergillus.

PROTOZOA

More complex than bacteria, protozoa are eukaryotic, relatively large, single-celled microorganisms. They have a tough outer cell membrane instead of a cell wall and ingest solid particles of food to obtain nutrients. Many have lifecycles involving only the functions of movement, nutrition, excretion, respiration and reproduction; they are considered to be the lowest form of animal life.

Protozoa like malaria have lifecycles that include sexual and asexual phases.

HELMINTHS

Helminths are parasitic worms that infest humans and other animals. The development of disease and its seriousness depends upon the type of worm, the intensity of infection, the exact site of infection and the patient's reaction to it. Types of infestation include tapeworms, hookworms, threadworms, roundworms and flukes. Millions of people across the world suffer from serious helminthic diseases such as schistosomiasis, bilharzia and strongyloidiasis, with many others having asymptomatic infestations due to worms like whipworms. It is important to remember that individuals can suffer from simultaneous multiple infestations with different types of worm. Prevention often relies upon personal hygiene, clean water supplies, quality of food and adequate cooking.

PRIONS

These are currently hypothesized as being the cause of the transient spongiform encephalopathies (TSE), for which there is no evidence of a conventional infectious agent and no DNA or RNA has yet been detected. Prions are an abnormal form of a constituent protein (PrP) in the brain. They are thought to be found in the central nervous system and also in other tissues such as the lymph glands, particularly the tonsils.

During the 1980s, new types of prion are thought to have evolved to cause bovine spongiform encephalopathy (BSE) in cattle and resulting in variant Creutzfeld–Jakob disease (vCJD) in humans.

INFECTION CONTROL IN RELATION TO HOST RISK FACTORS AND MICROORGANISMS OF CLINICAL SIGNIFICANCE

Infections develop because microorganisms capable of initiating an infectious reaction have found a favourable host. Both the host and the microorganisms possess certain inherent characteristics that allow this to happen. The human body becomes vulnerable because of underlying illness or because a prescribed treatment has increased its susceptibility.

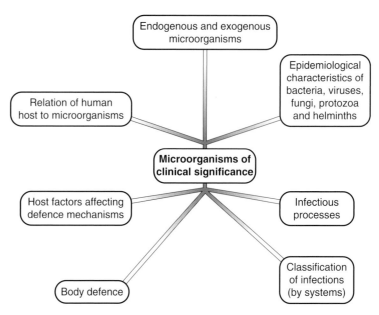

Figure 6.3 Factors involved in making microorganisms clinically relevant.

The microorganisms that display the ability to invade, spread throughout the tissues and cause disease and can be termed microorganisms of clinical significance. Figure 6.3 charts the link between microorganisms of clinical significance.

RELATION OF THE HUMAN HOST TO MICROORGANISMS AND THE INFECTIOUS PROCESS

Osterholm et al (1995) define the infectious process as an infection resulting 'from an encounter with a potentially pathogenic agent with a susceptible human host in conjunction with a suitable portal of entry'. The agent could already be residing on the human body (endogenous) or it could be from a source outside the host (exogenous). The outcome of this exposure could be a disease. Apart from the serious disease-causing microorganisms, people and microorganisms coexist in harmony most of the time. It is only when the equilibrium between the two is disrupted that microorganisms penetrate the body's defence mechanisms and cause infection. So the development of a disease depends upon the host and the agent. Microorganisms that cause infection have the capacity to enter the human body and spread throughout the tissues. They are also virulent enough to produce a disease in a susceptible host. For an infection to occur, six components have to come together:

1. the microorganism that is likely to cause infection
2. the reservoir where the infectious agent can survive and/or multiply

3. portals of exit, or a path by which the infectious agent can leave the reservoir
4. the mechanism for transfer of the infectious agent from the reservoir to the susceptible host
5. the portal of entry, or the path by which the agent enters the host
6. the susceptible person.

The risk of infection can be described in a formula:

$$\text{Risk of infection} = \frac{\text{dose} + \text{time} + \text{virulence (of microorganisms)}}{\text{Host susceptibility}}$$

The dose of some organisms required to cause an infection might be relatively low compared with the infective doses of other organisms. For example, a person suffering from *Shigella* dysentery might have been affected by only 100 organisms; whereas 100 000 *Salmonella* organisms are required before salmonellosis can occur.

The length of time for which an individual is exposed to the pathogen is also a contributory factor to the risk of infection.

The virulence, i.e. the capacity of the organism to produce a disease, plays a major role in the infectious process because it varies with each organism.

It is the vulnerability (susceptibility) of the human host that determines whether the above factors combine to produce an infection. The word 'virulence' is sometimes used to mean the combined effect of toxigenicity and invasiveness. Although it is necessary for a microorganism to gain entry into the host's body to produce disease, it can remain near the surface, as do ringworm fungi and *Neisseria meningitidis* in the pharynx. Similarly, for the organism to multiply and spread in the host, the host's tissues must supply the appropriate nutrients, atmospheric conditions and temperature that allow it to grow. Abnormal conditions in the host could enable an organism to thrive when this would not usually happen. Pathogenicity reflects the susceptibility of the host to disease as much as it does the ability of an organism to cause that disease.

A small minority of microorganisms live parasitic lives inside or on the surfaces of other living organisms. Such organisms live on the human body and can be referred to as commensal, symbiotic or pathogenic microorganisms. Commensals are those that take their nourishment from the host and do nothing else in return. Symbionts live in partnership with the host, taking the nutrients that the host provides and giving a service in return. The vitamin-synthesizing bacteria in the intestine are symbionts.

'Colonization' is the term used to describe microorganisms that are present on or in the body; growing and multiplying but without invading the surrounding tissues and causing damage. Normal skin is colonized by a stable population of microorganisms that assist the natural defence mechanisms of the body against infection. Colonization begins during the birth process and continues as contact is made with other people and the surrounding environment until a delicate balance of 'normal flora' is established.

Depending upon the length of time microorganisms coexist with the human body, they can be defined as resident or transient flora. Resident flora are found in certain areas of the body on a regular basis; transient flora inhabit the body for hours, days or weeks.

Microorganisms survive and multiply until they are removed by normal bodily functions such as handwashing. They do not normally cause disease in the host but are an important source of cross-infection in healthcare settings.

IDENTIFICATION OF MICROORGANISMS

Early and rapid identification of microorganisms is needed to prescribe correct treatment, prevent further complications or secondary infections and to start appropriate precautions to prevent cross-infection. The best use of the laboratory is to send only relevant specimens. To enable appropriate tests on each specimen, relevant information about the patient needs to be included on the accompanying form:

- relevant details of the main clinical condition
- date of onset of the illness
- information about recent/current/imminent antibiotic therapy
- history of recent travel abroad
- details of known antibiotic allergies.

Microbiological specimens

The value of laboratory investigation depends on the nature of the specimen. Although medical staff initiate the collection of specimens, the main responsibility for obtaining samples for laboratory investigation lies with the staff involved in direct 'hands-on' care. These staff should receive training in the correct procedure (Box 6.1).

Ideally, no specimen should be received by the laboratory more than 2 h after it has been taken. Transportation of specimens should be undertaken by portering staff. Specimens that cannot be delivered immediately should be stored in ward specimen fridges at 4°C to stop further multiplication of microorganisms (Parker 1999). Specimens from patients with known or suspected infections must be labelled with 'danger of infection' or 'biohazard' stickers (Health Service Advisory Committee 1991).

Postal transport of pathological specimens is available only to authorized medical or veterinary personnel. Specimens must be sent first class and clearly labelled 'Pathological Specimen – Fragile with Care'. The sender's name and address must be on the outer wrapping. New regulations came into effect from January 1999 to comply with UN 602 packaging requirements. The new regulations do not affect the type of substances that can be sent. Those substances that fall into WHO risk groups 1, 2 and 3 can be posted but risk group 4 is not carried by the Royal Mail (Advisory Committee on Dangerous Pathogens 1995, Health and Safety Commission 1996, Royal Mail 1999).

■ **BOX 6.1   Basic points to remember when collecting specimens**

- Use the appropriate container for the specimen. If unsure, check with the laboratory.
- Label the specimen container (not the lid) with the patient's details and date prior to collection. Number specimens sequentially.
- Always explain the procedure to the patient.
- Wash hands before and after taking a specimen.
- Prepare the skin whenever a specimen is obtained by needle or aspiration. Skin preparation should be with chlorhexidine or povidone–iodine in 70% alcohol, the alcohol being the essential element. Alcohol-impregnated swabs can be used.
- Collect an adequate amount of specimen. The greater the quantity of material, the higher the chance of detecting a causative organism, e.g. laboratory staff are more likely to incubate organisms from a sample of pus than from a swab from a wound that appears infected.
- It is advisable to moisten the bacteriology swab with sterile water or saline when taking swabs from dry wounds/body surfaces to allow for optimum 'pick-up' of organisms.
- Close the container tightly so that its contents do not leak or become contaminated in transport.
- If the container is soiled, change it for another.
- Specimens should be taken before the start of antibiotic therapy. If therapy is already in progress, specify the antibiotic on the request form.
- Complete the laboratory form, including the specimen site, diagnosis, date, time and requested test.
- Send specimens to the laboratory immediately to prevent overgrowth of non-pathogens and death of pathogenic organisms.
- Refrigerate (at 4°C) specimens that cannot be transported immediately. The refrigerator must not contain food or medicine.
- Blood cultures must be kept at body temperature and should be sent to the laboratory immediately. These must not be refrigerated or placed on radiators because heat or cold will destroy any organisms present. 'Out of hours' specimens should be stored in an appropriate laboratory incubator.

Patients collecting their own samples

Staff in outpatient clinics and general practice surgeries should instruct patients on how to collect samples themselves. The advice given in Box 6.2 will help staff working in these areas.

CONCLUSION

An understanding of microorganisms and their significance in clinical practice is the first stage in breaking the chain of infection.

■ **BOX 6.2**   **Advice for patients collecting their own specimens**

Collection of faeces for microbiology tests

- Write your name and the date on which the specimen has been taken on the label of the pot.
- The specimen required is a bowel motion. Instead of using a toilet, it might be easier if the sample is taken from a clean potty, chamber pot, commode or an old dish that can be thrown away.
- If you wish to take the sample from the toilet itself, it will be easier to cover the water surface with a small piece of newspaper, so that it will not sink. Do not put too much paper in the pan; it may block the drains.
- Unscrew the lid of the special specimen pot provided and, using the spoon attached to the lid, scoop up enough of your motion to cover the spoon well and place this inside the jar. Avoid contaminating the outside of the pot. Replace the lid firmly.
- *Wash and dry your hands.*
- Place the specimen pot in the sealable pocket of the plastic bag provided and close the pocket. Keep the specimen in a cool place (but not a refrigerator) and return with the request form without delay, for delivery to the laboratory.

Collection of midstream (clean-catch) urine

- Write your name and the date on which the specimen has been taken on the label of the bottle.
- Carefully wash external genitalia and dry with a clean towel. (Elderly and physically handicapped women might be advised to collect the specimen after a bath or shower.)
- Unscrew the top of the 30 ml container, being careful not to touch the inside of the bottle or lid.
- Start passing urine, allowing the first part to flow into the lavatory pan.
- Collect the next part of the specimen straight into the container (women should separate the labia with the fingers of the hand that is not holding the specimen container). The bottle should preferably be filled to the 20 ml mark (about ¾ full), although smaller amounts are usually adequate for testing. Try to avoid contaminating the outside of the container. Screw the lid on firmly.
- Dry any outside contamination of the bottle, if it has occurred, with toilet paper or tissue.
- Place the specimen bottle in the sealable pocket of the plastic bag provided and close the pocket.
- *Wash and dry your hands.*
- Keep the specimen cool and return it, within 2 h if possible, with the request form, for delivery to the laboratory. The specimen in its bag can be kept overnight in a refrigerator at 4°C (do not let it come into contact with food).

REFERENCES

Advisory Committee on Dangerous Pathogens 1995 Categorization of pathogens according to hazard categories of containment. HMSO, London

Health and Safety Commission 1996 The carriage of dangerous goods by road and rail (classification, packaging and labelling) and use of pressure receptacles regulations. HMSO, London

Health Service Advisory Committee 1991 Safe working and the prevention of infection in clinical laboratories. HMSO, London

Osterholm MT, Hedberg CW, McDonald KL 1995 Epidemiology of infectious diseases. In: Mandell GL, Bennett JE, Dolin R (eds) Principles and practice of infectious diseases, 4th edn. Churchill Livingstone, New York

Parker LJ 1999 Managing and maintaining a safe environment in the hospital setting. British Journal of Nursing 8(16):1053–1066

Royal Mail 1999 Pathological specimens. In: Handy guide to postal services. Royal Mail, London

Shanson DC 1999 Microbiology in clinical practice, 3rd edn. Butterworth Heinemann, Oxford

Appendix 6.1

Table of diseases

Safe infection control practice requires knowledge of microorganisms, the diseases they cause and how they spread between people. There are many textbooks available providing full scientific information about bacteria, viruses, fungi and helminths, and some of these are listed in the recommended reading list at the end of this appendix.

To assist practitioners to implement safe infection control practice, and to produce isolation policies in a disease-specific format if required, the diseases are listed in a familiar A–Z format. Although the list does not include every known infectious organism, it lists those responsible for the more common diseases and also some not often encountered in everyday practice. Information is given about the causative organisms, where they can normally be found, and any special features that might be of interest. Also included is the method by which transmission occurs from the organism's normal place of residence and how the organism gets into human beings, along with preventive measures to reduce the incidence of the disease.

Organisms causing disease in humans

Disease	Organism	Special features	Natural habitat	Mode of transmission	Prevention
Acquired immunodeficiency syndrome (AIDS)	Human immunodeficiency virus (HIV)	Retrovirus; types have been identified as HIV 1 and HIV 2	Humans	By blood, sexual transmission and vertical transmission (mother to baby)	Health education, needle exchange schemes, treatment of blood products and practice of safe sex, e.g. use of condoms. Hospital practices should include the disposal of sharps safely and care when in contact with blood and body fluids
Anthrax	Bacillus anthracis	Gram-positive, spore-forming encapsulated rods. The spores are only formed after the organism is shed from the body	An organism which can survive in soil for many years depending on temperature and humidity. It is a significant pathogen in both domestic and wild animals	Infection occurs in humans when spores enter abrasions on the skin or are inhaled by the lungs. Woolsorter's disease (respiratory or inhalation anthrax) is now rare. Internal anthrax remains a possibility as an aspect of biological warfare	Control measures include formalin decontamination of animal hides (this is no longer considered a legal requirement within the UK), strict control of domestic animals and the immunization of veterinary laboratory workers at risk
Argentinian haemorrhagic fever	Junin virus	Member of the arenaviruses	Wild rodents (bush mice) in cornfields	Airborne transmission via dust contaminated with infective rodent excreta; also laboratory infections occur and breaks in skin could be portals of entry for virus particles	Control of rodents. No vaccine is available
Ascariasis	Ascaris lumbricoides	Large intestinal roundworm; migratory stages pass through liver and lungs	World-wide, found mainly in tropical/ subtropical countries. Eggs found in soil	Ingestion of infected eggs from contaminated soil, food or water	Improved sanitation and hygiene
Aspergillosis	Aspergillus fumigantus, A. flavus and A. niger	Filamentous fungi causing opportunistic infections in immunocompromised patients	Occur widely in the environment especially in soil	Inhalation of airborne stages. Not transmitted from person to person	None known
Athlete's foot (see Ringworm)					
Blastomycosis	Blastomyces dermatitidis	Dimorphic fungus	Probably the soil. Found in America and parts of Africa	Inhalation of airborne spores which causes lung infections sometimes mistaken for tuberculosis; it can also produce abscesses	Unknown

Organisms causing disease in humans *(continued)*

Disease	Organism	Special features	Natural habitat	Mode of transmission	Prevention
Bolivian haemorrhagic fever	Machupo virus		Wild rodents	Airborne transmission by dust contaminated with excreta from rodents. Laboratory infections occur and virus can enter through breaks and abrasions on the skin	Control of rodents and isolation of humans
Botulism	*Clostridium botulinum*	Anaerobic Gram-positive rods producing a neurotoxin (the most potent toxins known). Eight immunologically distinct toxins produced by different strains of *C. botulinum*. Three most common in humans are A and B serotypes associated with meat, and E with fish	A major pathogen of birds and mammals but very rare in humans. Spores are common in soil	Botulism is acquired by ingestion of the preformed toxin. Intoxication is most often by ingestion of the toxin in foods that have not been adequately sterilized, e.g. home-preserved foods and improperly processed cans of food. Infant botulism results from ingestion of the organism and production of the toxin in the infant's gut. There is no person-to-person spread	Prevention is by encouraging good manufacturing practices. The toxin is not heat stable therefore adequate cooking of food before consumption will destroy it. Antitoxin is available from reference centres
Brucellosis (undulant fever)	*Brucella* spp.	Small Gram-negative rods	Three species are responsible for causing zoonotic infections in humans: *B. abortus* (cattle), *B. suis* (pigs), *B. melitensis* (goats)	Transmission is through consumption of contaminated milk or other unpasteurized dairy products and by direct contact in some occupations (vets, farmers, abattoir workers)	Recrudescence of infection is common. Prevention depends on eliminating the disease from domestic animals by selective slaughter and vaccination, and pasteurization of milk. Vaccination is available for people at risk in some countries but not the UK or US
Campylobacter infection	*Campylobacter jejuni*	Slender curved (seagull-shaped) Gram-negative rods	The normal reservoir is in a wide range of animals (especially cattle and poultry). The disease state is found in some domestic pets, e.g. puppies	Human disease is acquired from contaminated food and milk. Person-to-person spread is rare	Prevention is dependent on good hygiene practices. No vaccine is available
Candidiasis (thrush)	*Candida albicans*	Dimorphic fungus	Humans; occurs as yeast on mucosal surfaces as part of	Endogenous spread and by contact with secretions or excretions of the mouth,	Detection and treatment of vaginal candidiasis during pregnancy and treatment of other local

Disease	Organism	Reservoir	Transmission	Prevention/control
		normal flora (skin, mouth and intestine)	skin, vagina and faeces of patients and carriers. Also by mother to baby during childbirth	infections. Careful use of antibiotics should be considered
Chickenpox	Varicella-zoster virus	Member of the Herpesviridae family	Humans	Respiratory droplets and direct contact with vesicle fluid; infectivity is from 5 days before onset of rash to 5 days after its appearance	Checking of immune status for pregnant women who have been in contact with someone diagnosed with chickenpox. Specific immunoglobulin is available for contacts, vaccine not routinely available in UK but has been used in Japan and some European countries
Chlamydiosis	Chlamydia trachomatis	Obligate intracellular parasites with distinct life cycle	Humans; causes trachoma, urethritis and other infections of the genital tract	Sexual transmission; newborns may acquire conjunctival and pneumonic strains during birth from infected mothers	Health and sex education with emphasis on use of condoms during sexual intercourse. Vaccines are not available
Cholera	Vibrio cholerae	Curved Gram-negative rods	A human pathogen with no animal reservoir. Recent studies show the possibility of environmental reservoirs in coastal estuary waters	Infection is usually acquired from contaminated water or food	Prevention is by providing clean water supply and adequate sewerage disposal. A whole-cell vaccine is available but of limited use. New vaccines are now being developed
CJD (see Spongiform encephalopathies)					
Clonorchiasis	Clonorchis sinensis	Liver fluke	Larval stages in fish; complete cycle is human, snail, fish, human. Also infects other animals, e.g. cats, dogs and pigs	Ingestion of adult flukes when infected fish is eaten raw or undercooked	Cooking of fish and improved sanitation
Cold sores	Herpes simplex virus (HSV1)	Member of the Herpesviridae family	Humans	Contact with saliva, vesicle fluid, sexual contact and via the birth canal during birth	Health education and personal hygiene directed towards minimizing the transfer of infectious material
Colorado tick fever	Colorado tick fever virus	Orbivirus group	Infected ticks of small mammals, ground squirrel, porcupine, chipmunk	By bite of infected tick to humans, not person-to-person spread	Control of vectors as with Lyme disease

Organisms causing disease in humans (continued)

Disease	Organism	Special features	Natural habitat	Mode of transmission	Prevention
Common cold	Coronaviruses		Humans	Respiratory droplets, airborne and direct contact	No vaccine available. Improved personal hygiene and use of disposable tissues. Reduce overcrowding in living conditions
	Rhinoviruses	More than 100 serotypes are responsible for the common cold	Humans	By respiratory droplet spread	See above
Cryptococcosis	Cryptococcus neoformans	Yeast-like fungus	Common in soil where there are bird droppings	Inhalation of airborne cells	Removal of accumulation of pigeon droppings to prevent aerosolization of the organism
Cryptosporidiosis	Cryptosporidium spp.	Coccidian protozoan	Humans, cattle and other domestic animals	Via the faecal–oral route, person-to-person spread, transmission from infected animals and contaminated water is also important	Water treatment, education in personal hygiene and importance of effective hand hygiene practices. Safe disposal of faeces, especially from domestic pets. Guidelines required for educational farm visits by schools, youth clubs, etc.
CMV (cytomegalovirus) infection	Herpesvirus 5	Member of the Herpesviridae family	Humans; rarely causes symptomatic disease although infection is nearly universal throughout the world. Presence of antibodies varies in populations from 30–40% in developed countries to 100% in developing countries	Intimate contact with infectious tissues. Found in saliva, urine, semen, cervical secretions, milk, transplacental tissues and across the placenta	Observation of strict hand hygiene after changing nappies of babies and toileting of infants. Screening of blood donations for the immunosuppressed and organ donations
Dengue fever	Flavivirus	Severe disease only in second infection (i.e. rarely found in tourists who have not been previously infected)	Endemic in most tropical regions; humans and mosquitoes act as reservoirs	Bite of infected mosquitoes. No person-to-person spread	Education on prevention of bites by mosquitoes and eradication of vectors
Diarrhoea (antibiotic related)	Clostridium difficile	Slender Gram-positive spore-forming rods	Found as part of the normal gut flora in humans	Flourishes under selective pressure of antibiotics, can cause pseudomembranous colitis. It may be spread from person to person via the faecal–oral route and contamination of ward environments	Stopping of antibiotics if possible and attention to personal hygiene and cleaning of the environment

Diarrhoea (bacterial); other bacteria are also responsible for causing diarrhoeal illness	*Escherichia coli*	Gram-negative rods. Strains which cause diarrhoea can be divided into five major categories: (1) enterotoxigenic (2) enteroinvasive (3) enteropathogenic (4) enterohaemorrhagic (5) 'enteroaggregative'. Each category has different clinical symptoms, epidemiological patterns, virulence and set of O : H serotypes	Gut of humans and animals (cattle)	Spread is by contact and ingestion via the faecal–oral route. It may be food associated (e.g. poorly cooked meat or contaminated raw milk) and endogenous. Enterotoxigenic *E. coli* is a common cause of traveller's diarrhoea	Strict attention to personal and environmental hygiene
Diarrhoea (viral)	Rotavirus	Types A–D, of the Reoviridae family; only one type commonly causes human infection	Humans	Faecal–oral route and possibly airborne	Improved hygiene and sanitation
Diphtheria	*Corynebacterium diphtheriae*	Gram-positive, non-capsulate, non-sporing and non-motile rods	Usually found in the nasopharynx and occasionally on the skin of humans	Infection is usually spread by aerosol; focus of infection may be the throat or increasingly commonly the skin. Patients may carry toxigenic organisms for up to 2–3 months after infection	Immunization is effective in areas where herd immunity becomes sufficient to protect whole populations (85% or more). Babies acquire their immunity from their mothers for a few months after birth
Dysentery	*Shigella* spp.	Gram-negative rods	Normal reservoir is humans	Direct or indirect faecal–oral route. Human disease is acquired from contaminated food and milk	Prevention depends on good food hygiene and personal hygiene. No vaccine is available
Ebola and Marburg diseases	Ebola and Marburg viruses	Members of Filoviridae family	Unknown	Person to person by direct contact with infected blood and body fluids, including organs and semen	Restriction of sexual intercourse until semen free from virus. Control measures include isolation of cases and villages
Elephantiasis	*Wuchereria bancrofti* and *Brugia malayi*	Filarial nematodes, long thin worms living in the lymphatics with microfilaria larvae in blood	Humans; in SE Asia cats, civets and higher primates also act as reservoir	Microfilariae are taken up by blood-feeding insects (mosquitoes and blackflies), develop to the infective stage then are reintroduced to humans at the next blood meal	Avoidance of vectors and vector control
Food poisoning	*Bacillus cereus*	Gram-positive spore-forming rods	A soil organism found in low levels in raw, dried and processed foods	Spores are found on many foods especially pulses, rice and vegetables, surviving cooking and improper food storage which encourages	The majority of illnesses are short lived and self-limited. As with other food-borne illnesses, hygienic preparation of food is paramount. Cooked food should

Organisms causing disease in humans (continued)

Disease	Organism	Special features	Natural habitat	Mode of transmission	Prevention
Gas gangrene	Clostridium perfringens and other spp.	Anaerobic Gram-positive rods. Spore-forming but spores are rarely seen in infected material	Normal intestinal flora of humans and animals. Spores and vegetative organisms survive in soil	multiplication of vegetative organisms. Infection is acquired by ingestion of the organisms or toxins	be stored in a fridge and reheated thoroughly before serving
				Infection is acquired by contact; may be endogenous, e.g. wounds contaminated from the patient's own faecal flora, or exogenous, e.g. contamination of wounds with soil. Food poisoning is caused by ingestion of contaminated food	Gangrene requires rapid intervention with extensive debridement of the wound. Prevention of food poisoning is by hygienic preparation and thorough cooking
Genital herpes	Herpes simplex virus 2 or less commonly 1	Member of the Herpesviridae family	Humans	Sexual transmission	Health education and use of condoms during sexual intercourse
Glandular fever (mononucleosis)	Epstein–Barr virus	Member of the Herpesviridae family	Humans	Person-to-person spread via saliva	Education on personal hygiene (intimate contact only)
Gonorrhoea	Neisseria gonorrhoeae	Gram-negative diplococci	A human pathogen which may be carried in the genital tract, nasopharynx and anus	Infection is spread by sexual or intimate contact causing pelvic inflammatory disease and salpingitis in women and ophthalmia neonatorum in infants born to infected mothers	Prevention requires education and contact tracing. There is no vaccine available
Hand, foot and mouth disease	Coxsackievirus	An enterovirus	Humans	Direct contact with nose and throat discharges, and faeces	Reduce person-to-person contact and promote hand hygiene
Hepatitis A	Hepatitis A virus	Genus; Enterovirus member of the Picornaviridae family	Humans and rarely other primates, e.g. captive chimpanzees	Person to person by the faecal–oral route and common-source outbreaks related to food and water (considered infectious 1 week prior to the onset of jaundice)	Education in public hygiene, good sanitation and catering practices. Immunoglobulin and immunization are available
Hepatitis B	Hepatitis B virus	Hepadnavirus; antibody to surface protein protects against infection	Humans	Sexual transmission, via infected blood (needles, ear piercing, tattoos, etc.), vertical (mother to baby)	Vaccination of healthcare workers and babies born to mothers who are carriers of the virus. Safe disposal of needles
Hepatitis C	? Flavivirus		Humans; is the cause of most cases of 'non-A, non-B' hepatitis	Via blood through contaminated needles; transmission from mother to baby is uncertain	Health education and use of needle exchange schemes. Screening of blood donations

Disease	Agent	Characteristics	Reservoir/distribution	Spread	Prevention
Delta hepatitis	Hepatitis delta virus	Requires hepatitis B virus (HBV) to cause infection and either causes a co-infection or may be superimposed upon someone who is a carrier of HBV	Humans	Similar to hepatitis B	Prevention of hepatitis B infection
Hepatitis E		Can be severe or fatal in pregnant women	Humans and primates	Contaminated water and person-to-person spread by the faecal–oral route	Education in personal hygiene and improved sanitation
Histoplasmosis	*Histoplasma capsulatum*	Dimorphic fungus	Grows as hyphae in soil where there are bird droppings. Rare in Europe	Inhalation of airborne spores	Prevention of airborne inhalation by reducing levels of dust in contaminated environments, e.g. chicken coops
Hookworm	Two major species: *Ancylostoma duodenale* and *Necator americanus*	Small intestinal roundworms	Widespread in tropical/subtropical countries. Humans are reservoir	Eggs in faeces are deposited in the soil and develop into larvae which penetrate the skin when it comes into contact, or by ingestion of contaminated food	Improved hygiene and sanitation
Impetigo	*Staphylococcus aureus* and *Streptococcus pyogenes*	Gram-positive cocci	Humans and animals associated with them. Skin, especially the nose and perineum, with carriage rates higher in hospital patients and staff	Auto, direct contact, via hands	Prevention of spread is by attention to isolation techniques, hand hygiene and treatment of carriers in high-risk areas in hospital (these are dependent on local policies and protocols)
Influenza	Influenza virus types A and B		Humans, though animals have been thought to act as sources of new subtypes of influenza A	By respiratory droplets	Education in public hygiene especially related to unprotected coughing and sneezing. Immunization should be offered to those considered to be at particular risk
Kuru (see Spongiform encephalopathies)					
Lassa fever	Lassa virus	Arenavirus	Widely distributed over West Africa by wild rodents (bush rat)	Spread is by contact with rodent excreta. Person-to-person spread and laboratory infections occur by contact with infected body secretions	Specific rodent control. No vaccine available. Source isolation
Leishmaniasis	*Leishmania tropica* and *L. braziliensis*	Intracellular protozoon	Humans, wild rodents, marsupials and other unknown hosts in many areas	By the bite of infected sandflies	Education of the public in transmission and controlling of vectors

Organisms causing disease in humans (continued)

Disease	Organism	Special features	Natural habitat	Mode of transmission	Prevention
Legionnaires' disease	Legionella pneumophila	Gram-negative rods, which are a recent discovery in microbiological history	An environmental saprophyte that is found in water supplies and streams and ponds	Infection is acquired by inhalation of contaminated water from showers, air-conditioning, cooling towers, jacuzzis, etc. There is no person-to-person spread	Prevention depends on maintenance of hot water and air-conditioning systems, particularly in large buildings such as offices, hospitals and hotels. No vaccine is available
Leprosy (Hansen's disease)	Mycobacterium leprae	Aerobic rods which have a waxy cell wall which resists decolorization with acid and alcohol	A human pathogen	Droplet spread is aided by the ability of organisms to survive in the environment. Infection requires close prolonged contact through the upper respiratory tract and possibly through broken skin	Prevention is by education on the availability of drug therapy and detection of cases. Field trials show that prophylactic Bacille-Calmette-Guérin (BCG) vaccination reduces the incidence among contacts of cases
Leptospirosis (Weil's disease)	Leptospira interrogans	Finely coiled spirochaetes with hooked ends. There are many serovars with different animal hosts, e.g. L. interrogans serovar hardjo (cattle) and L. interrogans serovar icterohaemorrhagiae (rats)	A zoonosis, its usual hosts are rodents, bats, cattle, sheep, goats and other domestic animals	Leptospires are excreted in urine and contaminate food and water. Infection occurs by contact either through occupation (sewage workers, farmers and abbatoir workers); or by recreation activities on inland waters, e.g. canoeing, windsurfing, etc. on canals, rivers and reservoirs. Organisms may penetrate intact skin and conjunctiva	Prevention of disease after exposure can be by early treatment of symptoms with penicillin
Listeriosis	Listeria monocytogenes	Short Gram-positive rods	An enteric organism widely found in nature and survives well in the cold. It enters the food chain when silage is used as manure directly on to vegetables, also through contamination of soft cheeses, pâté, etc. Humans may carry the organism in their gut as part of the normal flora	Infection may be acquired by ingestion and via the placenta to the fetus in utero	Widespread distribution of the organism in nature makes prevention of acquiring the organism difficult. Pregnant women have been advised against eating uncooked food which is thought to be of particular risk, e.g. coleslaw, pâté, soft cheese and unpasteurized milk
Lyme disease	Borrelia burgdorferi	Finely coiled spirochaetes	A zoonosis transmitted to humans by hard ticks (Ixodes spp.) associated with deer	Ticks are found on bracken and in undergrowth and attach to exposed skin. Lyme disease is slowly	Prevention depends on avoiding contact with vectors by using protective clothing for walkers and forestry workers

progressive with 50% of cases having a characteristic skin lesion. Joint pains and fatigue are common

Malaria	Plasmodium falciparum	There are four human malaria species. Others are P. vivax, P. malariae and P. ovale and are generally not life threatening	A protozoon	By the bite of an infective female mosquito. Transfusion of infected blood	Improved sanitation to reduce vectors, window screens, clothing, etc. Screening of blood donors
Measles	Measles virus	Member of the family Paramyxoviridae. Significant mortality in babies, the immuno-suppressed and non-exposed populations	Humans	By respiratory droplets	Immunization
Meningitis: bacterial	Haemophilus influenzae	Gram-negative rods	Upper respiratory tract in humans	Person to person via the airborne route	Hib vaccine is given to children in US and UK
	Neisseria meningitidis	Gram-negative diplococci	Human pathogen carried in the pharynx with carriage rates higher in populations during epidemics	Droplet spread with several immunologically distinct capsular types (A, B, C)	A vaccine is available for types A and C but is ineffective in preventing infection with type B strains. Rifampicin is used for prophylaxis of close contacts
	Streptococcus pneumoniae	Gram-positive diplococci	See Pneumonia		
MOTT (mycobacteria other than tuberculosis)		Aerobic rods, which are acid fast (see Leprosy)	Ubiquitous in nature. Of the numerous species identified approximately 15 are recognized as being pathogenic to humans	With the exception of skin lesions there is no evidence of person-to-person spread. Host tissue damage and immunodeficiency may predispose to infection	
Mumps	Mumps virus	Genus Paramyxovirus, causes inflammation of salivary and other glands. Can cause meningitis or encephalitis	Humans	By respiratory droplets	Immunization
Necrotizing fasciitis	Streptococcus pyogenes (group A strep.)	Gram-positive cocci in chains	Found in the upper respiratory tract and on the skin of humans	Spread is by airborne droplets and contact. Survival in dust may be important	No vaccine available. Education in the mode of transmission

Organisms causing disease in humans (continued)

Disease	Organism	Special features	Natural habitat	Mode of transmission	Prevention
Ophthalmia neonatorum	Neisseria gonorrhoeae and Chlamydia trachomatis	Gram-negative diplococci	Human pathogen carried in the genital tract	Contact with the infected birth canal during childbirth in infants born to infected mothers	Through diagnosis and treatment of infected mothers
Paragonimiasis	Paragonimus westermanii	Lung fluke, thick fleshy worms living in pairs in cysts	Larval stages in crabs; adults infect humans and other animals, e.g. dogs, cats, pigs and wild carnivores	Ingestion of infected crab meat or other crustaceans eaten raw or undercooked	Cooking of crab meat and improved sanitation
Pharyngo-conjunctival fever	Adenoviruses	Types 3, 4 and 7 are most common. Type 3 is responsible for outbreaks associated with swimming pools. (Conjunctivitis more of a problem)	Humans	Via respiratory droplets or faeces and sometimes indirect contact on contaminated hands, towels, eyedroppers, etc.	Live oral vaccine has been used in military recruits
Pinworm	Enterobius vermicularis	Small roundworm found in the large bowel. Worms emerge from the anus at night to lay eggs	Humans (ubiquitous)	Ingestion of eggs carried from fingers and in dust. Eggs are infectious when laid so direct reinfection is common	Improved hand hygiene, treatment of cases and contacts
Pinta	Treponema carateum	Regularly coiled spirochaetes. Serology test reacts with T. pallidum	Humans	Person-to-person spread by prolonged direct contact with skin lesions	General health promotion measures
Pneumocystosis	Pneumocystis carinii	Previously classified as sporozoan protozoan, now classified as a fungus	Humans; found also in animals such as rodents, cattle and dogs	Assumed to be by droplet inhalation; causes a pneumonia-like condition in immunocompromised patients	None known
Pneumonia	Mycoplasma pneumoniae	Classified as mollicutes because they lack a true cell wall and consequent rigidity	Found in humans it is an important cause of atypical pneumonia	From person to person by the airborne route	Avoidance of crowded living conditions especially in institutions
	Streptococcus pneumoniae	Gram-positive coccus appearing in pairs (diplococci)	Found in the respiratory tract of humans with up to 4% of the population carrying it in small numbers	Transmission is by droplet spread	A vaccine is available (Pneumovax) composed of antigens of the most common serotypes

Disease	Organism	Classification	Reservoir/source	Transmission	Prevention
Polio	Poliovirus types 1, 2 and 3	Genus *Enterovirus*	Humans	Direct contact via the faecal–oral route, sewage contamination of drinking water	Immunization, education on the importance of hand hygiene
Prion diseases (see Spongiform encephalopathies)					
Pseudomonas infection	*Pseudomonas aeruginosa*	Gram-negative rod, opportunistic pathogen	Widespread in moist environments it is an opportunistic pathogen which can infect any body site. A small percentage carry the organism as part of their normal gut flora	Spread is by direct or indirect contact; endogenous infection may occur in compromised patients	Prevention depends on good aseptic technique in hospitals
Q fever	*Coxiella burnetii*	Rickettsiae, obligate intracellular parasites	Natural reservoirs are cattle, sheep, goats, cats and their ticks, fleas, mites and lice	Airborne dissemination of rickettsiae in dust and direct and indirect contact with infected animals and other contaminated materials	By avoidance of contact with vectors. Vaccines are available for at-risk groups, e.g. vets and farm workers
Rabies	Rabies virus	Rhabdovirus	Wild and domestic biting mammals including dogs, foxes, coyotes, wolves, jackals and bats	Via the bite or scratch of an infected animal. The virus is found in the saliva of the infected animal	Vaccination of pets, especially dogs and cats, education of the public and immunization of those whose profession is considered to be in a high-risk group, e.g. vets, staff of quarantine kennels. Post-exposure prophylaxis
Relapsing fever	*Borrelia recurrentis*	Spirochaete	Louse-borne disease in humans. Tick-borne disease in wild rodents	Vector-borne by the bite of lice or ticks. Person-to-person spread is by infected lice through sharing of clothes, bedding, unhygienic living conditions, etc.	Control of lice and ticks, education and improvement of living conditions and personal hygiene
Respiratory syncytial virus (RSV)	Respiratory syncytial virus	Member of the paramyxovirus family; causes severe pneumonitis in young children and the immunosuppressed	Humans	By respiratory droplets	Isolation of children in hospitals is desirable
Ringworm	Dermatophytes	Filamentous fungi invading the surface of keratinized structures of skin, hair and nails	Humans, rarely soil or animals	Contact with infected skin scales either by direct or indirect routes	Prevention is by improved skin care, hygiene and frequent cleaning of communal areas, e.g. showers and changing areas in public swimming baths, etc.

Organisms causing disease in humans (continued)

Disease	Organism	Special features	Natural habitat	Mode of transmission	Prevention
River blindness	Onchocerca volvulus	Long thin adult worms form subcutaneous nodules with microfilariae in the skin	Humans	By the bite of infected female blackflies	Avoidance of vectors and vector control
Rocky Mountain spotted fever	Rickettsia rickettsii	Rickettsiae, obligate intracellular parasites	Found in nature, rickettsiae are maintained in animal reservoirs and transmitted by the bites of ticks, lice, mites and fleas	Vector-borne by the bite of ticks, etc., not person-to-person spread	Infection is prevented by avoiding contact with vectors
Rubella (German measles)	Rubella virus	Togaviridae family; congenital infection causes severe fetal damage in first 16 weeks of pregnancy	Humans	By respiratory droplets	Immunization and screening for immunity
Salmonellosis	Salmonella spp.	Gram-negative, non-sporing rods	Widespread in animals in the food chain, affecting especially poultry, eggs, meat, milk and cream	Acquired by ingestion of contaminated food or person-to-person spread by the faecal–oral route	Prevention is by education of the need for cooking and handling of food adequately, strict hygiene and sanitation systems
Scarlet fever	Streptococcus pyogenes (group A strep.)	Gram-positive cocci in chains	Human respiratory tract and skin	Airborne droplet spread and direct contact	Exclusion of infected people from handling and preparing food. Adherence to the principles of asepsis
Schistosomiasis	Schistosoma spp.	Blood flukes with adult flukes found in blood vessels around the intestine and bladder	Humans and animals dependent on species	Larvae released from eggs infect aquatic snails. These release infective cercaria larvae which actively penetrate human skin	Avoidance of bathing, swimming, etc. in infected waters. Removal of snails and improved sanitation
Septicaemia	Streptococcus agalactiae (group B strep.)	Gram-positive cocci in chains. Causes neonatal septicaemia and meningitis	Human gut and vagina; carriage rate in pregnant women is 10–30%	Babies acquire the organism from colonized mothers at birth or by contact spread between babies in the nursery after birth	Screening of pregnant women is not reliable but prophylactic antibiotics may be given to babies of carriers

Disease	Agent	Characteristics	Reservoir	Transmission	Prevention/Control
Shingles	Herpes zoster (chickenpox virus)	Member of the Herpesviridae family, the virus remains latent after chickenpox and may erupt as shingles	Humans	Direct contact with vesicle fluid may cause chickenpox	Checking of immune status for pregnant women who do not know if they have previously had chickenpox
Spongiform encephalopathies (prion diseases)	Scrapie-type agents (slow viruses)	Probably not viruses, their structure and mode of replication is unknown. They contain little or no nucleic acid. A host-coded prion protein, in slightly altered form (protease resistant), is associated with infectivity. Highly resistant to heat, chemical agents and irradiation. Very slow replication with a very long incubation period	These agents infect a variety of mammals and can be transmitted to cows, mink, cats, mice, etc. when food contains infected material	Kuru: from infected human brain by contact during burial rites. CJD: in most cases unknown. Occasionally transmission is from infected human brain by medical or surgical procedures. Familial cases have a possible genetic transmission	Prevention of iatrogenic CJD when genetically engineered growth hormone was introduced. Discarding of surgical instruments used on cases
Staphylococcal diseases					
Boils, skin sepsis, postoperative wound infections	Staphylococcus aureus	Gram-positive cocci	Humans and animals associated with them. Skin, especially the nose and perineum, with carriage rates higher in hospital patients and staff	Spread is by contact	Prevention of spread is by attention to hand hygiene, isolation techniques, and treatment of carriers in high-risk areas in hospital (these are dependent on local policies and protocols)
Methicillin-resistant Staphylococcus aureus (MRSA)	See above	See above	See above	See above	Multiple resistance to antibiotics is of concern and antibiotic policies have been developed to address this issue
Toxic shock syndrome	Staphylococcus aureus	Syndrome caused by infection or colonization with toxin-producing strains	See above	Increased risk in high users of tampons and contraception devices, e.g. diaphragms and vaginal sponges	Education on use of vaginal tampons and vaginal sponges which are not to be left in place for more than 30 hours. Education of women that if symptoms of fever, vomiting or diarrhoea occur during menstruation they should discontinue tampon use immediately and consult a physician
Device-related infections	Staphylococcus epidermidis	Gram-positive cocci	Humans, skin with carriage rate 100%	An opportunistic pathogen; spread is by contact with self, other patients or hospital staff	Prevention is by care with invasive devices, attention to hand hygiene and principles of asepsis

Organisms causing disease in humans (continued)

Disease	Organism	Special features	Natural habitat	Mode of transmission	Prevention
Urinary tract infections (UTIs)	Staphylococcus saprophyticus	Gram-positive cocci	Humans, skin and genitourinary mucosa	UTIs in previously healthy women associated with sexual intercourse, endogenous spread to urinary tract in colonized women	Urination after intercourse helps to wash the organisms out of the bladder and so prevent infection
Strongyloidiasis	Strongyloides stercoralis	Minute intestinal round-worm living in humans only as larvae and parthenogenetic females	Humans, dogs, cats and primates	Infective larvae develop from eggs in faeces found in soil, from which infective larvae penetrate skin	Improved hygiene and sanitation
Syphilis	Treponema pallidum	Regularly coiled spirochaetes	Humans	Sexually transmitted requiring very close contact as it is extremely susceptible to heat and drying. It may also be transmitted vertically in utero to the unborn child and by blood transfusion	Prevention relies on detection and treatment of cases, contact tracing and serological testing of pregnant women
Tapeworms					
Beef and pork tapeworms	Taenia saginata and Taenia solium	Intestinal infection due to adult stage of the tapeworm	Humans are the definitive hosts with cattle and pigs acting as intermediate hosts	Transmission is by eating raw or undercooked meat from animals infected with larval stages of worms. T. solium eggs can hatch in humans allowing cysts to develop	Adequate cooking of meat. Prevention of human faeces contaminating grazing/feeding areas of cattle and pigs
Dwarf tapeworm (hymenolepiasis)	Hymenolepis nana	Small tapeworms; life cycle is direct or via insect	Humans; insects may act as intermediate hosts	Ingestion of eggs in contaminated food or water	Education in personal hygiene and sanitation
Fish tapeworm	Diphyllobothrium latum	Large tapeworms in fish	Humans; intermediate hosts are snails and fish	Eggs excreted in the faeces mature in water to larval stage in snails and fish (first and second intermediate hosts). Infection occurs when raw or undercooked fish are eaten by humans	Cooking of fish and improved sanitation
Hydatidosis	Echinococcus granulosus	Large fluid-filled (hydatid) cysts	Natural cycle is adult (dog), larvae (sheep)	Ingestion of eggs released from adult tapeworms in dogs	Hand hygiene after handling dogs
Tetanus (lockjaw)	Clostridium tetani	Anaerobic Gram-positive spore-forming rods	Organisms are widespread in the soil	Acquired by humans when contaminated soil enters wounds. The wound may be	Prevention is readily available and effective in the form of immunization with toxoid.

		with terminal round spore (drumstick)		major, e.g. war, road traffic accident (RTA), or minor, e.g. grazing of the knee from a fall or a rose thorn puncture whilst gardening. There is no person-to-person spread	It is usually given in childhood but if immunization status of the patient is unknown, toxoid is given in addition to antitoxin
Tinea (see Ringworm)					
Toxocariasis	Toxocara canis	Larvae of roundworm species	Eggs excreted in faeces of dogs	Ingestion of infective eggs by direct or indirect contact	Improved hygiene and routine deworming of puppies and pregnant bitches
Trichinosis	Trichinella spiralis	Minute roundworms living as adults in the intestine; causes muscle cysts in humans	It has a low host specificity–infects and matures in a wide variety of mammals	Acquired by eating raw or undercooked meat (usually pork) containing infected larvae	Improved hygiene and sanitation. Importance of adequate cooking of meat
Trichuriasis (whipworm disease)	Trichuris trichiura	Medium-sized roundworm in the large bowel	Humans, world-wide distribution	Ingestion of infective eggs in contaminated soil, food or water	Improved hygiene and sanitation
Tuberculosis	Mycobacterium tuberculosis complex	Aerobic rods, which are acid fast	Primarily humans, in some areas diseased cattle, rarely primates, badgers or other animals	Droplet spread is aided by the ability of the organisms to survive in the environment. Milk-borne spread to humans has been important in the past	BCG vaccination is valuable to those who are not exposed to heavy loads of mycobacteria early in life. Contact tracing of close contacts and public health measures. Pasteurization of milk and improved living conditions and diet have played a major role in prevention. Testing and slaughter of cattle
Typhoid and paratyphoid (enteric fevers)	Salmonella typhi and Salmonella paratyphi	Gram-negative non-sporing rods	Humans; a carrier state may follow acute illness, mild or subclinical infections. Carriers frequently have gall bladder pathology	Ingestion of contaminated food and water and by the faecal–oral route	Prevention is by education of the need for strict hygiene, sanitation systems and cooking of food adequately
Typhus	Rickettsia prowazekii	Obligate intracellular parasite	Humans are the reservoir; associated with unhygienic living conditions in times of war and famine	Not directly person-to-person transmission. Infection is spread when lice become infected after feeding on the blood of an infected person with acute typhus fever, excreting the infection in their faeces. In louse-infested communities humans become infected when	Improved living conditions with bathing and washing facilities. Use of insecticides can be made on clothes and people. Immunization is possible for susceptible people or groups, e.g. military personnel

Organisms causing disease in humans (continued)

Disease	Organism	Special features	Natural habitat	Mode of transmission	Prevention
				they rub the faeces or crushed lice into bites and superficial abrasions of the skin	
Urinary tract infections (UTIs)	Enterococcus	Gram-positive cocci	Gut of humans and animals	Infections are thought to be endogenously acquired, but cross-infection may occur in hospital patients	Strict application of the principles of asepsis
	Escherichia coli	Gram-negative rods	Gut of humans and animals; sometimes colonizes the lower end of the urethra and vagina	Spread is by contact and ingestion via the faecal–oral route	See above
	Enterobacter	Gram-negative rods	Gut of humans and animals and moist inanimate environments, especially soil and water	Infection may be endogenous or acquired by contact spread. Rarely associated with infection except as opportunists in immunocompromised hosts	See above
	Klebsiella	See above	See above	See above	See above
	Serratia	See above			See above
	Proteus	Gram-negative rods	Human gut, soil and water	Contact spread; infection is often endogenous	See above
Warts (skin and genital)	Papillomaviruses	Papovavirus group	Humans	By direct or indirect contact from skin to skin and by sexual intercourse	Prevention includes education about transmission, the wearing of shoes (plantar warts) and use of condoms for genital warts
Weil's disease (see Leptospirosis)					
Whooping cough	Bordetella pertussis	Small Gram-negative rods	Human pathogen; carriage by healthy individuals is not documented	Spread is by the airborne route from those already with the disease	Vaccine is administered to young children in three doses with diphtheria and tetanus toxoid
Yaws	Treponema pertenue	Regular coiled spirochaetes	Humans and possibly higher primates	Spread is by direct contact from infected skin lesions	Prevention is by general health promotion measures
Yellow fever	Flavivirus		Urban areas: humans and mosquitoes. Forest areas: primates, marsupials and mosquitoes	By bite from infected mosquitoes	Immunization of those at risk of exposure by residence, travel or occupation. Vector control of mosquitoes

RECOMMENDED READING

Baron S (ed) 1991 Medical microbiology: principles and concepts. Churchill Livingstone, Edinburgh

Boyd R 1995 Basic medical microbiology. Little Brown, Boston

Chin J (ed) 2000 Control of communicable diseases manual, 17th edn. American Public Health Association, Washington DC

Collee JG, Simmons A, Marmion BP, Fraser AG (eds) 1996 Practical medical microbiology, 14th edn. Churchill Livingstone, Edinburgh

Gillespie SH 1994 Medical microbiology illustrated. Butterworth-Heinemann, Oxford

Gillies RR 1997 Lecture notes on medical microbiology, 3rd edn. Blackwell Scientific Publications, Oxford

Gilligan PH, Shapiro D S, Smiley ML (eds) 1992 Cases in medical microbiology and infectious diseases. American Society for Microbiology

Greenwood D, Slack RCB, Peutherer JF (eds) 1992 Medical microbiology: a guide to microbial infections – pathogenesis, immunity, laboratory diagnosis and control. Churchill Livingstone, Edinburgh

Hentges DJ 1995 Medical microbiology and immunology. Little Brown, Boston

Holton JB, Bank N, Chiodini P 1994 Problems in medical microbiology. Blackwell Scientific Publications, Oxford

Jawetz E, Melnick JL, Adelberg EA, Brooks GF (eds) 1995 Medical microbiology, 20th edn. Appleton & Lange, Connecticut

McClean D 1990 Medical microbiology synopsis. Lea & Febiger

Mehtar S (ed) 1994 Guidelines for standards in laboratory practice in medical microbiology. Association of Medical Microbiologists

Miller J et al (eds) 1992 Medical microbiology: a short course. Wiley, Chichester

Mims CA, Zuckerman M, Urwin G 1994 Case studies in medical microbiology. Mosby Wolfe, London

Murray PR, Kobayashi G 1993 Medical microbiology, 2nd edn. Wolfe Publishing, London

Ross PW 1993 MCQs in medical microbiology and infectious diseases. Kluwer Academic Publishers, Netherlands

Sherris JC (ed) 1994 Sherris medical microbiology: an introduction to infectious diseases, international, 3rd edn. Appleton & Lange, Connecticut

Volk WA, Benjamin D, Robert K 1996 Essentials of medical microbiology. Lippincott, Philadelphia

Wilson J 2001 Infection control in clinical practice, 2nd edn. Baillière Tindall, London

Reservoirs

7

■ CONTENTS

SUMMARY

One of the aims of care organizations is the management of risk, both to patients and to staff. Hospitals are not the only place where groups of susceptible people congregate to receive care. Individuals in nursing and residential homes are equally compromised. Health centres and general practitioner (GP) surgeries, where the attendance is brief, can also pose some risks of infection. Play centres and children's nurseries have also been known to create a favourable setting for the spread of infections. Whatever the surroundings, the practitioners carry a professional and moral responsibility to ensure a safe environment and provide a high quality of care.

The dynamics of any care environment demand that the personnel remain vigilant to the risks associated with the ever-changing situations. Risks are inherent in patients (intrinsic) as well as associated with treatment and practices (extrinsic). The employing organizations carry the responsibility for ensuring that practitioners are adequately and appropriately

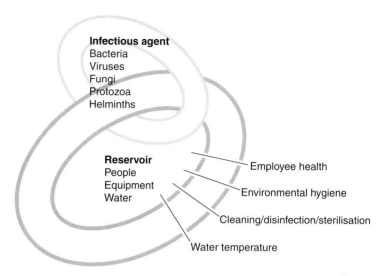

Figure 7.1 Breaking the chain of infection: reservoirs.

prepared in their role so that patients are not harmed by their actions or inactions.

The responsibility for creating a safe environment for patients and developing informed practitioners rests with both the infection control personnel and the managers of the organization. The Controls Assurance Standard for infection control (NHSE 2001a) set out clear organizational requirements to ensure that effective infection control measures are in place.

Adequately and appropriately prepared practitioners will have sufficient insight to enable them to identify the 'informed' element of each practice. They should be able to demonstrate a degree of understanding of the reasons for each action, actions taken by their employing organization and by themselves. This is the basis of 'informed care'. Choosing to ignore the application of certain basic steps can predispose patients to the risk of acquiring an infection. A failure to carry out safe practice knowingly can be interpreted as a desire to harm those receiving care. Quality care is assured when healthcare workers are able to make explicit the hazard associated with each practice (Fig. 7.1).

INTRODUCTION

'Safe environment' is a broad term used frequently in healthcare settings to signify a secure surrounding within which people are not harmed. In hospitals and other care institutions, the term refers to a process that results in the removal or destruction of any contamination that could reach a susceptible host. Decontamination procedures are an essential infection control measure.

The creation and maintenance of a safe environment rests both with employers and employees. Key legislation for managing a safe environment is the Health and Safety at Work Act (1974), which sets out the legal

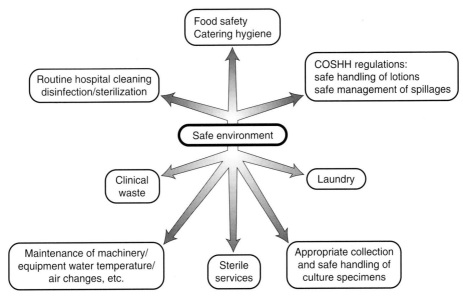

Figure 7.2 The principles of a safe environment.

responsibilities of employers and employees to health and safety in the workplace (Health Service Advisory Committee (HSAC) 1974). The regulations require employers to assess the risks to their employees. These principles are expanded in *The Management of Health and Safety at Work Regulations and Workplace Regulations* (Health and Safety Commission (HSC) 1992a,b,c). Employers are required to make a systematic assessment of the risks to the health and safety of their employees, and others, arising from work activities. Complementary guidance includes the *Control of Substances Hazardous to Health Regulations* (HSC 1999a) and the *Environmental Protection Act* (1990) (DoE 1990).

The *Control of Substances Hazardous to Health* (COSHH) came into force in 1988 and has been regularly updated since (HSC 1999a). Its main purpose is to ensure that employers systematically undertake risk assessment for all hazardous substances that are the result of work activity (chemical as well as biological). Staff must have an understanding of the chemical compatibility of the products that they use.

The components of a safe environment are depicted in Figure 7.2.

EMPLOYEE HEALTH

Patients and staff are at risk of contracting infections from each other. Staff members have more control over the circumstances that lead to these occurrences than their patients. This section examines the role and responsibility of the occupational health department, as well as of individual practitioners, in minimizing risks to both patients and staff.

Hazards are associated with practices as well as with exposure to microorganisms that are in abundance in healthcare settings. Patients and staff are at risk from practices and from each other. It is almost impossible to legislate for all eventualities when an exposure to infection may occur. By far the biggest reminder was the transmission of human immunodeficiency virus (HIV) in healthcare workers due to occupational exposures (Heptonstall et al 1993). A case of primary cutaneous tuberculosis was reported in a nurse following a needlestick injury from a patient with acquired immunodeficiency syndrome (AIDS) and undiagnosed tuberculosis (Kramer et al 1994). Such unfortunate episodes remind health professionals that many disease-producing microorganisms can be present in the blood, body fluids, secretions and excretions of a seemingly healthy and undiagnosed person. The accepted advice is that some basic precautionary steps need to be taken at all times when dealing with body excretions and secretions.

The role of the occupational health service in relation to infection control

The occupational health and infection control personnel work very closely to ensure that healthcare workers are neither at risk of contracting infectious diseases from patients or patient care practices nor transmit their infections to vulnerable patients in their care.

It is the responsibility of the employing authority to ensure that staff have access to an occupational health department (OHD) to 'help to prevent illness and injuries at work by ensuring that staff are appropriately trained, for example in infection control procedures, in lifting techniques or handling aggression' (National Health Service Management Executive (NHSME) 1994). Managers are also required under regulations known as RIDDOR to 'Report Injuries, Diseases and Dangerous Occurrences' (HSE 1995). The OHD should ensure that every staff member is fit to undertake duties in all healthcare settings. Careful consideration is given to employees with skin problems such as eczema and psoriasis. The carriage rate of many Gram-positive microorganisms in skin lesions can be substantial (Noble 1993) and can create problems in certain clinical areas.

All staff members' immune status to infectious diseases such as tuberculosis, rubella and polio must be assured. All healthcare staff involved in exposure-prone procedures should be immunized against hepatitis B, unless natural immunity to hepatitis B (HBV) as a result of infection has been documented (NHSME 1993a). The advisory group on hepatitis made further recommendations in 2000 (HSC 2000/020) as a consequence of an incidence of transmission of hepatitis B virus to patients from healthcare workers who were e-antigen negative (e-antigen is that part of the hepatitis B protein particle that denotes high infectivity). The working group stated that, in addition to the 1993 and 1996 guidance, hepatitis-B-infected healthcare workers who are e-antigen negative and who perform exposure-prone procedures should have their viral loads measured. Those whose viral loads exceeded 10^3 genome equivalents per ml should not perform exposure-prone procedures in the future (HSC 2000/020). There is also revised guidance on reducing the risk to patients from HIV-infected healthcare workers, which suggests that exposure-prone procedures can be divided into higher and lower risk categories (DoH 1998). The working group concluded that there was a real, though very low, risk of HIV transmission to patients from infected healthcare workers. Patients must be notified wherever practicable if they have undergone exposure-prone procedures by infected healthcare workers and offered testing. HIV-infected healthcare workers must continue to avoid performing all exposure-prone procedures and remain under regular medical and occupational health supervision while they continue to provide clinical care to patients (HSC 2000/020).

Hazards of needle-stick and sharps injuries

Collins & Kennedy (1987) provide a comprehensive review of occupational transmission of infections to healthcare workers from needlestick and sharps injuries. Infections include HIV, blastomycosis, brucellosis, cryptococcosis, diphtheria, Ebola fever, gonorrhoea (cutaneous), hepatitis B, herpes, leptospirosis, mycobacteriosis, mycoplasmosis, Rocky Mountain spotted fever, scrub typhus, sporotrichosis, *Staphylococcus aureus*, *Streptococcus pyogenes*, syphilis, toxoplasmosis, tuberculosis and malignancy.

Hepatitis B vaccination

Five cases of occupationally acquired hepatitis B infections in healthcare workers were reported in 1992 (Advisory Committee on Dangerous Pathogens (ACDP) 1995). An increased awareness of risk, safe practices and the widespread use of hepatitis B vaccination has helped reduce hepatitis B infection amongst healthcare workers. Any member of staff who might be at risk of acquiring hepatitis B occupationally by injury from bloodstained sharp instruments, contamination of surface lesions by blood or bloodstained body fluids or through deliberate injury or biting by patients should also be immunized (NHSME 1993a). Exposure-prone procedures are described as those where there is a risk that injury to the worker could result in the exposure of the patient's open tissues to the blood of the worker. These procedures include those where the worker's gloved hands are in contact with sharp instruments, needle tips and sharp tissues (spicules of bone or teeth) inside a patient's open body cavity, wound or confined anatomical space, and those where the hands or finger-tips are not completely visible at all times (BMA/NHSE 1995). It does not apply to 'the taking of blood, setting up and maintaining i.v. lines, minor surface suturing, the incision of abscesses or uncomplicated endoscopies or normal vaginal delivery' (BMA/NHSE 1995).

The British Medical Association document (BMA/NHSE 1995) suggests immunization for the following groups of staff:

- doctors in clinical areas
- nurses in clinical areas
- midwives in clinical areas
- operating theatre assistants
- podiatrists
- dentists
- dental surgery assistants and hygienists

- dental therapists
- radiologists
- pathologists
- mortuary staff
- laboratory staff
- staff working in institutions for the mentally handicapped
- porters, domestic staff, maintenance workers
- all GPs who undertake intrapartum care and/or minor surgery
- all practice nurses assisting with minor surgery who may be exposed to blood or sharps
- all general dental practitioners and dental surgery assistants engaged in clinical work
- all dental hygienists and dental therapists engaged in clinical work
- all medical academics who hold honorary clinical posts
- all nursing, medical, dental and podiatry students, including elective and visiting students, prior to undertaking work in clinical areas.

Course of hepatitis B vaccination

Hepatitis B vaccination is given over three doses at 0, 1 and 6 months. Annex A of the NHSME document HSG (93) 40 (NHSME 1993a) recommends an accelerated vaccine schedule (0, 1 and 2 months with a booster at 12 months) for non-immunized surgeons, junior doctors, medical and nursing students who rotate regularly between posts and might not complete a course of vaccination in one place of employment. This 'speeded-up' immunization carries an increased risk of non-response.

The antibody titre is checked 2–3 months after completion of the course to ensure vaccine uptake. Non-responders are given a fourth dose and the titre levels checked 2 months later. A titre level of <100 is followed by a fifth dose and checked after a further 2 months.

A booster immunization is given 3 or 5 years after the last injection, depending on the response to the vaccine.

Non-responders

Approximately 7 to 10% of people can be 'non-responders' despite a fourth or fifth dose. It is recommended that non-responders be tested for core antigen to check infectivity, as they might have been infected by the virus prior to immunization. It is also possible that non-responders could be carriers of the virus and therefore pose a risk to patients.

Non-responders without previous infection or exposure can themselves be at risk of infection and will require counselling on prevention. They should be referred to the steps listed in Box 7.1.

Current guidelines (NHSME 1993a) state that staff in post who are vaccine non-responders can continue without restriction of their practice provided that inoculation incidents are reported, treated and followed-up in accordance with standard guidelines outlined in Box 7.2.

A further recommendation is included in an executive letter EL (96) 77 entitled *Addendum to HSG (93) 40: Protecting Healthcare Workers*

■ BOX 7.1   Universal precautions

- Apply good basic hygiene practices with regular handwashing
- Cover existing wounds or skin lesions with waterproof dressings
- Avoid invasive procedures if suffering from chronic skin lesions on hands
- Avoid contamination of person by use of appropriate clothing
- Protect mucous membranes of eyes, mouth and nose from blood splashes and blood-stained fluids
- Prevent puncture wounds, cuts and abrasions in the presence of blood/blood-stained body fluids
- Avoid sharps usage wherever possible
- Institute safe procedures for handling and disposal of needles and other sharps
- Institute approved procedures for sterilization and disinfection of instruments and equipment
- Clear up spillages of blood and other body fluid promptly and disinfect surfaces
- Institute a procedure for safe disposal of contaminated waste.

■ BOX 7.2   Regimen for parenteral exposures

Immediate management

- The injured area should be encouraged to bleed (not by sucking) and washed liberally with soap and water. Wash under hot water to encourage vasodilation and bleeding
- If contaminated, the eyes, nose and mouth should be rinsed copiously with tap water.

Reporting and assessment of risk

- All accidents should be reported without delay to the individual's senior officer and the incident documented. Full details of the circumstances should be recorded, even where the patient is not suspected of infection or the used sharp instrument cannot be assigned to a particular patient.
- 10 ml of clotted blood should be collected from the staff member and, wherever possible, from the identified patient. This should be done with consent and, where necessary, appropriate counselling. Wherever possible, the consent obtained should be for the specimen to be 'stored' or 'to test and store'. The blood samples should be stored for at least 2 years as a starting point in case of illness developing.

and Patients from Hepatitis B (DoH 1996a), which suggests that health-care workers who are positive for hepatitis B surface antigen must cease exposure-prone procedures until their e-antigen status has been established.

Management of non-immune or non-vaccinated staff

Where exposure to HBV is likely or definite, blood samples from the source patient (if their recent serological status is not known) and the staff member should be obtained with consent and appropriate counselling. A clinical diagnosis could be made if the patient refuses a blood test. An initial treatment with specific immunoglobulin (HBIg) is recommended if given early. A course of hepatitis B vaccine should be started immediately. Thorough record keeping and subsequent medical follow-up are advised, as treatments given after an injury can fail.

Accidental exposure

The OHD, along with the infection control personnel, manage accidental parenteral exposure (i.e. direct inoculation into the bloodstream) of staff to infectious diseases. The viruses of the hepatitis and human immunodeficiency group are of concern. Significant parenteral exposure (see Box 7.3) to blood and body fluids that may be infectious requires prompt attention.

■ **BOX 7.3   Significant needlestick and other exposures**

- Pricking or cutting with a sharp instrument (such as a needle or scalpel) that has been used on a patient
- Swallowing, or splashing of blood or body fluids into the eye or nose
- Human bites (especially those that draw blood)
- Extensive spillage of blood or body fluids onto the skin (especially if there are pre-existing cuts, grazes, dermatitis).

Exposure to hepatitis C virus

A risk of contracting hepatitis C virus (HCV) of between 3 and 10% is reported for healthcare workers sustaining a needlestick injury involving hepatitis-C-infected blood (BMA 1996). Guidance on the risks and current management of occupational exposure suggests storage of serum from the source, if identified, and the testing of blood of the injured healthcare worker at 6 months after exposure. There is currently no effective routine postexposure treatment or protective vaccine available. The routine use of human normal immunoglobulin is not recommended (Heptonstall et al 1993).

Exposure to human immunodeficiency virus (HIV)

The risk of acquiring HIV infection following occupational exposure to HIV-infected blood is low. Epidemiological studies indicate that the average risk for HIV transmission after percutaneous exposure is about 3 per 1000 injuries in healthcare settings. After a mucocutaneous exposure, the average risk is less than 1 in 1000. There is considered to be no risk of HIV transmission where intact skin is exposed to HIV-infected blood (DoH 2000b).

The risk for HIV transmission after percutaneous exposures involving larger volumes of blood, particularly if the viral load of the source patient is likely to be high, exceeds the average risk of 3 per 1000 (Cardo et al 1997).

Four factors are associated with the increased risk of occupationally acquired HIV infection following exposure to HIV-infected blood:

- injury with a needle placed directly in a vein or artery
- deep injury
- visible blood on the device that caused the injury
- terminal HIV-related illness in the source patient.

Occupational exposure to HIV and other blood-borne viruses is quite common. Prevention of avoidable exposure is of prime importance. Many exposures are the result of a failure to follow recommended procedures, including the safe handling and disposal of needles and syringes, or wearing personal protective eyewear where indicated. Guidance is given by the Advisory Group on Hepatitis in *Guidance for Clinical Health Care Workers: Protection Against Infection with Blood-borne Viruses* (Health Service Circular 1998). The 1997 guidelines on occupational HIV postexposure prophylaxis (PEP) have been updated. They include new directions on the issues of healthcare workers seconded overseas (including medical and dental students) plus exposure to HIV outside the healthcare setting. Also included are recommended drug regimens, drug resistance, drug interactions and special considerations for healthcare workers who are, or might be, pregnant (DoH 2000b).

Any person significantly exposed to the risk of HIV infection in a healthcare setting (including domiciliary situations) should be assessed and managed according to the principles in the guidance, whether or not they are a healthcare worker. This includes relatives or friends providing care, and hospital domestic and waste disposal staff.

HIV postexposure prophylaxis

The administration of zidovudine prophylaxis to healthcare workers occupationally exposed to HIV is associated with an 80% reduction in the risk for occupationally acquired HIV infection (Cardo et al 1997).

If there has been a significant exposure and a source patient cannot be identified, risk assessment should be on an individual basis. Postexposure prophylaxis should be recommended to healthcare workers if they have had a significant occupational exposure to blood or another high-risk body fluid from a patient or other source, either known to be HIV infected or considered to be at high risk of HIV infection where the result of an HIV test has not or cannot be obtained for whatever reason.

For optimal efficacy, postexposure prophylaxis should be started as soon as possible after the incident and ideally within the hour. Starter packs of the recommended drugs should be kept in a number of readily accessible and well-advertised sites, including:

- the OHD
- the pharmacy

- the A&E department
- specific wards or departments.

Each pack should contain a 3-day course of the drugs sufficient to cover weekends and bank holidays. Training and clear protocols should be given to personnel who might be responsible for initial administration of drugs.

The Expert Advisory Group on AIDS (DoH 2000b) identifies three types of exposure in healthcare settings associated with significant risk:

1. percutaneous injury (from needles, instruments, bone fragments, significant bites that break the skin, etc.)
2. exposure of broken skin (abrasions, cuts, eczema, etc.)
3. exposure of mucous membranes, including the eye.

Combination drug therapy

In HIV-infected patients, combination drug therapy has proved more effective than zidovudine alone in reducing viral load. In theory, a combination of drugs could increase potency of postexposure prophylaxis and offer increased protection. This is thought to be especially relevant in view of the increased prevalence of resistance to zidovudine and other antiretrovirals.

Since 1997, the recommended drugs for postexposure prophylaxis starter packs have been zidovudine, lamivudine and indinavir taken for 4 weeks as follows:

- zidovudine 200 mg 3 times a day or 250 mg twice daily
  plus
- Lamivudine 150 mg twice daily
  plus
- Indinavir 800 mg 3 times a day.

The guidance provides alternative regimens should there be poor tolerability often considered attributable to indinavir.

Antiretroviral agents from at least three classes of drugs have been licensed for the treatment of HIV infection. Zidovudine is the only drug to date that has been studied and for which there is evidence of a reduction of risk of HIV transmission following occupational exposure (Cardo et al 1997).

There are local variations in the choice of regimen used. As newer antiretroviral drugs are developed, it is likely that other drugs will become the preferred regimen for postexposure prophylaxis.

Side-effects of drugs

All of the antiretroviral agents have been associated with side-effects, many of which can be managed symptomatically. They are mainly gastrointestinal (nausea, vomiting), although lethargy, insomnia and headaches have been reported with zidovudine (DoH 2000b). A more serious side-effect is bone marrow suppression, which can be found in patients receiving long-term treatment with zidovudine. Such side-effects are thought to be small in cases of prophylaxis lasting 1 month (Puro et al 1992).

Pregnancy does not exclude the use of HIV postexposure prophylaxis. The available evidence is that zidovudine and lamivudine are not contraindicated in the second and third trimesters of pregnancy. The British HIV Association has published guidelines for prescribing antiretroviral therapy in pregnancy (Taylor et al 1999).

Protease inhibitor drugs can have potentially serious interactions with other prescribed drugs.

Those providing advice on and protocols for prescribing postexposure prophylaxis should maintain awareness of advances in HIV therapeutics, potential side-effects, adverse drug reactions and drug interactions and seek further expert advice where necessary.

HIV-infected healthcare workers

The UK Advisory Panel for HIV-infected healthcare workers (DoH 1998) has set out a number of key recommendations on the management of infected healthcare workers. The guidance considers the need to 'protect patients, to retain public confidence and to provide safeguards for confidentiality and employment rights of HIV infected healthcare workers'.

Other significant exposures

Meningitis

Meningitis, especially meningococcal meningitis, generates anxiety amongst healthcare staff. Much of the concern is due to the publicity given to this disease, especially its sudden onset and sometimes rapid fatal outcome.

The person-to-person transmission of the organism *Neisseria meningitidis* is by droplets from the upper respiratory tract (De Voe 1982). The carriage rate of the organism is high, with approximately 10% of the general population normally carrying one of a number of strains in the nasopharynx, most of which cause very few problems (Cartwright et al 1987).

The risk of transmission of infection to healthcare workers is thought to be very low. Prophylactic antibiotics and vaccination could be considered if exceptionally close contamination occurs, such as in mouth-to-mouth resuscitation (Communicable Disease Report (CDR) 1995a).

Where prophylaxis is necessary, rifampicin is the drug of choice. Staff receiving rifampicin should be informed that it might lead to:

- reduction in the efficacy of hormonal contraceptives
- red colouration of urine, sputum and tears
- permanent staining of soft contact lenses
- occasional rash
- gastrointestinal disturbances.

The vaccines available in the UK provide protection against serogroups A and C. Vaccine against serogroup B is not yet available. The identity of the strain of the offending meningococcus is unlikely to be known when prophylaxis is commenced but vaccination can be given once the serogroup is known.

Since the autumn of 1999 there has been an immunization programme of meningococcal vaccine group C. This has been given to children aged from

2 months to 18–19 years. It is hoped that this programme of immunization will have a major impact on group C meningococcal disease, which is responsible for 40% of cases of meningococcal disease within the UK (Donaldson et al 1999). Short-term efficacy of the vaccine showed 97% for teenagers and 92% for toddlers in the first 9 months since its introduction (Ramsey et al 2001).

Scabies

Ectoparasites such as head, body and pubic lice are relatively rare in healthcare establishments. However, scabies is common and has a potential to be transmitted to and from patients and staff in an outbreak.

The mite *Sarcoptes scabiei* causes scabies – a parasitic infection of the skin. The transmission of scabies usually occurs from person to person by skin-to-skin contact. The unpleasant feature of scabies is itching and scratching, which is the result of sensitization to the mite antigens (Maunder 1992). The characteristics of classical scabies include intense pruritus and cutaneous tracks (burrows) over the distal extremities, waist and axillae. About 15 mites are harboured by the individual with symptomatic classical scabies, whereas thousands of mites can be present on the skin of patients diagnosed with Norwegian or crusted scabies. While the risk of transmission is thought to require approximately 20 min of direct skin-to-skin contact in classical scabies, in the case of Norwegian scabies, transmission is higher and requires less time due to the numbers of mites present on the individual.

Treatment of scabies

The majority of healthcare establishments will have written protocols on who should be treated and what products are effective in each situation. Products include 1% lindane (Quellada M) malathion (Derbac-M) and permethrin (Lyclear). Lindane is effective but relatively toxic and is not advised for children under the age of 2 years, for pregnant or breastfeeding women and in people with low body weight or a history of epilepsy; malathion lotion is safe for this group of people. Permethrin has very low toxicity, high cure rates and short treatment time (Maunder 1992). The general advice on treatment is as follows:

- Hospital staff contacts and other patients might require treatment even if currently asymptomatic. The decision is based on the degree of skin-to-skin contact exposure and mite density of the source patient. Everyone should be treated at the same time.
- The compound must be applied to all parts of the body, including the scalp and paying particular attention to the fingernails, wrists, anogenital area and between the toes. The lotion is washed off after 24 h, although it is important to reapply the lotion to the hands each time they have been washed.
- Personal clothing and bed linen must be changed after treatment and washed at a temperature in excess of 50°C (Lettau 1991).

- Patients' clothing and bed linen must be bagged and labelled as infected. Transmission of scabies from infected linen to laundry workers has been documented (Thomas et al 1987).

The allergy and itching can persist for a period of time after treatment has been given. Occasionally, an overuse of treatment lotions can lead to irritant dermatitis. An element of persistent psychogenic pruritus has also been described. Lettau (1991) suggests reassurance, follow-up skin scrapings and trials of symptomatic therapy until the problem is resolved.

Tuberculosis

The guidelines of the Joint Tuberculosis Committee of the British Thoracic Society (2000) entitled *Control and Prevention of Tuberculosis in the United Kingdom: Code of Practice* have recently been reviewed and include guidance on infection control, bovine tuberculosis and the risks of transmission of tuberculosis during air travel. The epidemiology of tuberculosis in the UK has continued to change in recent years. Numbers of notified cases in England and Wales in 1987 were 5058, rising to 6087 in 1998, with the increases greatest in urban areas. In 1998, 56% of reported cases were in people not born in the UK. At least 3% of cases were estimated to be HIV infected. Drug resistance remains an important issue, although rates have not risen in recent years (Irish et al 1999).

Control of tuberculosis in healthcare workers

Staff at potential risk of contracting tuberculosis are:

- staff in regular contact with patients
- laboratory workers handling specimens.

Staff protection includes:

- Recording:
  - any symptoms of tuberculosis
  - details of previous BCG vaccination
  - the presence or absence of a BCG scar
- Tuberculin skin testing (only necessary in new employees who do not have a definite BCG scar)
- BCG vaccination for negative or grade 1 tuberculin skin (Heaf) reaction and site inspected 6 weeks later
- A further tuberculin test and a second vaccination if still negative
- Chest X-ray where indicated, i.e. negative or low skin reaction and careful enquiry
- Referral to a chest physician.

Healthcare workers who are grade 2, 3 or 4 tuberculin-test-positive might have encountered tubercle bacilli in the past. They do not require BCG vaccination but must report any future suspicious symptoms. A chest X-ray is indicated if the worker is from a country where tuberculosis is common.

BCG vaccination is not recommended for individuals known or suspected to be infected with HIV.

Treatment of staff members

Once the diagnosis is confirmed, treatment is with a combination of anti-microbial drugs. Sputum specimens are examined regularly.

Follow-up of staff members

The OHD will contact those members of staff identified as having been in contact with a potentially infective person. Members of staff will have their immune status checked for tuberculosis and vaccination will be provided if necessary.

Management of close contacts

Close contacts of patients with smear-positive pulmonary disease are defined as staff undertaking:

- mouth-to-mouth resuscitation
- prolonged care of a high-dependency patient
- repeated chest physiotherapy.

Investigation should include:

- inquiry into BCG vaccination status
- tuberculin skin testing
- chest radiography.

The treatment and follow-up should be as discussed above.

Compulsory treatment of tuberculosis is not allowed but, in exceptional circumstances, it might be necessary to consider compulsory admission of a patient who is causing serious risk of infection to others under the Public Health (Control of Diseases) Act (1984). If the person has to be detained it will be necessary to obtain a magistrate's order for admission and another order for detention.

Contact tracing

Contact tracing and examination is undertaken to detect associated cases, to detect persons infected but without evidence of disease, to identify candidates for BCG vaccination and to detect a source case and other co-primary cases. Contact tracing can also identify geographical linkage of cases and prompt cluster investigation.

BCG immunization

National policy is that BCG vaccination should be offered to all children between the ages of 10 and 14 years and to certain groups at higher risk of exposure to tuberculosis. These include infants and children born to adults born in the UK but from ethnic groups originating in high prevalence countries. Neonates and infants up to the age of 3 months who have no known contact with tuberculosis can be offered BCG immunization without prior tuberculin testing. Older infants and children should undergo tuberculin testing before BCG immunization.

Control of tuberculosis in hospitals

Although the treatment of tuberculosis should be in the patient's home whenever possible, some patients will need admission to hospital because of the severity of illness, because of adverse effects of chemotherapy, for investigations to establish the diagnosis or for social reasons. Risk assessments need to be done into the likelihood of infectiousness and multidrug resistant tuberculosis (MDR-TB) and to take into account the immune status of other patients on the ward.

Adults with non-pulmonary tuberculosis can be nursed on a general ward but patients with suspected pulmonary tuberculosis should initially be isolated in a single room, vented to the outside, until their sputum status is known and risk assessments have been made.

Children with tuberculosis, and their visitors, should be segregated until their visitors have been screened to exclude them as a source of infection. Only those, including children, who have been in contact with the patient before diagnosis should be allowed to visit while the child is considered infectious.

Tuberculosis in prisons

Tuberculosis was not common in prisons in the early 1990s and transmission within prisons had not been recorded until 1993 (HM Prison Report 1993). The majority of prisoners and prison officers should be protected by BCG vaccination. New staff should be screened as for at-risk healthcare workers. Prisoners are entitled to the same level of care and investigation as the general population. Diagnosed cases should have directly observed therapy (DOT) supervised by a chest physician and should be isolated as for other patients. Notification of cases to the local centre for communicable disease control (CCDC) is essential to enable contact tracing.

Particular risks

Probation officers, police officers, community workers and volunteers who work with patients and prisoners are not normally at risk of developing tuberculosis. Normal contact-tracing procedures apply if contact with undiagnosed infectious tuberculosis occurs inadvertently.

Elderly people in long-stay care should have their previous history of tuberculosis noted on admission. Residents developing symptoms suggestive of tuberculosis should be investigated. If a resident is diagnosed as having infectious tuberculosis, normal contact-tracing procedures should apply.

Schoolteachers and others working with children are no longer screened to exclude active tuberculosis routinely before taking up a post. It is important that those working with children should be aware of the symptoms of tuberculosis and attend for early medical examination should they develop possible symptoms. Transmission of tuberculosis within schools has been reported in the UK. Providing information to pupils, teachers and parents is the most important element of the management of tuberculosis in schools, so that diagnosis can be made early.

Accurate estimates of the level of tuberculosis among homeless people are difficult to obtain because of problems with the definition of homelessness and the mobility of the population. All available studies point to tuberculosis being a particular problem in this group.

Potentially infectious cases of tuberculosis are occasionally identified among people who have recently travelled by air. However, follow-up of passengers exposed to infectious cases has shown no case of active tuberculosis. Exposure on long-haul flights appears to carry a very small risk of transmission. The World Health Organization (WHO) has published guidance intended to apply to all domestic and international airlines (WHO 1998).

Tuberculosis in cattle is becoming more common in the UK. There is negligible risk of transmission to the British population because of milk pasteurization. Cattle tuberculosis is almost entirely due to infection with *Mycobacterium bovis*. Surveillance of human *M. bovis* infection has been enhanced. Where studies of human contacts of cattle have been undertaken, little evidence of transmission and no clinical disease has been found (Cawthorne et al 1997).

Varicella-zoster (chickenpox and shingles)

The varicella-zoster virus is highly communicable as it causes chickenpox and can reappear many years later as shingles. Once seen predominantly in children, chickenpox is now seen more frequently in adults (Miller et al 1993a,b). As chickenpox is highly contagious, its spread amongst non-immune staff and susceptible patients remains problematic. It can cause serious illness in immunosuppressed patients, including those taking corticosteroids (Rice et al 1994) premature and critically ill infants, adults and pregnant women.

An attack of disseminated shingles and superimposed chickenpox can prove fatal in compromised patients (Chin 2000). Maternal varicella affects both the woman and the fetus. The severe maternal morbidity includes varicella pneumonia in 10–20% of infected women, with around 40% mortality. Intrauterine infection can result in congenital varicella syndrome or stillbirth, and maternal varicella at the end of pregnancy or 2 days after delivery can result in neonatal varicella, which is associated with high mortality (Katz et al 1995, Paryani & Arvin 1986).

Chickenpox is highly contagious and difficult to control because the period of infectivity lasts from 2 or 3 days before the appearance of the rash until the lesions crust (Jones & Reeves 1997). Jones and Reeves recommend prompt identification of non-immune staff members, because they can transmit the infection to susceptible patients while incubating the disease themselves. To avoid transmission, non-immune staff contacts should be excluded from work from the 10th to the 21st day after exposure. Non-immune pregnant staff should be advised to avoid all contact with the disease. Miller & Hopkinson (1986) suggest passive immunization with anti-varicella-zoster immunoglobulin for pregnant women who have come into contact with chickenpox and who have no history of previous infection. Vaccine against chickenpox is not routinely available in the UK.

Exposure to cadavers

Risks of infection from infected dead bodies remain a hazard to people who handle them. Healing et al (1995) have identified a number of infectious conditions and pathogens in recently deceased humans. These include tuberculosis, group A streptococcal infection, gastrointestinal organisms, the agents that cause transmissible spongiform encephalopathies (such as Creutzfeldt–Jakob disease), HBV and HCV, HIV and possible meningococcal meningitis and septicaemia. Cadavers present a risk to nurses when performing last offices, and to medical staff, especially pathologists, technical staff in pathology, morticians, funeral directors, embalmers and members of the emergency services.

Protection of staff when handling cadavers

Until the advent of universal precautions, sealed or zipped plastic body bags were used mainly for cases thought to be infective to handlers. Now, body bags or plastic sheets are used routinely as a universal precaution against infection or to transport leaking or offensive bodies. According to Healing et al (1995), only a very small proportion of deaths are attributable to transmissible infections and funeral directors must be informed of the cases that present real risks of infection to their staff.

Practices and precautions in post-mortem rooms are based on the guidance in the Health Service Advisory Committee Report (DoH 1991b) and building notes from the DoH (1991c). The basic recommendations centre on:

- covering of cuts and lesions with waterproof dressings
- handwashing after every procedure and before eating or smoking
- careful cleansing of any injuries sustained during procedures
- using appropriate protective clothing for procedures
- cleaning the environment with phenolic disinfectant
- washing of instruments in a washer–disinfector, autoclaved or immersed in a phenolic disinfectant for 20 min.

Appropriate protective clothing for handling cadavers

- Latex examination gloves for handling bodies and hazardous material. Hands should be washed after use. Latex gloves provide short-term (10 min) protection against formaldehyde
- Chemically protective gloves (nitril) for protection from longer-term exposure to chemicals, such as formaldehyde
- Filter mask for respiratory protection against lead dust, fungi, spores and aerosols
- Face visor to prevent splashes onto the eyes, nose and mouth
- Plastic apron to protect the body from splashes from the cadaver
- Rubber boots to protect feet against wet situations and contamination by body fluids
- A gown, coat or coverall with a hood to provide whole body protection against splashes and to protect clothes and hair from impregnation with dust and spores

- Safety helmet, boots, safety glasses and work gloves to protect against mechanical injury (Healing et al 1995).

Gastroenteritis

A considerable area of concern regarding exposure, both from patient to staff and vice versa, is gastrointestinal infection. Causes of intestinal infection can be viral, bacterial or parasitical. All cases of gastroenteritis should be regarded as potentially infectious and healthcare workers displaying symptoms of gastroenteritis should normally be excluded from work (CDR 1995c, Scottish Centre for Infection and Environmental Health (SCIEH) 1994). The guidance document *Food Handlers: Fitness to Work* (DoH 1995a) states that healthcare workers with symptoms of gastrointestinal infections such as 'feeling queasy', abdominal pain or cramps, nausea, vomiting, diarhoea, etc. could contaminate food and the environment and must stop working and report to their senior officer.

Returning to work

The Working Party of the PHLS Salmonella Committee (CDR 1995c) suggests that the decision to allow infected staff to return to work should depend on whether they belong to a group that poses an increased risk of spreading infection.

People who pose an increased risk are:

- food handlers whose work involves touching unwrapped foods to be consumed raw without further cooking
- staff of healthcare facilities who have direct contact, or contact through serving food, with susceptible patients or persons in whom an intestinal infection would have particularly serious consequences.

The CDR review recommends that the circumstances of each case, excretor, carrier or contact should be considered individually. Other factors, such as type of employment, provision of sanitation facilities at work, school or other institution, and standards of personal hygiene, should also be taken into account. It might be possible to transfer the staff member to other duties, or it could be necessary to recommend temporary exclusion from work.

People who do not pose an increased risk can return to work 48 hours after their bowel habits have returned to their normal pattern. It is the absence of symptoms rather than the absence of a causative organism that is the main deciding factor as to whether someone remains excluded from work (DoH 1995a). Infections with notifiable organisms of special public health significance will require consideration by the infection control department and the Consultant for Communicable Disease Control (CCDC). These include:

- *Salmonella typhi* or *S. paratyphi* A, B or C (DoH 1995a)
- verotoxin-producing *Escherichia coli* (CDR 1995b)
- cholera and bacillary dysentry.

Food handlers with hepatitis A are advised to remain off work for 7 days after the onset of symptoms (CDR 1995c). Also of concern are food handlers who:

- are carriers of the disease
- are household contacts of a case of enteric fever
- are household contacts of a continuing asymptomatic carrier
- have been in contact with a known case or outbreak, at home or abroad.

The Department of Health guidance document (DoH 1995a) entitled *Food Handlers: Fitness to Work* details the advice for such cases.

A formal exclusion from work, microbiological follow-up before return and possible examination of social and household contacts might be necessary in all or some of the cases of gastrointestinal infections. Most health-care establishments follow the Public Health Laboratory Services (PHLS) recommendations for gastrointestinal infections (CDR 1995c) and the DoH (1995a) guidance.

Other infections in relation to food handlers

Infected lesions of the skin, eyes, ears and mouth could contaminate food with *Staphylococcus aureus* or streptococci. Food handlers who have a scaling, weeping or discharging lesion on an exposed part of their skin that cannot be adequately covered must cease work that involves the handling of food. This guidance also applies to any food handler who has weeping or pustular lesions of the eyes, mouth and gums (DoH 1995a).

ENVIRONMENTAL HYGIENE

The home environment

General home hygiene is based on risk assessment. It is necessary to identify those sites and surfaces that are most frequently contaminated with potentially infectious organisms and that are most likely to spread contamination.

Table 7.1 Categorizing reservoir sites in the home

Category	Type of site
Reservoirs	Toilet bowls, all sink U-bends, plastic washing bowls, draining boards, nappy buckets
Reservoirs/disseminators	Wet cleaning utensils, dishcloths, dish sponges, floor cloths, mops, washing-up brushes, scouring pads, face cloths, bath sponges and cloths, nail brushes, toothbrushes, showerheads, humidifiers
Contact surfaces	Toilet flush handles, toilet seats, door handles, tap handles, basin and bath surfaces. Other household objects touched frequently by more than one person, e.g. telephones
Other surfaces	All floors carpeted and non-carpeted, walls, bedroom and other living room surfaces, furniture, etc.

It is important that these areas are given priority in applying hygiene procedures. In some cases cleaning is sufficient, although sometimes disinfectants should be used.

Reservoirs

Although the probability of contamination at these sites is high, indications are that the risk of transfer under normal conditions is low. Transfer is through direct contact with contaminated reservoir site surfaces. There is some evidence of cross-contamination from toilets and sink U-bends by splashing or aerosol formation, however, this is conflicting and further studies are needed. Reservoir sites must be:

- cleaned regularly, the frequency depending upon the amount of use, number of occupants in the home, general conditions in the home
- cleaned hygienically, the use of a chemical disinfectant might be necessary, depending on risk assessment.

Reservoir/disseminators

In the home, these represent a situation that has the highest risk of transfer. If cleaning cloths or cleaning utensils in the kitchen or bathroom are left in damp conditions they can support the growth of microorganisms. Use of disposable cloths should be encouraged. For reuseable wet-cleaning items, the following procedures should be applied:

- All items must be decontaminated after contact with any contaminated surface or material (e.g. after wiping raw food, wiping up spills, cleaning nappy buckets)
- Used wet-cleaning cloths should be decontaminated at least once a day
- Ensure all cloths are hygienically clean, not just visibly clean, before use in risk-handling procedures (e.g. preparing food to be eaten raw)
- Decontamination can be achieved by use of hot machine-washing, (cloths in washing machines, utensils in dishwashers), by boiling or by use of a chemical disinfectant
- After decontamination, cloths must be dried as quickly as possible
- Mops used to clean up heavily contaminated areas of faeces or vomit should be cleaned, rinsed with a disinfectant solution and dried as quickly as possibly
- There is some evidence that aerosols generated from showerheads and humidifiers can cause infection, although this is only likely with 'at risk' groups. Showerheads should be maintained to avoid the accumulation of stagnant water. Humidifiers should be emptied regularly, disinfected and refilled with fresh water.

Home hygiene in emergency situations

Following emergency situations and natural disasters, such as flooding, the home can become dangerously contaminated and the risk of infection increases. In these situations, local authorities will usually provide advice and support for affected homes and make provision in the case of loss of power and running water.

The hospital environment

Hospital environments become contaminated with dust, soil, chemical residues, debris, etc., as well as with organic matter and potentially infectious organisms. A safe environment is achieved by removing or destroying contamination and thereby preventing microorganisms or other contaminants reaching a susceptible site in sufficient quantities to initiate infection or any other harmful response (MDA 1996a). The term 'decontamination', which is used to describe this process, consists of cleaning, disinfection and sterilization.

Microorganisms and the environment

Humans, microbes and the environment are intricately intertwined; microbes will be present in any environment occupied by humans (Collins 1988). It is neither practical nor desirable to produce microbe-free surroundings, especially in areas of concentrated gatherings. However, it is desirable to 'minimize the number of organisms present and to favour those least likely to cause human infection, and to make it hostile to those most likely to be harmful' (Collins 1988). The number and type of microbes present will depend on the:

- number of people in the environment
- amount of activity in the environment
- amount of moisture present in the environment
- presence of material capable of supporting microbial growth
- rate at which organisms suspended in the air are removed (Collins 1988).

Counts of microbes are also influenced by the type and condition of the environment. These will be much higher on horizontal than on vertical or inverted surfaces, and very low from smooth intact walls and ceilings (Ayliffe et al 1990).

Collins (1988) describes the cleaning of hospitals as having two functions:

1. Non-microbiological:
   - to improve or restore appearance
   - to maintain function
   - to prevent deterioration.
2. Microbiological:
   - to reduce the number of microbes present
   - to remove substances that support their growth or interfere with subsequent disinfection or sterilization.

Microbiological contamination of hospital environment

The organisms most commonly found in a dry environment, free from substances likely to support microbial growth, are coagulase-negative staphylococci, thought to originate from patients' skin. Organisms causing hospital-acquired infections in patients have frequently been found from the patient's surroundings (Sanderson & Rawal 1987, Sanderson & Weissler 1992). A study by Sanderson and Alshafi's (1995) found that although the organisms were recovered mainly from both the top and bottom sheets of 10 out of 33 patients investigated, streptococcus group B and *Candida tropicalis* were also recovered from the floor and bedside chair of the 2 patients with these organisms in their urine and bedlinen. Coliforms were recovered from the floor samples of 5 patients whose urine samples yielded unrelated organisms.

The ability of some organisms to survive in the environment for long periods has been established. Enteropathogenic strains of *Escherichia coli*, which had not been excreted by patients on a ward for 16 months, were isolated from the dust trapped in the cracks of poorly maintained parquet floors (Rogers 1963). Also recovered were non-enteropathogenic strains of *E. coli* from perforations in linoleum caused by stiletto heels. This would suggest that organisms infecting a patient can also contaminate that patient's wider environment. According to Sanderson & Alshafi (1995), the contamination of the environment by both urine and faecal organisms could be widespread.

Whether these environmental organisms are an unrecognized source of infection is open to debate (Ayliffe et al 1967, Fisher et al 1993, Rogers 1963). Chadwick & Oppenheim (1996), however, noted that a thorough and systematic cleaning of a ward that had had a continuing problem with glycopeptide-resistant enterococci and a substantial increase in the number of newly colonized patients, led to a decrease in both the number of newly colonized patients and the level of environmental contamination with the organism. The authors describe hospital environmental cleaning as 'evidence-based' and 'a cost effective method of infection control'. Furthermore, clean care establishments inspire confidence in patients and their relatives, as well as in staff.

In recent years, patients' perceptions have been that standards of cleanliness have fallen. It is recognized that how people perceive their environment determines their views about the quality of care they will receive from the organisation. The NHS Plan (DoH 2000a) announced a new investment of £30 million in Trusts to improve the cleanliness of the patient environment. Assessment of Trusts was carried out by Patient Environment Action Teams (PEATs). The teams consisted of individuals from the NHS, private sector and patient organizations and included estates staff, members from hotel services and infection control nurses (ICNs).

National cleaning standards have been developed (NHS Estates 2000) against which performance can be measured. For the first time since the 1970s, the NHS Plan makes clear that there will be year-on-year improvements in the cleanliness of hospitals.

Routine cleaning

Much of the routine cleaning process centres on maintaining the appearance of the place by removing debris and dirt. This can be adequately achieved by cleaning with neutral detergent and water. It is more difficult to produce an environment that is microbe-free. According to Collins (1988), organisms in the environment reach a plateau in which rates of deposition and death are in equilibrium. Cleaning will only temporarily change the numbers present. This suggests a constant presence of microbes in the environment. However, if not cleaned regularly, there will be a build-up of substances likely to support the growth of microbes. The hospital environment needs to be clean enough not to cause concern to patients and it should be microbiologically safe (Collins 1988).

Cleaning schedules

Bibby (1982) claims that the frequency and method of cleaning is unlikely to have a major effect on the number of patients who become infected. Yet cleaning schedules should continue to remain an integral part of hospital practice because there is no guarantee that infection rates would not rise if standards were allowed to drop.

The limited resources, both financial as well as (domestic) manpower, demand that the frequency of cleaning should take note of possible risks of infection likely to be associated with each area/room or specific item of equipment. The cleaning schedule can then be prioritized as high, medium or low, as suggested here.

High priority

Daily cleaning plus regular checks and further cleaning as required. Examples include:

- beds, bedside lockers and tables, patient chairs
- lavatories, baths and showers – including floors
- commodes
- sluice rooms – including floors
- treatment rooms – including floors
- ward kitchens – including floors
- patient area ward floors (dust-attracting mops) wet mopping as necessary.

Medium priority

Once or bi-weekly cleaning. Examples include:

- bed and curtain frames
- other floor areas in a ward area.

Low priority

1-, 2- or 3-monthly cleaning. Examples include:

- high dusting
- floor polishing
- office cleaning.

Additional cleaning is necessary during outbreaks. The cleaning schedule requires flexibility to incorporate the changing circumstances of a clinical situation. The domestic supervisors and assistants require basic training and understanding of the what, why and how of cleaning hospitals, because, as stated by Collins (1988) 'defining cleaning frequency is not entirely the answer to maintaining standards, for if any item is dirty it needs cleaning again regardless of when it was last cleaned, and if it is already clean there is little point in cleaning it again'.

Cleaning materials and methods

1. Cleaning with household detergent and warm water remains by far the best, most effective and most commonly accepted method of removing both the contamination and microbes
2. Dry dust-mopping is effective and removes the need for wet mops and buckets of water
3. The use of disinfectant solutions is justified in some instances, e.g. spillage of body fluids, where the environmental contamination could contribute to the indirect transmission of pathogenic microorganisms (DoH/PHLS 1994a,b, Lancet 1992, Madge et al 1992, Working Party Report 1998).

Colour-coded cloths

Most establishments operate a system of colour coding to ensure, for example, that cloths used for cleaning a sluice area are not used for bedside tables and lockers or in the ward kitchen. Cleaning materials can easily become contaminated and will then increase the microbial count rather than reduce it. Detergent and other cleaning fluids can be heavily contaminated with Gram-negative bacilli, thus Gram-positive cocci in the area being cleaned will be replaced by Gram-negative bacilli (Collins 1988).

Steps to prevent contamination of cleaning materials include:

- Using disposable cloths. Non-disposable cloths should be decontaminated after each use. Floor mops have been found to be heavily contaminated with Gram-negative bacilli (Ayliffe et al 1967, Maurer 1985)
- Discarding (and not refilling) empty detergent containers
- If practising 'spray-cleaning', the spray bottle must be emptied and the bottle and nozzle washed and rinsed thoroughly and allowed to dry between use
- Discarding used fluid, including water used with mops, immediately after use and rinsing the bucket and mop thoroughly under running hot water. Invert the bucket and stand the mop upright to facilitate drying. Used fluids and wet equipment encourage the growth of Gram-negative bacilli. Floor mops can be sent to the laundry but, if this is not possible, they should be disinfected using chlorine-releasing agents (Babb 1996)
- Removing organic material with a detergent-based solution before applying disinfectants. Disinfectants are readily inactivated by organic material (Ayliffe et al 1993)

- Cleaning spillages of human secretions and excretions promptly. These are likely to be contaminated with human pathogens and can support the growth of more sensitive organisms.

The role of infection control in standards of cleaning

Many healthcare settings employ external cleaning agencies that operate under the umbrella of 'hotel services management' of the employing authority. The frequency of cleaning, materials and methods are defined in a contract and are difficult to alter. The involvement of the local infection control personnel is crucial to discussions when contract specifications are written. They can ensure that:

- The schedule takes account of high, medium and low-risk items of equipment and areas
- Flexibility exists within the contract to take account of changing (cleaning) needs and of outbreaks
- All supervising personnel, whether belonging to the contractors or to the health organization, understand the basic theory underlying every practice and product and are trained to judge cleanliness by the same standards as the infection control personnel
- There is a basic minimum training for all cleaning staff.

Most ICNs are also associated with audit activities that incorporate an audit of the cleaning standards. The West Midlands branch of the Infection Control Nurses' Association has developed a comprehensive audit package that incorporates all environments (ICNA West Midlands Group 1995).

As stated earlier, national cleaning standards have been developed by the ICNA and the Association of Domestic Managers (ADM) and endorsed by the DoH (NHS Estates 2000). These include an audit tool specifically for measuring the cleanliness of the environment. The new standards describe what a 'clean' hospital looks like and define the term 'clean' within a building. NHS Trusts have been required to comply with the standards since April 2001 and they will form part of the Performance Assessment Framework for the NHS. Performance will be assessed regularly and league tables will be published nationally.

CLEANING, DISINFECTION AND STERILIZATION – DECONTAMINATION PROCESSES

Decontamination is the combination of processes, including cleaning, disinfection and sterilization, used to render a reuseable medical device safe for further use. Today, decontamination is an issue of public health importance because of the concerns about preventing hospital-acquired infection and minimizing the theoretical risk of iatrogenic transmission of transmissible spongiform encephalopathies (TSE), especially variant Creutzfeldt–Jakob disease (vCJD).

Latest guidance on decontamination of medical devices (NHSE 2001b) exhorts the chief executives of NHS Trusts and health authorities to implement the standard on the cleaning and sterilization of medical devices.

The Medical Devices Agency (MDA) has been given the responsibility, on behalf of the government, to carry out the requirements of the directives in the UK. The definition of a medical device includes not only the device but also any accessories that might be used with it (MDA 2000a):

...A medical device can be defined as any instrument, apparatus, appliance, material or healthcare product, excluding drugs, used for a patient or client for the purpose of:

- *Diagnosis, prevention, monitoring, treatment or alleviation of disease.*
- *Diagnosis, monitoring, treatment, or alleviation of, or compensation for, an injury or handicap.*
- *Investigation, replacement or modification of the anatomy or of a physiological process.*
- *Control of conception.*

Rehabilitation aids, prostheses, continence aids, contact lenses, hospital beds and wheelchairs are also medical devices. The document 'Equipped to care: the safe use of medical devices in the 21st century' (MDA 2000a) includes an extensive list of products that fall into the definition of a medical device. Cleaning is an essential preparation when decontaminating equipment, and must precede disinfection and sterilization.

Definitions (MDA 1996a)

- *Cleaning*: a process that physically removes contamination but does not necessarily destroy microorganisms. The reduction of microbial contamination is not routinely quantified and will depend upon many factors, including the efficiency of the cleaning process and the initial bioburden. Cleaning removes microorganisms and the organic material on which they thrive. It is a necessary prerequisite of effective disinfection or sterilization.

- *Disinfection*: a process used to reduce the number of viable microorganisms but that might not necessarily inactivate some microbial agents, such as certain viruses and bacterial spores. Disinfection might not achieve the same reduction in microbial contamination level as sterilization.

- *Sterilization*: a process used to render an object free from viable microorganisms, including viruses and spores. Sterilization is required where small numbers of residual organisms on an item could be sufficient to cause disease, where exceptionally virulent organisms are suspected or where surviving organisms might multiply on an item and reach an infective dose before its use.

For the purpose of rendering an item safe for patient use, it should be cleaned, disinfected or sterilized. The process used depends on the risk of infection involved in the use of the item (BMA 1989, Rutala 1990, Spaulding 1968). Items are classified in relation to risk, as shown in Table 7.2.

Table 7.2 Assessment of patient care items (Babb 1992)

Category	Treatment	Method	Items
High risk In contact with a break in the skin or mucous membrane or introduced into a sterile body area (if sterilization is not practical, high level disinfection may be adequate)	Cleaning and sterilization	*Heat-tolerant:* Autoclave Hot air oven *Heat-sensitive:* Single use Ethylene oxide Low-temperature steam and formaldehyde Sporicidal disinfectants, e.g. glutaraldehyde	Surgical instruments, laparoscopes arthroscopes, cardiac catheters, implants, infusions, injections, needles, syringes, swabs, surgical dressings, sutures
Intermediate risk In contact with intact mucous membranes, body fluids, or contaminated with particularly virulent or readily transmissible organisms, or if the item is to be used on highly susceptible patients or sites	Cleaning and disinfection (or sterilization)	All the above and *Heat-tolerant:* Boiling Pasteurization Low-temperature steam washer/disinfectors *Heat-sensitive:* Disinfectants, e.g. glutaraldehyde, chlorine-releasing agents, alcohol, clear soluble phenolics	Respiratory and anaesthetic equipment, gastrointestinal endoscopes, bronchoscopes, thermometers, vaginal speculae, body fluid spillage, dirty instruments prior to reprocessing, bedpans
Low risk In contact with normal and intact skin	Cleaning usually adequate, disinfection if known infection risk	Manual cleaning with detergent Automated cleaning/disinfection Disinfectants	Trolley tops, operating table, wash-bowls, lavatory seats, baths, washbasins, bedding, patient supports
Minimal risk Remote, not in direct contact with patients or immediate surroundings. Unlikely to be contaminated with a significant number of pathogens or be transferred to a susceptible site	Cleaning alone	Manual or automated cleaning, damp dusting, wet mopping, dust-attractant mops, vacuum cleaners	Floors, walls, furniture, ceilings, drains

Decontamination of equipment before service or repair

All medical devices and equipment being sent for examination, inspection, service or repair must be safe to handle (DoH 1987, MDA 1995b, NHSME 1993b). The responsibility for ensuring the development and rigorous enforcement of a written policy for such items rests with the users. There is a risk of infection in handling items that have been in contact with patients or their body fluids (such as those in clinical areas, service departments, laboratories, dentistry, post-mortem rooms) or which are contaminated by hazardous chemicals (such as those in laboratories and in the pharmacy ultraclean cabinets). The Safety Notice MDA SN 9516 *Decontamination of Medical Devices and Equipment Prior to Investigation, Inspection, Service or Repair* (MDA 1995b) details the actions to be taken by all those involved with the return of medical devices to the Medical Devices Agency, manufacturers/suppliers or other departments. A written certificate or statement of decontamination should accompany the item: methods of decontamination are given in NHSME (1991).

The failure of healthcare establishments to implement the decontamination of equipment prior to service exposes staff to biological contamination (MDA 1996a). Devices and equipment sent to various agencies require the following considerations:

- Devices and equipment should be made safe to handle: cleaning alone will suffice if they have been in contact with a patient, but not body fluid. Disinfection or sterilization is necessary in the latter case
- The recipient should be contacted prior to the item being dispatched if it is impractical for all parts of the equipment to be made safe
- In cases where cleaning or decontamination could destroy vital evidence, the item should be labelled, placed in quarantine and the intended recipient contacted at the earliest convenience
- A written statement identifying the contamination status of the equipment should accompany the item. This should contain full details of the decontamination method used.

Single-use items

There might be a temptation on the part of healthcare workers to reuse single-use items in an effort to protect the environment and cut costs. An advisory document from the Medical Devices Agency (MDA 2000a) explains the hazards and responsibilities associated with the reuse of medical devices supplied for single use only. The Medical Devices Agency has also produced a bulletin explaining the symbols associated with medical devices and their packaging that includes a symbol for 'do not reuse' (MDA 2000b).

Although most healthcare professionals are aware of the risks associated with reuse of single-use items, Castille (1999) highlighted the concerns of retaining other items for recirculation. Items identified included open packs of wound-care products; saving unused swabs and dressings; sharing topical creams and lotions between patients; reusing nebulizers, oxygen masks, breathing circuits and masks; and failing to change sheets, pillowcases, blankets and duvet cases between patients. All of these acts increase the risk of cross-contamination. If a product has been designated by a manufacturer as being for single-patient use then it should be treated as such (Parker 1999a).

The decontamination of reuseable medical devices is the combination of processes that, if not correctly undertaken (individually or collectively), might increase the likelihood of microorganisms being transferred to patients or staff. Guidance is based on the reuseable medical device life-cycle and comprises the processes of: acquisition, cleaning, disinfection, sterilization, transportation and storage before use.

The guidance given in health technical memoranda (HTM), MDA, device bulletins (DB) and the CD-ROM issued with Health Service Circular HSC 1999/179 (NHS Estates 1999), has been designed to ensure that the hazards are minimized and that decontamination procedures comply with legislative requirements and good practice. HTM 2030 (NHSE 1999) suggests that it is likely that civil action could be taken against a hospital for supplying, for example, 'disinfected' products that were not in fact disinfected and caused the infection of a patient (NHSE 1999).

High-risk items

These are items that come into close contact with a break in the skin or mucous membrane or which are introduced into sterile body areas. Surgical instruments, cardiac or urinary catheters, implants, needles, and so on are included in this 'high-risk' category. High-risk items must be sterilized.

Methods of sterilization

Sterilization can be achieved by physical methods, irradiation and chemical methods. Certain solutions, such as glutaraldehyde, are capable of achieving sterilization but only under controlled conditions and over prolonged exposure times. These methods are less reliable than physical methods and, wherever possible, sterilization by autoclave is the best option. Sterilization can be achieved by:

- high temperature moist heat sterilization
- high temperature dry heat sterilization
- low temperature steam and formaldehyde sterilization
- ethylene oxide sterilization
- gamma irradiation
- low temperature plasma diffusion.

Moist heat sterilization

A temperature higher than that of boiling water (i.e. 134–138°C) is achieved by steam under a pressure of 32 lb per square inch. Time of exposure is 3 min.

Types of autoclave

A porous load steam sterilizer is suitable for wrapped goods. The sterilizing cycle incorporates vacuum-assisted air removal before the introduction of steam. The steam can penetrate the goods through the wrapping material.

A downward displacement sterilizer is suitable for unwrapped goods. The air is removed by displacement with steam rather than by vacuum. A complete removal of air is not possible and hence the steam might not penetrate trapped air in wrapped goods.

A fluid-cycle steam sterilizer is suitable for fluids in sealed containers. Temperatures of 121–124°C can be maintained for 15 min, or 115°C for 30 min.

Low temperature steam and formaldehyde (LTSF) can be used for heat-sensitive instruments. A temperature of 73°C should be maintained for 3 h.

Hot air sterilization

Hot air sterilization is used for instruments that might be damaged by steam, e.g. non-stainless metals, hollow needles, glass syringes. It is also used for non-aqueous liquids, oils and powders. Temperatures of 160°C should be maintained for 2 h, 170°C for 1 h and 180°C for 30 min.

Ethylene oxide sterilization

This is used for heat-sensitive equipment, both wrapped and unwrapped. It is mainly an industrial process. Temperatures of 20–60°C should be maintained for times ranging from 2 to 24 h.

Benchtop sterilizers

Benchtop steam sterilizers are intended for the sterilization of unwrapped instruments and utensils for use in the immediate patient environment.
[MDA 1996a]

The guidance bulletin on the sterilization, disinfection and cleaning of medical equipment (MDA 1996a) provides comprehensive information on the purchasing, maintenance and inspection of benchtop sterilizers. It also includes regulatory and legal aspects, technical aspects and safety consider-ations, and sources of further information. It gives particular consideration to the procedures that are *not* recommended in a benchtop sterilizer, namely:

- The processing of wrapped loads, which could result in a failure to sterilize the load through:
  - inadequate removal of air and hence inadequate steam penetration of load
  - inadequate drying of load
- The processing of instruments and utensils with lumens, which should not be carried out in benchtop sterilizers because air removal and steam penetration might be impaired
- The processing of porous material, e.g. swabs, towels, dressings, gowns and drapes, which should not take place in benchtop sterilizers for the reasons cited above.

A code of practice on the sterilization of instruments and infection control in GP surgeries has been produced by the British Medical Association (1989) and there are similar directives for dental surgeries (Glenwright & Martin 1993).

Monitoring sterilizers and the sterilization process

The responsibility for maintenance rests with the user as well as with the organization's Estates department. HTM 2010 (MDA 1993, 1996a) provides the necessary guidance for the appropriate functioning and management of equipment and machinery. The responsibilities are summarized in the Medical Devices Agency guidance documents parts 1 and 2 (MDA 1993, 1996a).

Medium- or intermediate-risk items

Medium-risk items are items that come into contact with mucous membranes, damaged skin, infected lesions, blood and other body fluids, or which are contaminated with particularly virulent or readily transmissible organisms. The category also applies to items that are to be used on immunocompromised patients (MDA 1996a). These items are made safe by disinfection.

Methods of disinfection

As with sterilization processes, disinfection must be preceded by cleaning. Disinfection can be achieved by physical methods and chemical disinfectants. Whenever heat disinfection can be used, this should be the first option over chemicals.

COSHH and disinfection

Only products accompanied by the manufacturer's safety datasheet and that have undergone a COSHH risk assessment prior to their use should be disinfected. Protective clothing must be worn when making up and using solutions, according to the risk assessment, and exposure limits must be adhered to. The expiry dates of solutions and powders should be checked prior to use. Any sensitivities or reactions must be reported to the Occupational Health Department and to Health and Safety representatives, and should also be documented by the department where it occurred.

Low temperature steam

This is a moist heat disinfection/pasteurization process that kills most vegetative microbes and viruses. The process works by removing air and introducing dry saturated steam at a pressure below atmospheric level. A temperature of 73°C should be maintained for 10 min.

Boiling water

Disinfection is achieved by exposure of items to boiling water. Important measures include complete removal of trapped air from tubing and the total immersion of items in boiling water. This method is not suitable for:

- hollow or porous items where hot water cannot penetrate the lumen
- tubes longer than 1 m (MDA 1993).

A temperature of 100°C should be maintained for 5 min. Timing should start after the water starts to boil following immersion of the item.

Washer–disinfectors

Washer–disinfectors can be used to clean and disinfect (or make safe) surgical instruments prior to packaging and sterilization. They can also be used to make non-invasive items (such as anaesthetic equipment, flexible endoscopes and human waste receptacles) free of infection risk and safe to use without additional treatment. Currently, of particular importance is the removal of prions of vCJD, which tolerate conventional thermal and chemical sterilization processes.

The preferred method of disinfection is to use heat, but some items are heat sensitive and must be disinfected by chemical means. Automated processing in a purpose-built washer–disinfector is more effective and reliable than manual cleaning because cycle parameters can more easily be monitored. The principal stages in the process are cleaning, disinfection, rinsing and drying. The European Community is currently producing a series of washer–disinfector standards for machines intended to clean and disinfect medical devices and other articles used in the context of medical, dental, pharmaceutical and veterinary practice (Babb & Bradley 2001). These standards will cover general requirements, definitions and tests (Part 1), processes for surgical instruments, anaesthetic equipment, hollow-ware, etc. (Part 2), human waste containers (Part 3) and thermolabile reusable devices, e.g. endoscopes (Part 4).

Cleaning failures are usually due to dried excretions and secretions following lengthy delays before processing, the temperature of the initial wash being above protein coagulation temperature (45°C), misdirection of jets, failed ultrasonic transducers, and blocked cleansing jets. The use of unsuitable processing chemicals, failure to irrigate lumened devices or badly placed instruments also contribute to cleaning failures.

Thermal disinfectors: types and purpose

- Cabinet washer–disinfectors are loaded and unloaded manually and are used for items such as bedpans, urinals and suction bottles. The machine will empty these containers before processing. It can also be used to disinfect anaesthetic accessories, theatre clogs, hollow-ware and other theatre equipment, theatre instruments, glass and metal hollow-ware from laboratories and instrument trays
- Ultrasonic washer–disinfectors are used for surgical instruments
- Tunnel washer–disinfectors are used for theatre instruments.

Temperatures of 71°C should be maintained for 3 min, 80°C for 1 min or 90°C for 12 s.

HTM 2030 (NHSE 1995) provides guidance on washer–disinfectors in healthcare settings.

Chemical washer–disinfectors

These are used for heat-sensitive endoscopes and accessories. Their action is as follows (MDA 1996a):

- Cleaning is achieved by soaking, spraying, irrigating channels, deluging with water and compatible detergent or exposure to ultrasonic

cleaning during a timed cycle. The temperature of the cleaning stage should be at or below 35°C
- Disinfection is achieved by exposure to an approved disinfectant for a predetermined period. This is followed by one or more rinses in water to remove disinfectant residues. The final stage of the cycle includes fluid expulsion from the lumens by air pressure and an optional air dry or alcohol rinse.

Chemical disinfection

This is the use of a chemical compound that destroys vegetative bacteria, fungi and most viruses (Ayliffe et al 1993). Chemical disinfectants are used when alternative methods of processing heat-sensitive items are not available. It also includes liquid chemical immersion.

Numerous disinfectants, e.g. glutaraldehyde, are available for chemical immersion; the efficacy varies with each disinfectant and is not discussed here.

Immersion time varies from 4 min (British Society of Gastroenterology (BSG) 1998) and depends on the nature of the contamination. Most viruses and non-sporing bacteria are destroyed in 10 min. Disinfectants that are effective against mycobacteria and spores can take several hours to produce the required result (Griffiths et al 1998).

The process of disinfection

A successful disinfection process will include a:

- chemical with appropriate antimicrobial property
- chemical of accurate dilution and strength
- chemical that is stable
- chemical that is compatible with the items processed
- good contact between the disinfectant and item to be disinfected for a predetermined minimum time.

The chemical also needs to be user friendly and cost effective (Ayliffe et al 1993).

Some disinfectant chemicals, such as glutaraldehyde and chlorine-releasing agents, are irritant to the skin, eyes and respiratory tract. They can also be corrosive and flammable. The Department of Health Safety Action Bulletin SAB (94) 21 *Use and Management of Glutaraldehyde Solutions* (DoH 1994a) recommends risk assessment as laid down in the Health and Safety Regulation entitled *The Control of Substances Hazardous to Health* (COSHH) (HSC 1999). Further safety precautions include:

- containment of toxic vapours and adequate ventilation
- use of waterproof clothing, robust rubber (nitril) gloves and eye protection if splashing is likely
- thorough washing and drying of hands on completion of the task
- the covering of immersion tanks
- thorough rinsing of instruments following immersion.

Choosing disinfectants

The ideal disinfectant is effective against a wide range of clinically significant microorganisms, including pathogenic spores. Selecting disinfectants for hospital use is the responsibility of the Infection Control Team (ICT). It is unlikely that a single disinfectant will be found that meets all the preferred criteria. A careful appraisal is necessary to choose the product and the process that meets the local requirements.

Glutaraldehyde

Glutaraldehyde was first introduced as an instrument disinfectant in 1963, when it replaced the widespread use of formaldehyde. The most widely used glutaraldehyde preparations in the UK are the 2% activated alkaline glutaraldehydes such as Cidex. Its major benefit is its wide spectrum of activity, even under moderate soiling conditions. However, it is a recognized irritant to the skin, eyes and respiratory tract. It is also listed as a skin and respiratory sensitizer. The Health and Safety Executive (HSE) has published mandatory maximum exposure limit (MEL) as 0.05 p.p.m. over a short (15 min) and long (8 h) time weighted average (Babb & Bradley 1995).

Quaternary ammonium compounds (QAC) and peroxygen compounds

QACs such as Dettox and peroxygen compounds such as Virkon were introduced as safer alternatives to the glutaraldehydes in the 1980s. Their spectrum of activity is poor, particularly against spores, mycobacteria and enteroviruses (Broadley et al 1993, Griffiths et al 1999, Tyler 1990). Virkon has been found to be damaging to some endoscope components and consequently is not recommended for the disinfection of endoscopes (Babb & Bradley 2001).

Alcohols

Seventy per cent isopropanol, ethanol and industrial methylated spirit (IMS) are very popular and, although ineffective against spores, are rapidly tuberculocidal (Griffiths et al 1999). They are widely used for disinfecting trolley tops, work surfaces, thermometers, scissors, dropped instruments, probes, monitors, transducers and electrical equipment. Being flammable, they cannot be used in large amounts in automated washer–disinfectors because of the fire risk. Alcohols can be used for the manual disinfection of endoscopes and other heat-sensitive items and for drying lumened devices.

If the microbiological quality of the water cannot be assured, alcohol can be used for post-rinse disinfection because it evaporates, leaving surfaces dry.

Peracetic acid

This is the most popular alternative to glutaraldehyde. It is available in a number of different forms. These include Steris system, NuCidex, Perascope and Perasafe. Except for Steris, which is used in a dedicated processor, the other products can be reused provided they are within the use dilution range and are compatible with the washer–disinfector.

Efficacies vary slightly between formulations. Although peracetic acid is not currently listed as an irritant, it is composed of hydrogen peroxide and acetic acid, both of which are irritants.

Peracetic acid is less stable and more damaging to instruments and processors than glutaraldehyde. In most cases this damage is superficial.

Chlorine dioxide

This has similar properties to peracetic acid and has a broad spectrum of activity. Chlorine dioxide is listed as an irritant and also is known to damage some instrument and processor components. Lower concentrations are less damaging and less irritant, but they are also less effective, especially when organic matter is present. Thorough cleansing and single use of the disinfectant is preferred (Babb & Bradley 2001).

Superoxidized water

There is a new system where an instrument disinfectant is generated at the point of use by the electrolysis of salt solution (NaCl). The solution collected from the positive terminal contains a mixture of radicals with strong oxidizing properties. These are highly effective as a disinfectant against spores, mycobacteria, fungi and viruses (Selkon et al 1999, Shetty et al 1999). The disinfector generator is placed close to the endoscope washer–disinfectors. The Sterilox generation criteria are critical to efficacy and microprocessor controlled and if not met, Sterilox generation will stop.

Ortho-phthalaldehyde (OPA)

Cidex OPA 0.55% was introduced into the UK at the start of 2001. Its main benefits are similar to Cidex but it does not require activation (Alfa & Sitter 1994). It is more stable and produces little or no odour because it has low vapour properties. It is not yet listed as a respiratory sensitizer, although product data identifies it as a skin irritant. It does not appear to damage instrument components but it stains protein and, like other aldehydes, is a fixative (Babb & Bradley 2001).

Making choices

The following advice should be followed before changing disinfectants used for instrument processors (Babb & Bradley 1995, MDA 1996d):

- inform and involve your ICT or ICC
- review manufacturers' efficacy data and other claims
- consult instrument and processor manufacturers about compatibility
- cost the change, bearing in mind the use life of the disinfectant and its stability
- establish what is required to meet health and safety legislation, e.g. COSHH assessment, and cost this
- ensure items are thoroughly cleaned before immersion and that the disinfectant manufacturer's stated contact times and processing temperatures are achieved.

Failure of disinfection

Disinfection can fail because disinfectants (MDA 1993):

- can be inactivated by a variety of substances, e.g. blood and other body fluids, incompatibly charged detergents, wood, cork, plastics, rubbers and some inorganic chemicals
- cannot penetrate organic material and kill microorganisms. Also, some disinfectants coagulate proteins and so hamper their own penetration
- can decay and lose their efficiency. This can happen at any time but mainly when they are diluted. Elevated temperatures and the presence of impurities can also lead to the decay of disinfectants.

Disinfection can also fail because:

- insufficient time is allowed
- there is an inadequate concentration of the disinfectant
- there is organic material providing protection to target organisms
- there is recontamination of equipment such as endoscopes as a result of inadequate cleaning and disinfection of the tank's fluid pathways and endoscope washer–disinfectors (DoH 1992, 1993b).

Specialist items

Suction apparatus

Suction apparatus can become contaminated with microorganisms found in body fluids. The apparatus, receptacles, lids, tubings and connections have all been found to be contaminated (Bassett et al 1965, Creamer 1993). Contamination of the apparatus can be high; 11.5% of the pieces of suction apparatus examined have been found to be bacteriologically contaminated during an investigation by Creamer (1993). Outbreaks and incidents of infections linked to heavily contaminated suction apparatus and tubing have been reported from wards, operating theatres, intensive care units, special-care baby units and endoscopy units: some have resulted in fatalities (Beecham et al 1979, Blenkharn & Hughes 1982, Ip et al 1976, Khan et al 1991, Rahman 1980, Rubbo et al 1966, Stiver et al 1979).

Ideally, the process should include disinfection or sterilization, but access to washer–disinfectors or autoclaves could be limited. In most care situations, emptying, dismantling and cleaning of the apparatus occurs at a ward or department level. Staff should be made aware of the risk of hand contamination and the importance of handwashing following contact with the apparatus. The advice should stress the:

- wearing of plastic aprons and gloves
- removal and careful disposal of tubing and catheter
- dismantling of the lid from the receptacle
- careful emptying of the aspirate to avoid splashing
- thorough cleaning with detergent, hot water and appropriate cleaning and bottle brushes (reusable brushes should be washed and hooked to dry)
- thorough drying of the accessories and the receptacle using disposable paper towels.

Disposable suction liner systems are now available and are the preferred option of disposal. They are currently used in areas such as special-care baby units, intensive care units, critical care units, accident and emergency (A&E) and theatres.

Ophthalmic instruments

Ophthalmic instruments such as tonometer prisms and examination contact lenses carry a risk of cross-infection in ophthalmic departments. Contact lenses given to patients for trial purposes must not be re-used and disposable contact lenses are recommended. Also available are disposable tonometer prisms for use as an alternative to decontamination. Infections such as herpes and adenoviruses, Gram-negative bacilli and fungi can be transmitted via contaminated eye instruments. HIV and hepatitis B are also of concern, although no cases of such transmissions have been reported (Austin et al 1992, Dart et al 1995). Government advice issued in 1999 (MDA 1999a) following concern about the risk of transmission of variant Creutzfeld–Jakob disease (vCJD) advises that those components of ophthalmic instruments and medical devices that touch the surfaces of the eye should be restricted to single patient use wherever this is practicable and does not compromise clinical practice. When they are to be reused, they should be:

- wiped clean
- immersed in 20 000 p.p.m. available chlorine for 1 h.

Hands are thought to cause cross-infection more often than contaminated instruments and Austin et al (1992) recommend handwashing between patients and the use of disposable gloves where convenient and especially if the skin is broken or inflamed.

Ineffective sterilization of handpieces and reusable accessories used in Phaco microsurgical procedures has been linked with cases of eye infection (MDA 1995a). The hazard note provides the following guidance for decontamination and sterilization of these items:

- separate the irrigation sleeve, needle and tubing from the Phaco handpiece
- separate all other reusable accessories
- flush and clean in accordance with the manufacturer's instructions
- sterilize in autoclaves equipped with air removal (i.e. sterilizers for wrapped and porous loads).

Instruments and appliances used in the vagina and cervix

Viable papilloma virus has been found on used vaginal speculae (McCance et al 1986, Skegg & Paul 1986). Decontamination of instruments used in the vagina and cervix is incorporated in the Department of Health Safety Action Bulletin (SAB (94) 22) *Instruments and Appliances Used in the Vagina and Cervix: Recommended Methods for Decontamination* (DoH 1994b). Moist heat, dry heat sterilization or boiling water disinfection is recommended; chemical disinfection is not advised. The decontamination requirement for complex equipment such as endoscopes used in gynaecology may not withstand these methods of decontamination and will require local consideration.

Low-risk items

Low-risk items are items that are in contact with healthy skin or mucous membrane or which do not come into close contact with susceptible individuals. Low-risk items are washed with detergent and warm water and stored dry.

Stethoscopes

Stethoscopes have been known to be colonized with organisms (Breathnach et al 1992, Wright et al 1995). Wright et al (1995) found a high proportion of stethoscopes in the neonatal intensive care unit to be contaminated with coagulase-negative staphylococci, which are the main cause of infection in very low birthweight infants. Both studies highlighted the lack of stethoscope cleaning and recommended regular cleaning with an alcohol-impregnated swab.

Tourniquets

Reuseable tourniquets have been shown to pose a potential risk of cross-infection. Golder et al (2000) found that a number of tourniquets, taken randomly from different wards and departments, grew *Escherichia coli*, *Pseudomonas aeruginosa*, *Enterococcus faecalis* and methicillin-sensitive *Staphylococcus aureus* (MRSA). The study recommended that disposable tourniquets should be introduced.

Ice-making machines

Ice cubes have been reported to be a recognized source of infection (DoH 1993a, Newsome 1968). The organism *Xanthomonas maltophilia*, which caused the outbreak of septicaemia in leukaemia patients that was reported by Newsome (1968), was thought to originate from ice cubes. The source was identified as the storage cabinet of the ice-making machine on the ward. The infected patients had been given ice to suck or in cool drinks. Ice cubes are used for many purposes: patients' drinks, ice packs for inflamed joints, for cooling fans, to cool transplant kidneys, for patients on restricted fluids, and so on (Burnett et al 1994). These authors isolated a few organisms of significance from most of the samples tested. It is important to remember that in the *Food Safety (General Food Hygiene) Regulations* (DoH 1995b), ice is classified as a food. The hazard notice HN (93) 42 (DoH 1993a) makes the following recommendations:

- ice should be made from drinking-quality water
- freshly cleaned containers or single-use ice cube bags should be used
- ice should be preferably made in a domestic freezer or the ice-making compartment of a refrigerator
- reusable containers should be washed in a dishwasher with a high temperature rinse/disinfection cycle, or by an equally effective method

- ice should be handled with care to avoid contamination
- ice should be stored for the shortest practicable time
- the ice-making machine should be cleaned in accordance with the manufacturer's instructions. A visible record of defrosting and cleaning should be available at all times
- ice may be removed only by using a plastic scoop that is designated solely for that purpose
- any ward or department wanting to purchase a machine should first contact the infection control department for advice
- immunocompromised patients must not be given ice from these machines; they should be given only sterile ice
- staff must be encouraged to wash their hands before handling ice for patients
- the environment around the ice-making machines must be kept sufficiently clear to allow for air circulation and prevent contamination
- ice must not be transported between wards or between departments for consumption.

The Estates department is responsible for ensuring that the:

- water supply to the ice-making machine is not taken from the dead-end branch of the cold water service system
- warm air exhaust from the ice-making machine is not allowed to impinge directly onto taps or pipes supplying cold water
- machine is installed in accordance with the guidance contained in HTM 2040 *The Control of Legionellae in Health Care Premises: a Code of Practice* (HSE 2001).

A further approved code of practice (HSC (G) 70) has been issued to provide practical guidance on risk management, record keeping and the duties on suppliers of products and services. It also includes new guidance on testing for legionella in water systems and maintenance requirements (HSE 2001).

Lancing devices

Lancing devices for multipatient capillary blood sampling have been implicated in outbreaks of hepatitis B and their use should be restricted to one person (DoH 1990).

In-house spirit levels

The hazard notice MDA HN 9609 (MDA 1996b) draws attention to an outbreak of multiresistant *Pseudomonas aeruginosa* in an intensive care unit that infected a number of patients and led to the death of one. The same organism was isolated from an 'in-house' manufactured spirit level used in central venous pressure (CVP) measurement. The hazard notice suggests that only commercially available spirit levels should be used and that suitable infection control procedures are followed at all times (MDA 1996b).

Blood gas analysers

A Medical Devices Agency safety notice (MDA 1996c) draws attention to an association between infections in immunocompromised patients and the near-patient location of blood gas analysers. The importance of regular decontamination using locally agreed procedure and good hygiene practices, including handwashing after each use, is emphasized. The responsibility rests with the user of the equipment and the infection control personnel.

Safety notice MDA SN 9619

This safety notice (MDA 1996d) draws attention to the damage to some components of medical devices, e.g. endoscopes and reprocessing units, caused by certain decontaminant agents. The agents are not named but the user is advised to follow the 'instructions for use' and to consult equipment manufacturers for advice regarding the compatibility of the decontamination regimen with their products. The decontamination agent/decontaminant incorporates detergents, disinfectants and sterilants.

Care of mattresses and pillows

The necessity of cleaning mattresses between patient use has been questioned (Walsh & Foord 1993). Hospital bed mattresses have been recognized both as a reservoir of pathogens and as a source of outbreaks of infection (Fujita et al 1981, Loomes 1988, Moore & Williams 1991, Ndwala & Brown 1991). Hospital mattresses have been found to be wet with leaking covers (Larcombe 1988). Damaged mattresses and waterproof covers can harbour microorganisms. O'Donoghue & Allen (1992) isolated a range of organisms from damaged mattresses and found that the same organisms were also isolated from 10 infected patients who had undergone clean, orthopaedic operative procedures. Discarding a number of damaged and contaminated mattresses terminated the outbreak.

Nurses are responsible for checking mattresses and mattress covers and Peto & Calrow (1996) provide a 'water test' to check the integrity of hospital mattresses and plastic covers. A regular programme of inspecting, turning and replacing mattresses is recommended in the DoH safety action bulletin entitled *Hospital Mattress Assembly: Care and Cleaning* (DoH 1991a):

- The mattress cover must be cleaned on discharge of patients, or periodically in long-term care
- A thorough cleaning with a solution of neutral detergent and hot water and a single-use wipe is adequate
- Cleaning should be followed by thorough drying with a paper towel. The mattress should be allowed to dry before remaking the bed.

Further advice has been issued on the maintenance of foam mattresses and their covers (MDA 1999b).

Feather pillows have been identified as a source of *Acinetobacter* (Weernick et al 1995). The organism was isolated from a number of patients in a hospital in the Netherlands and was associated with severe infections. The use of feather pillows should be discouraged.

Toys

Toys are an essential accompaniment in many healthcare settings: in GP surgeries, health centres, outpatient and A&E departments, paediatric wards and maternity units. Similarly, the sharing of toys amongst toddlers in child daycare centres is a matter of routine. Both well and unwell children handle toys. The problem of infection in children is aggravated, according to Schuman (1983), by the normal behaviour of the children themselves:

- toddlers between the ages of 2 and 4 years have been observed to put a hand or an object in the mouth every 3 min
- close contact of young children is almost constant unless the children are specifically segregated
- younger children are incontinent of faeces before toilet training
- younger children lack proper personal hygiene because of their age.

A number of environmental items, including toys, have been implicated in the transmission of microorganisms in a burns unit (Wormold 1970). Viruses can be excreted in huge numbers in respiratory secretions and stools, and their persistence on surfaces for hours and days is common. Increased environmental contamination has been described during an outbreak of diarrhoea in daycare settings (Weniger et al 1983). Toys may be important vectors in these circumstances.

A survey of inanimate surfaces and of the hands of staff and children in five day centres in Houston, US, during outbreaks of diarrhoea revealed faecal coliforms on the hands and on classroom objects, including toys. Contaminated hands and objects were thought to play a role in the spread of enteric bacteria (Ekanem et al 1983). Laboratory studies have shown viable rotaviruses to survive on environmental surfaces for up to 10 days (Kumarsinghe et al 1982). According to Swaffield (1983), diarrhoea is one of the top five reasons for infant hospital admission, and each year GPs see 1 million children under 4 years old with diarrhoea and enteric upsets.

Pseudomonas aeruginosa was reported to have been recovered from dried sputum over 1 week old from sinks, soap, baths, tables, brushes, clothes, and toys in a cystic fibrosis clinic (Zimakoff et al 1983). The Teddy (T.) Bears, introduced by the National Institute of Health in the US to encourage handwashing by hospital personnel, and also presented to hospitalized children, were found to be colonized with bacteria, fungi or both within 1 week of hospitalization. The organisms cultured from T. Bears included *Staphylococcus epidermidis* and *S. aureus,* alpha-streptococci, *Corynebacterium acnes, Micrococcus* spp., *Klebsiella pneumoniae, Pseudomonas aeruginosa, Escherichia coli, Bacillus* spp., and species of *Candida, Cryptococcus, Trichosporon, Aspergillus* and others. Concomitant cultures from the patients revealed similar isolates (Hughes-Walter et al 1986).

Hygienic management of toys in communal settings

Wherever possible:

- Toys should be made of heat-tolerant materials, i.e. capable of thermal disinfection by hot cycles in a washing machine or they should have impervious surfaces suitable for chemical disinfection. Stuffed toys should be discouraged; if allowed, they should not be shared
- Children with impaired immunity should avoid contact with communal toys
- Toys should be stored in clean plastic containers
- It might be useful for donated toys to be received by an appointed person and distributed as appropriate.

Toys at home

When there are young children in a home, such as crawling toddlers, a number of the surfaces they come into close contact can become contaminated. These can include toys that children put into their mouths and parents must be made aware that these can sometimes act as a means of transfer of infection, particularly where they are shared between different children. Ideally, toys should be washed and disinfected between uses by different children (Hale & Polder 1996).

Specialist equipment and facilities

Whirlpool baths, spa and hydrotherapy pools

Hydrotherapy equipment has traditionally been used to treat patients with medical conditions, which include (but are not limited to) burns, septic ulcers, lesions, amputations, orthopaedic impairments and injuries, arthritis, and kidney lithotripsy (CDC 2001). Potential routes of infection include incidental ingestion of the water, sprays and aerosols, and direct contact with wounds and intact skin. Risk factors include the age and sex of the patient, the underlying medical conditions, the length of time spent in the hydrotherapy water and portals of entry.

Whirlpool baths, spa and hydrotherapy pools have been associated with skin, ear, eye, chest and urinary tract infections (Brett & Du Vivier 1985, Hollyoak et al 1995, Insler & Gore 1986, Ratnam et al 1986, Ringham 1989, Rose et al 1983, Salmen et al 1983, Schlech et al 1986).

Healthcare facilities should maintain stringent cleaning and disinfection practices in accordance with the manufacturer's instructions and with relevant scientific literature until data supporting more rigorous infection control measures become available.

Many disciplines are involved in hydrotherapeutic equipment, including ward staff, engineers, domestic staff, physiotherapists and infection control personnel. The Public Health Laboratory Service (PHLS) has produced comprehensive guidelines covering hydrotherapy and spa pools entitled *Hygiene for Hydrotherapy Pools* (PHLS 1999) and *Hygiene for Spa Pools* (PHLS 1994). The PHLS (1999) recommends that, before a patient enters a pool, ward staff should ensure:

- that the patient has a clean face and teeth
- safe bladder drainage – emptying of condoms, if worn
- bowel evacuation if the patient is incontinent.

Infected patients and patients with wounds likely to become infected from the use of the pool should be excluded until infection control advice has been sought.

Physiotherapy staff engaged in preparing patients for the pool should ensure:

- voiding of the bladder
- an aseptic technique when spiggoting condoms/catheters from drainage bags.

In case of contamination of pools (PHLS 1999):

- *with formed stool*: close the pool to bathers, remove the stool, hyperchlorinate, and reopen the pool when the normal disinfectant level is established
- *with loose stool dispersed*: close the pool to bathers, empty the pool and hose down, refill and commence circulation, hyperchlorinate, brush the pool surfaces and maintain circulation for three turnover cycles. Backwash the filter and reopen the pool when the normal disinfectant level has been re-established
- *with vomit*: actions as for loose stool. Backwashing of filters might be necessary.

Paddling pools

Paddling pools easily become contaminated and, unlike larger systems, have no proper chlorination arrangements to prevent infection:

- water sprinklers are preferable for water play instead of pools
- children who have diarrhoea and vomiting must not be allowed into the pool
- time allowed in the pool should be restricted and stopped immediately if faecal soiling occurs
- children in nappies should be cleaned before being allowed into the pool.

Therapeutic beds

There is a vast proliferation of specialist beds for pressure relief and pressure ulcer management within all inpatient establishments. Often, beds are rented and many are purchased. Most manufacturers provide an infection control policy that they recommend or operate. These policies are generally produced in collaboration with infection control nurses.

Whether rented or purchased, the beds should receive thorough cleaning between patient use, after heavy contamination and before returning the bed at the end of the rental period. In most instances, a basic thorough cleaning with detergent and warm water followed by thorough drying of the bed is adequate. It might be necessary to use a disinfectant such as sodium hypochlorite solution at 1000 p.p.m.

Beds might need to be sent to a dedicated processing centre to be thoroughly decontaminated and disinfected. The infection control personnel using the centre should consider on-site visits and vetting of their decontamination procedures.

Points to consider

Therapeutic beds, especially fluidized microsphere beds, are useful for nursing compromised patients. The manufacturers' literature describes these beds as 'self-sterilizing' owing to their high pH. They have, however, been associated with the nosocomial spread of *Enterococcus faecium* and *Enterococcus faecalis*. Gould & Freeman (1993), investigating the first strain of vancomycin-resistant *Enterococcus faecium* in a hospital, isolated the organism from the dirty mattress cover used for the infected patient, as well as from a clean, unused, cover that was carefully removed from its sealed bag. The authors recovered one isolate of vancomycin-resistant *Enterococcus faecium* and several isolates of vancomycin-sensitive *Enterococcus faecium* from other mattress covers. Further isolates of vancomycin-sensitive *Enterococcus faecium* and *Staphylococcus aureus* were grown from a second 'clean' wrapped cover. The only common link between the three vancomycin-resistant *Enterococcus-faecium*-colonized and infected patients during this investigation was that they had been nursed on therapeutic beds supplied by the same manufacturer.

Vancomycin-resistant enterococci are becoming increasingly common in the UK and are spreading rapidly in hospitals in the US (CDR 1995b). If therapeutic beds have become a potential reservoir, it might be cost effective to sample mattress covers at random and after use by an infected patient.

Birthing pools

Water births are greatly favoured by both mothers and midwives. Although considered to be a safe and effective form of pain management during labour, their safety with regard to infection control has not been fully established. It is not unusual for the bowel contents of the mother to be discharged during delivery. Although the discharge in water births is removed with a sieve and the remaining discharge is diluted substantially, organisms such as *Escherichia coli* and group B streptococci could get into the newborn lungs with increased risk of neonatal infection (Zimmermann et al 1993).

Contamination of pools and accessories has also been reported. Loomes and Finch (1990) isolated *Pseudomonas aeruginosa* and *Klebsiella pneumoniae* from the water pumps and heating systems of birthing pools. Rawal et al (1994) have described pseudomonas sepsis in a baby after water birth. The organism was isolated from the baby's ears and umbilicus and was the same serotype as that cultured from the birthing tub, disposable lining, filling hose, taps and exit hose. Positive cultures from ears, necessitating antibiotics, and raised respiratory rate and grunting requiring admission into the special-care baby unit have been described by Coombs et al (1994) in a number of babies delivered under water.

Ridgeway & Tedder (1996) suggest that contamination of the birthing pool surfaces with large quantities of maternal bacteria and viruses is inevitable. This contamination will be from amniotic fluid, blood and faeces. They recommend that only women uninfected by the blood-borne viruses should be allowed to use the pool in their establishment.

National guidelines on the effective management of birthing pools do not exist. A thorough cleaning after use is vital but sterility cannot be guaranteed. National guidelines on birthing pools would be welcome but the recommendations by Coombs et al (1994) for plumbed pools in their establishment serve as a useful guide for other areas. They suggest that:

- taps are opened for 5 min each day to reduce the risk of contamination from water that might otherwise remain static and tepid in the dead leg
- the water is allowed to flow for 2 min before filling the pool
- the pool is cleaned and dried thoroughly after each use.

Rawal et al (1994) suggest a regular microbiological surveillance of birthing tub systems. They have shortened the filling and exit hoses and these are heat disinfected after each use.

Breast pumps

Mothers of premature infants who cannot be breast-fed are often encouraged to provide expressed breast milk. Breast pumps are often used to do this, both in hospital or in the mother's own home. Breast pump apparatus has been implicated in an outbreak of *Klebsiella* bacteraemia in a newborn intensive care unit (Donowitz et al 1981). The milk can become contaminated during collection or storage. The mother should be free of infection and receive instructions on how to dismantle, decontaminate, reassemble and express milk without contaminating the equipment or the feed. This should include handwashing and hygiene of breasts. The pump should be disinfected between each patient use. Single-use disposal systems are now available.

RESERVOIRS OF BUILDINGS AND ESTATE

Within the controls assurance standards there is recognition of the role of the physical environment, which is usually the responsibility of the Estates department. This remit includes the management of land, buildings, plant and non-medical equipment. It is a government requirement that all NHS Trusts have a strategy for such management, which includes infection control. An effective and well-run physical environment will help ensure that patients, staff and visitors are safe and comfortable.

Legionnaire's disease

An area of responsibility for engineers in relation to infection control is the prevention of Legionnaire's disease. The *Legionella* species are encountered in natural environments such as lakes, rivers and mud, and in man-made water systems such as piped water and air-conditioning systems. Water-cooled air-conditioning systems and industrial evaporative cooling towers, where large bacterial loads can build up with extensive aerosol formation, have been associated with outbreaks in hotels and hospitals. Planned prevention is said to be the most important defence against the disease. All healthcare settings are required to follow the guidance set out in the government and Health and Safety Commission approved code of practice on the prevention and control of Legionnaire's disease (HSE 2001). Apart from regular draining and cleaning of water storage tanks, the recommendations include the storage and circulation of hot water at a minimum of 60°C. There are hazards associated with this high water temperature, especially in areas where the elderly, the mentally ill and children are nursed. The temperature of the water at the tap should be 45–50°C. However, the hot water at the tap often discourages staff from washing their hands appropriately or adequately. Only mixer taps should be installed in clinical areas.

Control and prevention of *Aspergillus* species

Aspergillus species are environmental organisms found in soil, water and decaying vegetation. They have been isolated from unfiltered air, ventilation systems, false ceiling dust, contaminated dust dislodged during hospital renovation and construction, food, spices, dried flowers and plants. Other reported reservoirs include contaminated fireproofing material and damp wood. Due to their size, the *Aspergillus* spores remain suspended in the air for long periods of time and, once introduced into the environment, can last for many months.

Acquisition of aspergillosis is by inhalation of the fungal spores. Patients with severe prolonged granulocytopenia, especially bone marrow recipients, are at the highest risk. Non-immunocompromised hospital patients and staff are rarely, if ever, infected with this organism.

A formal risk assessment needs to be carried out prior to any renovation or construction work in healthcare institutions in consultation with the infection control department (NHS Estates 2001). The following issues need to be considered:

- Construction and renovation policy
- Planning, design and preconstruction:
  - design and structure
  - preparation for demolition and construction
  - dust and debris control
  - ventilation and environmental control
  - contamination of patient rooms, supplies, equipment and related areas
  - impact on special areas
  - patient location and transport
  - interruption of utility services
  - worker risk assessment and education

- Postconstruction clean-up
- Monitoring of activities during construction
- Environmental emergencies and remediation
- Contamination of ventilation in surgical suites or other invasive areas:
  - sealing and air intakes
  - operating room ventilation
  - air handlers, ducts and filters
- Water contamination:
  - general remediation procedure after water contamination
- Surfaces: design or disruption/damage issues:
  - design
  - flooding accidents
  - ceiling tiles/porous materials
  - walls
  - floors
  - carpeting
- Furnishings, fixtures and equipment:
  - furniture
  - handwashing facilities/sinks
  - whirlpool/spa/birthing pools
  - eyewash stations
  - showers
  - potable water.

Operating room environment

The majority of postoperative infections in wounds, other than clean wounds, appear to be from endogenous sources. The operating room environment can influence some surgical wound infection, which suggests that a degree of environmental control is necessary (Holton & Ridgeway 1993).

Design

In 1962, the Medical Research Council (MRC 1962) recommended six basic design requirements for the control of infection in operating theatres. These were:

1. Separation of the department from the general traffic and movement of the hospital
2. A sequence of increasingly clean zones from the entrance to the operating and sterilizing areas
3. Easy movement of staff from one clean area to another without passing through 'dirty' areas
4. Removal of dirty materials from the suite without passing through clean areas
5. Airflow from clean to less clean areas
6. Heating and ventilation to ensure safe and comfortable conditions for patients and staff.

These design considerations are still incorporated in the health building notes (HBN 26 1990) for operating theatres today. Most theatres today are now designed in 'zones' (DoH/NHSE 1991):

- aseptic (operative zone): theatre and lay-up rooms
- clean (restricted access zone): anaesthetic and scrub rooms
- protective (limited access zone): entrance, recovery, changing rooms
- disposal (general access zone).

There are basically three 'circuits of hygiene' within the operating theatre. These refer to the physical movement of surgical staff, surgical instruments and patients (Parker 1999b).

Ventilation

The operating room ventilation system serves a dual purpose: to prevent infection of the patient's wound and to provide a comfortable atmosphere for the surgical team.

The primary source of bacteria in the operating room is the people. Microbial contamination in the form of skin scales is generated through the physical activities of staff and the concentration of bacteria. This has been found to be proportional to activity and numbers of people in the room (Hambraeus & Laurell 1980, Lidwell et al 1967). Although most people disperse bacteria of low pathogenicity, around 10% of males and 1% of females also disperse *Staphylococcus aureus*, the organism commonly associated with wound infection from exogenous sources. It is generally accepted that microorganisms in the air of operating rooms are associated with infections in prosthetic joint surgery (Lidwell et al 1983). The air movement in operating rooms is designed to curtail the transfer of bacteria from less clean to clean areas and to reduce the airborne bacterial contamination. However, only a small number of bacteria are required to produce deep infections in orthopaedic surgery. Here an ultraclean air system that allows a further reduction of airborne contamination is generally used.

Current national guidance on all aspects of operating theatre ventilation including performance testing is contained in HTM 2025 (NHS Estates 1994).

Most standard theatres are plenum ventilated at 20 air changes per hour in the aseptic zone without recirculating the air. Ultraclean ventilation is achieved by laminar airflow from a diffuser or filter bank directly downward over the operating site. Recirculation of air is by using high efficiency particulate air (HEPA) filters and is essential to reduce running costs (McCulloch 2000).

Pets

Animals in healthcare facilities have historically been limited to laboratories and research areas. Their presence in patient-care areas is now more frequent both in acute and long-term care settings. Although dogs and cats are the most commonly found in healthcare settings, other animals include fish, birds, rabbits, rodents and reptiles. These animals, like humans, can be host for a wide variety of organisms that are potential pathogens for people and other animals. There is minimal evidence that outbreaks of infectious diseases have occurred as a result of contact with animals by immunocompetent patients. However, zoonoses can be transmitted from animals to humans either directly or indirectly by bites, scratches, aerosols, ectoparasites, accidental ingestion, or via contact with contaminated soil, food, water or unpasteurized milk.

The idea of pet therapy arose from the observation that patients with pets at home appear to recover from surgical and medical procedures more rapidly than patients without pets. Known as pet-assisted therapy (PAT), it is an intervention that includes an animal into the treatment process. Animals participating in such schemes should have up-to-date vaccinations, be routinely screened for enteric parasites, be free of ectoparasites (e.g. fleas and ticks) and should have no obvious dermatological lesions associated with bacterial, fungal, viral or parasitic infestations. The animals should be clean and well-groomed, the visits should be supervised and the area cleaned after visits according to standard cleaning procedures.

Immunocompromised patients are recommended to avoid:

- animal faeces or soiled litter tray material
- animals with diarrhoea
- very young animals <6 months of age and <12-month-old cats
- exotic animals and reptiles.

In the US, healthcare facilities are introducing the 'Eden alternative' where children, plants and animals are part of the daily care setting. The use of resident animals has not been scientifically evaluated and the following issues should be considered before starting similar projects:

- Will animals come into direct contact with patients?
- Will animals be allowed to roam freely in the facility?
- How will staff provide care for the animals?
- How will staff manage allergies, asthma and phobias?
- How will staff prevent bites and scratches?
- How will staff prevent soil and environmental contamination by enteric parasites (*Toxoplasma*, *Toxocara* and *Ancylostoma*)?

As a general preventive measure, resident animal programmes are advised to restrict animals from the following areas:

- food preparation kitchens
- laundries
- central sterile supply and storage areas for clean supplies
- medication preparation areas
- isolation and protective environments
- operating rooms
- patient eating areas.

The *Guidelines on the Control of Infection in Residential and Nursing Homes* (Public Health Medicine and Environment Group (PHMEG) 1996) offer the following points for keeping pets in healthcare settings:

- a member of staff should be designated as responsible for care
- handwashing should always follow handling
- the animal should have a clean feeding space, away from the kitchen or food preparation area, and its own dishes should be washed separately
- the animal should be checked regularly for signs of infection and taken to a vet promptly when unwell. It should have all the relevant inoculations and be wormed every 6 months
- the animal should not lick or jump-up at residents or staff
- claws should be trimmed regularly
- open containers of food, purchased from a commercial enterprise, should be stored separately from human food
- the animal should be allowed 20 min to eat its food, which should then be discarded
- the animal should be exercised before meeting residents
- bedding and the animal's coat (especially dogs and cats) should be cleaned regularly. Insecticides might be necessary for both the pet and its environment to prevent infestation with fleas
- litter boxes should be cleaned on a daily basis, by healthy staff who are not pregnant. They should wear protective clothing for the procedure. Washing litter trays with hot water and detergent every week will remove most germs.

Child daycare centres often keep pets such as terrapins, lizards and mice, all of which have been associated with the carriage of salmonella. Direct transmission to humans is thought possible (Gilbert & Roberts 1990). Staff should carefully supervise the handling of pets by children. Children's hands should be washed and dried thoroughly after handling.

Hygiene issues for homes with pets

Owners of pets need to be made aware of the potential infection hazards associated with their pets. There is evidence to show that the presence of pets in the home is associated with increased levels of contamination in the kitchen and bathroom (Scott 1981). Domestic cats, dogs and other types of pets, although apparently healthy, can act as carriers of enteric pathogens such as *Salmonella* and *Campylobacter*. Pets such as cats and dogs can also bring pathogens into the home on their paws and contaminate kitchen food preparation surfaces as well as floor surfaces. In addition to the hygiene measures described above, pet owners should be advised to:

- avoid cleaning pet cages and tanks in the kitchen sink
- avoid contact of pets with food preparation surfaces
- decontaminate pet feeding utensils using a hygienic cleaner or by application of a disinfectant
- make sure children always wash their hands after handling their pets, especially before eating
- make sure spills from pet faeces, urine and vomit are cleaned immediately and that any contaminated surfaces are cleaned and disinfected.

Pest control

Infestation remains a problem in many healthcare establishments, especially in old buildings. Infestation can occur in any part of a hospital building but is commonly found in boiler rooms, ducts, drains and kitchens where shelter, warmth, food and water are in abundance. The creatures infesting hospitals range from cockroaches and Pharaoh's ants to rodents (Edwards & Baker 1981). Cockroaches have been known to carry Gram-negative bacilli mechanically (Burgess et al 1973) and to be reservoirs of drug-resistant salmonella.

All hospitals are required to operate a pest control policy. The health service management document *Food Hygiene and Pest Control in the Health Service* (DoH 1986) recommends that all healthcare establishments 'must eradicate, so far as is reasonably possible, any risk of infestation by pests from their premises both in food handling areas and elsewhere'. Pest control policies generally follow the advice detailed in this circular.

REFERENCES

Advisory Committee on Dangerous Pathogens 1995 Protection against blood-borne infections in the workplace: HIV and hepatitis. HMSO, London

Alfa MJ, Sitter DL 1994 In-hospital evaluation of ortho-phthalaldehyde as a high level disinfectant for flexible endoscopes. Journal of Hospital Infection 26:15–26

Austin MW, Clark DI, Moreton CA 1992 Disinfection of tonometer prisms and examination contact lenses in ophthalmic departments (Letter). Eye 6:115–116

Ayliffe GAJ, Collins BJ, Lowbury EJL et al 1967 Ward floors and other surfaces as reservoirs of hospital infection. Journal of Hygiene (Cambridge) 65:85–93

Ayliffe GAJ, Collins BJ, Taylor LJ 1990 Hospital acquired infection. Principles and practice, 2nd edn. Butterworth, London

Ayliffe GAJ, Coates D, Hoffman PN 1993 Chemical disinfection in hospitals. PHLS, London

Babb J 1992 Action of disinfectants and antiseptics and their role in surgical practice. In: Taylor EW (ed) Infection in surgical practice. Oxford University Press, Oxford, UK

Babb JR 1996 Application of disinfectants in hospitals and other health care establishments. Infection Control Journal of South Africa 1(1):4–12

Babb JR, Bradley CR 1995 A review of glutaraldehyde alternatives. British Journal of Theatre Nursing 5(7):20–24

Babb JR, Bradley CR 2001 Choosing instrument disinfectants and processors. British Journal of Infection Control 2(2):10–13

Bassett DCJ, Thompson SAS, Page B 1965 Neonatal infections with *Pseudomonas aeruginosa* associated with contaminated resuscitation equipment. Lancet i:781

Beecham HJ, Cohen ML, Parkin WE 1979 *Salmonella typhimurium* transmission by fibreoptic upper intestinal gastrointestinal endoscopy. Journal of the American Medical Association 241:1013–1015

Bibby BA 1982 Mathematical modelling of patient risk. PhD Thesis: Aston University, Birmingham

Blenkharn JI, Hughes VM 1982 Suction apparatus and hospital infection due to multiply-resistant *Klebsiella aerogenes*. Journal of Hospital Infection 3:173–178

Breathnach AS, Jenkins DR, Pedler SJ 1992 Stethoscopes as a possible vector of infection by staphylococci. British Medical Journal 305:1573–1574

Brett J, Du Vivier A 1985 *Pseudomonas aeruginosa* and whirlpools. British Medical Journal 290:1024–1025

British Medical Association (BMA) 1989 Code of practice for sterilization of instruments and control of cross infection. BMA Publications, London

British Medical Association (BMA)/National Health Service Executive (NHSE) 1995 A code of practice for implementation of hepatitis B immunization guidelines for the protection of patients and staff. BMA/NHS Executive, London

British Medical Association (BMA) 1996 A guide to hepatitis C. BMA Publications, London

British Society of Gastroenterology 1998 Working party report: cleaning and disinfection of equipment for gastrointestinal endoscopy. Gut 42(4):585–593

British Thoracic Society 2000 Control and prevention of tuberculosis in the United Kingdom: code of practice 2000 of the Joint Tuberculosis Committee of the British Thoracic Society. Thorax 55:887–901

Broadley SJ, Furr JR, Jenkins PA, Russell AD 1993 Antimycobacterial activity of Virkon. Journal of Hospital Infection 23:189–197

Burgess NRH, McDermott SN, Whitting J 1973 Laboratory transmission of enterobacteriacae by oriental cockroach *Blatta orientalis*. Journal of Hygiene 71:9–14

Burnett IA, Weeks GR, Harris DM 1994 A hospital study of ice-making machines: their bacteriology, design, usage and upkeep. Journal of Hospital Infection 28:305–313

Cardo D, Culver DH, Ciesielski CA et al 1997 A case control study of HIV seroconversion in health care workers after percutaneous exposure. New England Journal of Medicine 337:1485–1490

Cartwright KAV, Stuart JM, Jones DM, Noah ND 1987 The Stonehouse survey: nasopharyngeal carriage of meningococci and *Neisseria lactamica.* Epidemiology and Infection 99:591–601

Castille K 1999 To reuse or not to reuse – that is the question. Nursing Standard 13(34):48–52

Cawthorne D, Raashed M, Synnott M et al 1997 Contact tracing in bovine TB. European Respiratory Journal 11:1388

Centers for Disease Control and Prevention (CDC) 2001 Draft guideline for environmental infection control in healthcare facilities. Recommendations of the Healthcare Infection Control Practices Committee (HICPAC)

Chadwick C, Oppenheim BA 1996 Cleaning as a cost effective method of infection control. Lancet 347(9017):1776

Chin J (ed) 2000 Control of communicable diseases control, 17th edn. American Public Health Association, Washington DC

Collins BJ 1988 The hospital environment: how clean should a hospital be? Journal of Hospital Infection 11(suppl A):53–56

Collins CH, Kennedy DA 1987 Microbiological hazards of occupational needlestick and 'sharps' injuries. Journal of Applied Bacteriology 62:385–402

Communicable Disease Report (CDR) 1995a Review. Control of meningococcal disease: guidance for consultants in communicable disease control. PHLS, London

Communicable Disease Report (CDR) 1995b Vancomycin resistant enterococci in hospitals in the United Kingdom. CDR 5(50):281

Communicable Disease Report (CDR) 1995c Review. The prevention of human transmission of gastrointestinal infections, infestations, and bacterial intoxications. PHLS, London

Coombs R, Silby H, Norman P 1994 Water birth and infection in babies. British Medical Journal 309:1098

Creamer E 1993 Decontamination quality: suction equipment. Journal of Infection Control Nursing/Nursing Times 89:65–68

Dart CR, Goddard SV, Cooke RPD 1995 Audit of decontamination procedures for specialist opthalmic equipment. Journal of Hospital Infection 29:297–300

Department of Health (DoH) 1986 Food hygiene and pest control in the health service (HC(86)31). DoH, London

Department of Health (DoH) 1987 Decontamination of healthcare equipment prior to inspection, service or repair (HN(87)22). DoH, London

Department of Health (DoH) 1990 Lancing devices for multi-patient capillary-blood sampling: avoidance of cross infection by correct selection and use (SAB(90)78). DoH, London

Department of Health (DoH) 1991a Hospital mattress assembly: care and cleaning (SAB(91)65). DoH, London

Department of Health (DoH) 1991b Safe working and prevention of infection in the mortuary and post-mortem room. HMSO, London

Department of Health (DoH) 1991c Mortuary and post-mortem room (Health Building Note 20). HMSO, London

Department of Health (DoH) 1992 Endoscope washer disinfectors: recontamination of equipment (SAB(92)1). DoH, London

Department of Health (DoH) 1993a Infections caused by *Xanthomonas maltiphilia* (Hazard(93)42). DoH, London

Department of Health (DoH) 1993b Endoscope washer disinfectors (SAB(93)32). DoH, London

Department of Health (DoH) 1994a Use and management of glutaraldehyde solution (SAB(94)21). DoH, London

Department of Health (DoH) 1994b Instruments and appliances used in the vagina and cervix: recommended methods for decontamination (SAB(94)22). DoH, London

Department of Health (DoH) 1995a Food handlers; fitness to work. Guidance for food businesses, enforcement officers and health professionals. HMSO, London

Department of Health (DoH) 1995b Food safety (general food hygiene) regulations. HMSO, London

Department of Health (DoH) 1996a Addendum to HSG (93) 40: protecting healthcare workers and patients from hepatitis B (EL(96)77). DoH, London

Department of Health (DoH) 1996b Guidelines for pre-test discussion on HIV testing (PL/CMO(96)1). HMSO, London

Department of Health (DoH) 1998 AIDS/HIV infected health care workers: guidance on the management of infected health care workers and patient notification. HMSO, London

Department of Health (DoH) 2000a The NHS plan. A plan for investment, a plan for reform. HMSO, London

Department of Health (DoH) 2000b HIV post-exposure prophylaxis: guidance from the UK Chief Medical Officers' Expert Advisory Group on AIDS. HMSO, London

Department of Health (DoH) 2000c Guidance on the management of the public health consequences of tuberculosis in cattle. HMSO, London

Department of Health/Public Health Laboratory Service Joint Working Group (DoH/PHLS) 1994a *Clostridium difficile* infection. Prevention and Management. Health Publication Unit, Heywood, Lancashire

Department of Health/Public Health Laboratory Service Joint Working Group (DoH/PHLS) 1994b *Clostridium difficile* infection. Prevention and Management. PHLS, London

Department of the Environment (DoE) 1990 Environment Protection Act (1990). Waste management – the duty of care: a code of practice. HMSO, London

De Voe IW 1982 The meningococcus and mechanisms of pathogenicity. Microbiology Review 46:162–190

Donaldson L, Moores Y, Howe J 1999 Introduction of immunization against group C meningococcal infection. DoH, London

Donowitz LG, Marsik FJ, Fisher KA, Wenzel RP 1981 Contaminated breast milk: a source of *Klebsiella* bacteraemia in a newborn intensive care unit. Review of Infectious Diseases 3:716–720

Edwards JP, Baker LF 1981 Distribution and importance of the Pharaoh's ants *Monomorium pharaoris* (L) in national health service hospitals in England. Journal of Hospital Infection 2:249–254

Ekanem EE, Dupont HL, Pickering LK, Selwyn BJ 1983 Transmission dynamics of enteric bacteria in day care centres. American Journal of Epidemiology 118:562–572

Fisher MC, LiPuma JJ, Dassen SE et al 1993 Source of *Pseudomonas cepacis*: ribotyping of isolation from patients and from the environment. Journal of Paediatrics 123:745–747

Fujita K, Lilly HA, Kidson A, Ayliffe GAJ 1981 Gentamycin resistant *Pseudomonas aeruginosa* infection from mattresses in a burns unit. British Medical Journal 283:219–220

Gilbert RJ, Roberts D 1990 Foodborne gastroenteritis. In: Parker MT, Collier LH (eds) Topley and Wilson's principles of bacteriology, virology and immunity. Edward Arnold, London

Glenwright HD, Martin MV 1993 Infection control in dentistry – a practitioner's guide. Occasional Paper, issue no. 2. British Dental Association, London

Golder M, Chan CL, O'Shea S et al 2000 Potential risk of cross-infection during peripheral-venous access by contamination of tourniquets. Lancet 355(9197):44

Gould FK, Freeman R 1993 Nosocomial infection with microsphere beds. Lancet 342:241–242

Griffiths PA, Babb JR, Fraise AP 1998 *Mycobacterium terrae*: a potential surrogate for *Mycobacterium tuberculosis* in a standard disinfection test. Journal of Hospital Infection 38:183–192

Griffiths PA, Babb JR, Fraise AP 1999 Mycobactericidal activity of selected disinfectants using a quantitative suspension test. Journal of Hospital Infection 41:111–121

Hale CM, Polder JA 1996 The ABCs of safe and healthy childcare. A handbook for childcare providers. US Public Health Service, CDC, Atlanta

Hambraeus A, Laurell G 1980 Protection of the patient in the operating suite. Journal of Hospital Infection 1:15–30

Healing TD, Hoffman PN, Young SEJ 1995 The infection hazards of human cadavers. Communicable Disease Report. CDR/PHLS, London

Health Building Notes 1990 26 Operating departments. HMSO, London

Health Service Advisory Committee (HSAC) 1974 Health and Safety at Work Act (1974). HMSO, London

Health Service Advisory Committee (HSAC) 1996 Safe working and prevention of infection in the mortuary and post-mortem. HMSO, London

Health and Safety Commission (HSC) 1992a The management of Health and Safety at Work Regulations (SI 2051). HMSO, London

Health and Safety Commission (HSC) 1992b The management of Health and Safety at Work Regulations (1992). Approved code of practice. HMSO, London

Health and Safety Commission (HSC) 1992c Workplace (Health, Safety and Welfare) Regulations (1992). Approved code of practice (L24). HMSO, London

Health and Safety Commission (HSC) 1999 The control of substances hazardous to health regulations (amendments). HMSO, London

Health and Safety Executive (HSE) 1995 Reporting of injuries, diseases and dangerous occurrences. HMSO, London

Health and Safety Executive (HSE) 2001 Legionnaire's disease: the control of legionella bacteria in water systems. Approved code of practice. HMSO, London

Health Service Circular (HSC) 1998 Guidance for clinical health care workers: protection against infection with blood-borne viruses (HSC 1998/063)

Health Service Circular (HSC) 2000 Hepatitis B infected health care workers (HSC 2000/020)

Heptonstall J, Gill ON, Porter K et al 1993 Health care workers and HIV: surveillance of occupationally acquired infection in the United Kingdom (CDR Review 3 (11)). PHLS, London

HM Prison Report 1993 The first report of the Director of Health care of Prisoners. HMSO, London

Hollyoak V, Allison D, Summers J 1995 *Pseudomonas aeruginosa* wound infection associated with a nursing home's whirlpool bath. CDR Review 5(7):R100–R105

Holton J, Ridgeway GL 1993 Commissioning operating theatres. Journal of Hospital Infection 23:153–160

Hughes-Walter T, Williams B, Pearson T 1986 The nosocomial colonization of T bear. Infection Control 7(10):495–500

Infection Control Nurses Association (ICNA) 1995 West Midlands Group. Infection control audit pack. Infection Control Nurses Association, West Midlands Branch, Birmingham

Insler MS, Gore H 1986 *Pseudomonas* keratitis and folliculitis from whirlpool exposure. American Journal of Ophthalmology 101:41–43

Ip HMH, Sin WK, Chali PY et al 1976 Neonatal infection due to *Salmonella worthington* by a delivery room suction apparatus. Journal of Hygiene 77:307–314

Irish C, Herbert J, Bennett D et al 1999 Database study of antibiotic resistant tuberculosis in the United Kingdom. British Medical Journal 318:497–498

Joint Tuberculosis Committee of the British Thoracic Society 2000 Control and prevention of tuberculosis in the United Kingdom: Code of Practice 2000. Thorax 55:887–901

Jones EM, Reeves DS 1997 Controlling chickenpox in hospitals. British Medical Journal 314:4–5

Katz VL, Kuller JA, McMahon MJ et al 1995 Varicella during pregnancy. Maternal and fetal effects. Western Journal of Medicine 163:446–450

Khan MA, Abdur-Rab M, Israr N et al 1991 Transmission of *Salmonella worthington* by oropharyngeal suction in hospital neonatal unit. Pediatric Infectious Diseases Journal 10:668–672

Kramer F, Sasse SA, Simms JC, Leedom JM 1994 Primary cutaneous tuberculosis after a needlestick injury from a patient with AIDS and undiagnosed tuberculosis. American Journal of Infection Control 22:374

Kumarsinghe G, Hamilton WJ, Gould JDM et al 1982 An outbreak of *Salmonella muenchen* infection in a specialist paediatric hospital. Journal of Hospital Infection 3:341–344

Larcombe J 1988 One good turn deserves another. Nursing Times 84(11):36–39

Lancet (Leading article) 1992 Nosocomial infection with respiratory syncytial virus. Lancet 340:1071–1072

Lettau LA 1991 Nosocomial transmission and infection control aspects of parasitic and ectoparasitic diseases. Part III Ectoparasites/summary and conclusions. Infection Control and Hospital Epidemiology 12(3):179–185

Lidwell OM, Lowbury EJL, Whyte W et al 1983 Airborne contamination of wounds in joint replacement operations: the relation to sepsis rates. Journal of Hospital Infection 4:111–131

Lidwell OM, Richards IDG, Polakoff S 1967 Comparison of three ventilating systems in an operating theatre. Journal of Hygiene 65:193–205

Loomes S 1988 Is it safe to lie down in hospital? Nursing Times 84(49):61–63

Loomes AS, Finch R 1990 Breeding grounds for bacteria (letter). Nursing Times 86(6):14–15

McCance DJ, Campion MJ, Barham A, Singer A 1986 Risk of transmission of human papilloma virus by vaginal specula. Lancet i:816–817

McCulloch J (ed) 2000 Infection control, science, management and practice. Whurr Publishers, London

Madge P, Paton JY, McColl JH, Mackie PLK 1992 Prospective controlled study of four infection control procedures to prevent nosocomial infection with respiratory syncytial virus. Lancet 340:1079–1083

Maunder JW 1992 Pharmacology update: the scourge of scabies. Chemist and Druggist 54–55

Maurer IM 1985 Hospital hygiene, 3rd edn. Edward Arnold, London

Medical Devices Agency (MDA) 1993 Sterilisation, disinfection and cleaning of medical equipment: guidance on decontamination from the Medical Advisory Committee to the Department of Health Medical Devices Directorate. MDA, London

Medical Devices Agency (MDA) 1995a Handpieces used in Phaco microsurgical procedures and their reusable accessories (Hazard notice MDA HN 9503). MDA, London

Medical Devices Agency (MDA) 1995b Decontamination of medical devices and equipment prior to investigation, inspection, service or repair (safety notice MDA SN 9516). DoH, London

Medical Devices Agency (MDA) 1995c Symbols on medical devices and their packaging (MDA DB 9505). MDA, London

Medical Devices Agency (MDA) 1996a Sterilisation, disinfection and cleaning of medical equipment: guidance on decontamination from the Microbiology Advisory Committee. Part 1: Principles; Part 2: Protocols. HMSO, DOH, London

Medical Devices Agency (MDA) 1996b 'In-house' manufactured spirit levels used in central venous pressure (CVP) monitoring (MDA HN 9609). MDA, London

Medical Devices Agency (MDA) 1996c Need for decontamination of blood gas analysers used in near-patient testing (Safety notice MDA SN 9612). MDA, London

Medical Devices Agency (MDA) 1996d Compatibility of medical devices and their accessories and reprocessing units with cleaning, disinfecting and sterilizing agents (Safety notice MDA SN 9619). MDA, London

Medical Devices Agency (MDA) 1999a Single patient use of ophthalmic medical devices: implications for clinical practice (MDA AN 1999 (04)). MDA, London

Medical Devices Agency (MDA) 1999b Foam mattresses: prevention of cross-infection (MDA SN 1999 (31)). MDA, London

Medical Devices Agency (MDA) 2000a Equipped to care: the safe use of medical devices in the 21st century, safeguarding public health. MDA, London

Medical Devices Agency (MDA) 2000b Single use medical devices; implications and complications of reuse (MDA DB 2000 (04)). MDA, London

Medical Research Council (MRC) 1962 Design and ventilation of operating room suites for control of infection and for comfort. Lancet ii:945–951

Miller E, Hopkinson WM 1986 Use of anti-varicella zoster immunoglobulin for the prevention of chickenpox in neonates and pregnant women. Communicable Disease Report 86(14):3–4

Miller E, Vurdien J, Farrington P 1993a Shift in age in chickenpox. Lancet 341:308–309

Miller E, Marshall R, Vurdien J 1993b Epidemiology, outcome and control of Varicella-zoster infection. Review of Medical Microbiology 4:222–230

Moore EP, Williams EWA 1991 Maternity hospital outbreak of methicillin resistant *Staphylococcus aureus.* Journal of Hospital Infection 19(1):5–15

National Health Service (NHS) Estates 1994 Ventilation in healthcare premises. (HTM 2025). DoH, London

National Health Service (NHS) Estates 1999 Controls assurance in infection control: decontamination of medical devices (HSC 1999/179). NHS Estates/DoH, London

National Health Service (NHS) Estates 2000 Standards for environmental cleanliness in hospitals. DoH, London

National Health Service (NHS) Estates 2001 Infection control in the built environment – design and planning. HMSO, London

National Health Service Executive (NHSE) 1994 Ventilation in healthcare premises (HTM 2025). DoH, London

National Health Service Executive (NHSE) 1995 Management policy on washer disinfectors 30/80 (HTM 2030). NHSE Estates, London

National Health Service Executive (NHSE) 1998 Guidance on the management of AIDS/HIV infected health care workers and patient notification (HSC 1998/228). NHSE, London

National Health Service Executive (NHSE) 2001a Controls assurance standard in infection control 1999 (Rev 02). HMSO, London. Available: http://tap.ccta.gov.uk/doh/rm5.nsf/b7546ce4a0608579002565c4003bf709/9bd9b4beb414923100256a5400615b0b?OpenDocument

National Health Service Executive (NHSE) 2001b Controls assurance standard – decontamination of single-use medical devises (Rev 02). HMSO, London. Available: http://tap.ccta.gov.uk/doh/rm5.nsf/b7546ce4a0608579002565c4003bf709/ed0073a14114f65200256a5400603d8b/$FILE/Decontamination.PDF

National Health Service Management Executive (NHSME) 1991 Decontamination of equipment, linen and other surfaces contaminated with hepatitis B and/or human immunodeficiency virus (HC(91)33). DoH, London

National Health Service Management Executive (NHSME) 1993a Protecting health care workers and patients from hepatitis B (HSG(93)40). DoH, London

National Health Service Management Executive (NHSME) 1993b Decontamination of equipment prior to inspection, service or repair (HSC(93)26). DoH, London

National Health Service Management Executive (NHSME) 1994 Occupational health services for NHS staff (HSG(94)51). DoH, London

Ndwala EM, Brown L 1991 Mattresses as a reservoir of epidemic methicillin resistant *Staphylococcus aureus*. Lancet 337:488

Newsome SWB 1968 Hospital infection from contaminated ice. Lancet 14:620–622

Noble WC (ed) 1993 The skin microflora and microbial skin disease. Cambridge University Press, Cambridge

O'Donoghue MAT, Allen KD 1992 Costs of an outbreak of wound infections in an orthopaedic ward. Journal of Hospital Infection 22:73–79

Parker L 1999a Managing and maintaining a safe environment in the hospital setting. British Journal of Nursing 8(16):1041–1116

Parker L 1999b Rituals versus risks in the contemporary theatre environment. British Journal of Theatre Nursing 9(8):341–345

Paryani S, Arvin A 1986 Intrauterine infection with varicella-zoster virus after maternal varicella. New England Journal of Medicine 314:1542–1546

Peto R, Calrow A 1996 An audit of mattresses in a teaching hospital. Professional Nurse 11(9):623–626

Public Health (Control of diseases) Act 1984

Public Health Laboratory Service (PHLS) 1994 Hygiene for spa pools. PHLS, London

Public Health Laboratory Service (PHLS) 1999 Hygiene for hydrotherapy pools, 2nd edn. PHLS, London

Public Health Medicine Environmental Group (PHMEG) 1996 Guidelines on the control of infection in residential and nursing homes. DoH, London

Puro V, Ippolito G, Guzzanti E 1992 Zidovudine prophylaxis after accidental exposure to HIV infection. AIDS 6:963–969

Rahman M 1980 Mycobacteria from suction apparatus (letter). Journal of Hospital Infection 1:85–86

Ramsey ME, Andrews N, Kaczmarski EB, Miller E 2001 Efficacy of meningococcal serogroup C conjugated vaccine in teenagers and toddlers in England. Lancet 357:195–197

Ratnam S, Hogan K, March SB, Butler RW 1986 Whirlpool associated folliculitis caused by *Pseudomonas aeruginosa*: report of an outbreak and review. Journal of Clinical Microbiology 23:655–659

Rawal J, Shah A, Stirk F, Mehtar S 1994 Water birth and infection in babies. British Medical Journal 309:1098

Rice P, Simmons K, Carr R, Banatvala J 1994 Near fatal chickenpox during prednisolone treatment. British Journal of Medicine 309:1069–1070

Ridgeway GL, Tedder RS 1996 Birthing pools and infection control. Lancet 347:1051–1052

Ringham S 1989 A whirlpool of bacteria. Nursing Times 85:77–80

Rogers KB 1963 Epidemiology of hospital coliform enteritis. In: Williams REO, Shootes R (eds) Infection in hospitals: epidemiology and control. Blackwell, Oxford

Rose HD, Franson TR, Sheth NK et al 1983 Pseudomonas pneumonia associated with the use of home whirlpool spa. Journal of the American Medical Association 250:2027–2029

Rubbo SD, Gardner JF, Frankin JC 1966 Source of Pseudomonas aeruginosa infection in premature infants. Journal of Hygiene 64:121–128

Rutala WA 1990 APIC guidelines for selection and use of disinfectants. American Journal of Infection Control 18:99–117

Salmen P, Dwyer DM, Vose H, Kamse W 1983 Whirlpool associated Pseudomonas aeruginosa urinary tract infection. Journal of the American Medical Association 250:2025–2026

Sanderson PJ, Alshafi KM 1995 Environmental contamination by organisms causing urinary-tract infection. Journal of Hospital Infection 29:301–303

Sanderson PJ, Rawal P 1987 Contamination of the environment of spinal cord injured patients by organisms causing urinary-tract infection. Journal of Hospital Infection 10:173–178

Sanderson PJ, Weissler S 1992 Recovery of coliforms from hands of nurses and patients: activities leading to contamination. Journal of Hospital Infection 21:85–93

Schlech WF, Simonson N, Sumarah R, Martin RS 1986 Nosocomial outbreak of Pseudomonas aeruginosa folliculitis associated with a physiotherapy pool. Canadian Medical Association Journal 134:909–913

Schuman SH 1983 Day care associated infections: more than meets the eye. Journal of the American Medical Association 249:76

Scott E 1981 Bacteriological contamination in the domestic environment and its control. MPhil Thesis, University of London

Scottish Centre for Infection and Environmental Health (SCIEH) 1994 Guidelines for bacteriological clearance following gastroenteritic infection. Communicable Disease (Scotland) Weekly Report (Edinburgh) 28(26):8–13

Selkon J, Babb JR, Morris R 1999 Evaluation of the antimicrobial activity of a new super-oxidised water, Sterilox®, for the disinfection of endoscopes. Journal of Hospital Infection 41:59–70

Shetty N, Srinivasan S, Holton J, Ridgway GL 1999 Evaluation of microbicidal activity of a new disinfectant: Sterilox 2500, against Clostridium difficile spores, Helicobacter pylori, vancomycin-resistant Enterococcus species, Candida albicans and several Mycobacterium species. Journal of Hospital Infection 41:101

Skegg DCG, Paul C 1986 Viruses, specula, and cervical cancer. Lancet i:747

Spaulding EH 1968 Chemical disinfection of medical and surgical materials. In: Lawrence CA, Block SS (eds) Disinfection, sterilization and preservation. Lea & Febiger, Philadelphia

Stiver HG, Clarke J, Kennedy J, Cohen M 1979 Pseudomonas sternotomy wound infection and sternal osteomyelitis complication after open heart surgery. Journal of the American Medical Association 241:1034–1036

Swaffield L 1983 Clean babies. Nursing Times Community Outlook 79(51):369–371

Taylor GP, Lyall EGH, Mercey D et al 1999 British HIV Association guidelines for prescribing antiretroviral therapy in pregnancy. Sex Transmission Infection 75:90–97

Threlkeld AB, Froggatt JW 3rd, Schein OD, Forman MS 1993 Efficacy of disinfectant wipe method for the removal of adenovirus 8 from tonometer tips. Ophthalmology 12(100):1841–1845

Thomas MC, Giedinghagen DH, Hoff GL 1987 Brief report: an outbreak of scabies among employees in hospital-associated commercial laundry. Infection Control 8:427–429

Tyler R, Ayliffe GAJ, Bradley C 1990 Virucidal activity of disinfectants: studies with the poliovirus. Journal of Hospital Infection 15:339–345

Walsh M, Foord P 1993 Nursing ritual research and rational action. Butterworth-Heinemann, Oxford

Weernick A, Severin WP, Tjernberg I, Dijkshoorn L 1995 Pillows, an unexpected source of *Acinetobacter*. Journal of Hospital Infection 29(3):189–199

Weniger BA, Futtenbur AJ, Goodman RA et al 1983 Faecal coliforms on environmental surfaces in two day care centres. Applied Environmental Microbiology 45:733–735

Working Party Report 1998 Revised guidelines for control of epidemic methicillin resistant *Staphylococcus aureus*. Journal of Hospital Infection 39:253–290

World Health Organization (WHO) 1998 Tuberculosis and air travel: guidelines for prevention and control (Report WHO/TB/98, 256). WHO, Geneva

Wormold PJ 1970 The effect of a changed environment on bacterial colonization rates in an established burns unit. Journal of Hygiene 68:633–645

Wright IMR, Orr H, Porter C 1995 Stethoscope contamination in neonatal intensive care unit. Journal of Hospital Infection 29:65–68

Zimakoff J, Hoiby N, Rosendal K, Guilbert JP 1983 Epidemiology of *Pseudomonas aeruginosa*: infection and the role of contamination of the environment in a cystic fibrosis clinic. Hospital Journal of Infection 4:31–40

Zimmerman R, Huch A, Huch R 1993 Water birth – is it safe? Journal of Perinatal Medicine 21:5–11

Portals of exit

■ CONTENTS

SUMMARY

This chapter considers the safe management of microbes once they have left their reservoir.

INTRODUCTION

Recent published guidelines in the UK for Infection Control (DoH 2001) included standard principles for the use of personal protective equipment. The recommendations are based upon current available evidence and are applicable to all healthcare practitioners. They cover the use of aprons, gowns, gloves, eye protection and face masks and also indicate where the wearing of such equipment is indicated under current Health and Safety requirements (HSE 1992).

The primary use of personal protective equipment is to protect staff and to reduce the possibility of transmission of microorganisms. There has been an attempt, since the 1980s, to eliminate the unnecessary wearing of protective clothing in general care settings where evidence does not support its effectiveness against hospital-acquired infections.

The general consensus is that the wearing of protective clothing must be based on the level of risk of transmission of microorganisms associated

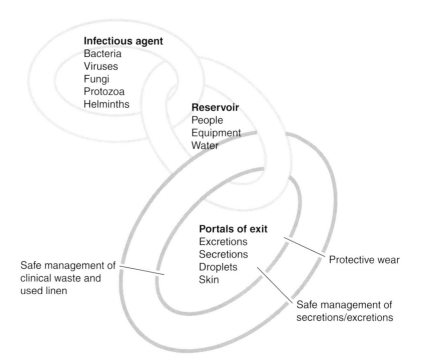

Figure 8.1 Breaking the chain of infection: portals of exit.

with a specific care activity. This is either to protect the patient from organisms by staff, or to protect staff from the risk of contamination from a patient's blood, body fluids, secretions or excretions (Fig. 8.1).

PROTECTIVE WEAR

Gloves

Most organizations advocate the use of gloves to protect health professionals from microbiological hazards when handling body excretions and secretions. The gloves also prevent the transfer of organisms already present on the hands of staff to vulnerable patients.

Gloves should not be worn unnecessarily because prolonged and indiscriminate use can cause adverse reactions and skin sensitivity (Burke et al 1995, Medical Devices Agency (MDA) 1996, 1998, Yassin et al 1994). Gloves should be removed after each care activity to prevent cross-infection to other sites of the body on a patient and between patients. Washing gloves rather than changing them is not a safe practice (Centers for Disease Control (CDC) 1988).

Because of the problem of glove leakage, standards have been revised for the manufacture of single-use gloves (British Standards Institution (BSI) 1994a,b,c). The integrity of gloves is not perfect and a number of studies have shown that gloves do leak (De-Groot Kosolchar & Jones et al 1989, Korniewicz et al 1990, Richmond et al 1992). Hands can also be contaminated on removing gloves, so handwashing is still an essential requirement because, although gloves reduce the risk of contamination, they cannot eliminate it completely. Hands are not necessarily clean because gloves have been worn.

Plastic or polythene gloves (ethylene co-polymer)

Once used commonly, plastic gloves have heat-sealed seams that predispose them to splitting. Up to 85% of plastic gloves were found to be permeable within the first 10 min of use (Gerhardt 1989). Personal and protective equipment (PPE) regulations at work (HSE 1992) state that personal and protective equipment is not suitable if it does not fit the wearer correctly. Plastic gloves are often ill-fitting and, as such, fall into this category. Smock & Shiel (1990), the British Medical Association (1989) and the Infection Control Nurses Association (1999) all suggest that plastic gloves have no place in clinical application.

Vinyl or PVC gloves

Gerhardt (1989) found vinyl gloves to be as permeable as plastic gloves. However, leakage rates from 4 to 63% have been reported in some studies (De-Groot Kosolchar & Jones 1989, Korniewicz et al 1990). Fogg (1989) suggests that vinyl gloves can be used for activities requiring general cleanliness or for brief, superficial contact with potentially infectious materials that would not stress the glove.

It has been suggested that vinyl gloves produce toxic substances and hydrochloric acid when incinerated, and that, for this reason, they should not be used. However, vinyl gloves have a place in clinical practice and should be used on the basis of risk management.

Glove sensitivity reactions have also been documented to vinyl (Burke et al 1995).

Nitrile (acrylonitrile)

These are now the gloves of choice when a latex-free environment is needed. They provide a biological barrier to organisms and are effective for handling glutaraldehyde. They contain the same chemicals as latex and release cyanide when incinerated (Brehler 1996).

Latex gloves (natural latex rubber)

Natural latex rubber remains the material of choice because it allows the wearer to maintain dexterity. Latex gloves are not prone to splitting and are generally recommended for tasks requiring handling of blood and body fluids, as stated in current standard precautions. A leakage rate of between 3 and 52% has been reported with latex gloves (De-Groot Kosolchar & Jones 1989, Korniewicz et al 1989).

There are increasing reports of latex allergy (MDA 1996) and staff members complaining of allergy should consult their occupational health department.

There is now a considerable body of evidence that the use of cornstarch powder to assist in applying gloves is harmful. It is associated with adhesions, latex allergy and an increased risk of infection associated with invasive devices contaminated with the cornstarch (Haglund & Junghams 1997). As such, powdered gloves are no longer recommended for use in healthcare settings (ICNA 1999).

Gloves and the operating room

Gloves are worn to prevent skin bacteria from the operator's hands entering the wound, and to protect the operator from contamination by blood and exudate from the patient. Damage, in the form of minute holes, to gloves during surgery is well known. This can place both the patient and surgeon at risk of acquiring infection. In theatre, double-gloving has been recommended as a means to reduce hand injury during surgical procedures (Korniewicz et al 1994). This risk of glove perforation during surgery makes it important that fresh gloves are applied for each new procedure. The use of a coloured underglove makes it easier to detect when fluids enter the space between the outer and inner glove. It permits instant detection of the perforation and gives healthcare workers a chance to change their gloves (Parker 2000). A recent study in Denmark recommended that double gloves should be used for all types of gastrointestinal surgery, including laproscopic surgery (Lars et al 2000). It is already a recommended practice for orthopaedic surgery (Cole & Gault 1989, Eckersley & Williams 1990).

Reusing disposable gloves

Washing of gloved hands between procedures and reusing disposable gloves is hazardous, so is the practice of decontaminating the hands with alcohol handrubs. Adams et al (1992) showed that microorganisms were not always removed from gloves despite mechanical friction using handwashing agents. Micropunctures were also detected in a percentage of all types of used gloves tested.

Microbial contamination of hands through gloves and possible transmission of infection has been reported by Doebbeling et al (1988) and Olsen et al (1993).

The wearing of gloves does not remove the need for thorough handwashing on removing the gloves.

Masks

The use of masks to reduce postoperative wound infection remains controversial (Berger et al 1993, Mitchell & Hunt 1991, Orr 1981, Orr & Bailey 1992, Tunevall 1991, Tunevall & Jorbeck 1992). Face masks were introduced into operating rooms on the premise that bacteria in the form of droplet nuclei from the nose and mouth of surgical staff contributed to postoperative wound infections (Romney 2001). However, only a few organisms are dispersed when speaking (Duguid 1946), and these can be removed with forced ventilation. Prosthetic orthopaedic operations are more susceptible to organisms of low pathogenicity, and the inoculum required to initiate infection is low because of the presence of a foreign body. Masks are recommended here because these organisms are frequently found in the mouth (Whyte 1988). Masks for general surgery are considered unnecessary

(Orr 1981, Orr & Bailey 1992) but, if worn, should be changed after each operation. Careful manipulation of masks is essential to prevent contamination of hands.

Nowadays, masks are taking on a greater role of protecting the wearer from blood and body fluid splashes from patients during surgery (Romney 2001). Revised guidelines for tuberculosis by the British Thoracic Society (Ormerod 2000) recommend that staff attending to patients suspected of or diagnosed with multidrug-resistant tuberculosis should use dust mist-fume masks that meet the 1992 Personal Protective Equipment (EC Directive) Regulations (DoH 1998a, HSE 1992).

Eye protection

Eye protection must be readily available in any clinical area where procedures likely to produce splashing to the eyes are performed. A variety of goggles, masks with visors and headgear with visors are available. Current guidelines found that protective eyewear offered protection against the physical splashing of infected substances into the eyes. It is recommended that eye protection, along with face masks, should be worn where there is a risk of blood, body fluids, secretions/excretions splashing into the face and eyes (DoH 2001).

Aprons and gowns

The systematic review undertaken by the DoH when producing the guidelines for standard principles on infection control showed no supporting evidence for the routine use of gowns in general or specialist clinical settings (DoH 2001). However, the guidelines recommend that all healthcare workers wear protective clothing when contamination with blood, body fluids, secretions and excretions (excluding sweat) is anticipated. Their use is also recommended when there is to be close contact with a patient, materials, or equipment resulting in contamination of clothing with microorganisms (DoH 1998b, Ward et al 1997). Plastic aprons are recommended for general use and full body gowns should only be worn when there is a risk of extensive splashing of blood, body fluids, secretions or excretions; these gowns should be fluid repellent (DoH 1998b).

Plastic aprons should be considered a single-use item for one procedure or episode of patient care, and then discarded and disposed of as clinical waste.

Operating room clothing

There is a constant shedding of microorganisms from exposed skin and from mucous membranes. Use of barrier clothing in operating rooms is needed to minimize the contamination of the air as well as of the wound.

Shedding from skin is increased by friction from clothes during activity. Dispersal of bacteria-carrying particles amongst theatre personnel can be profuse, especially from the perineal area. Clothing made of ordinary cotton fabric is ineffective in preventing airborne bacterial dispersal from the skin of the operating team (Duguid & Wallace 1948). Non-woven fabric is more effective. Total body exhaust suits are recommended for the scrub team during elective joint replacement surgery (Charnley 1979). It is recommended that, because microorganisms can penetrate cotton surgical gowns, with penetration increasing when the gown is wet, gowns should be chosen according to the task and the expected degree of exposure to blood (Belkin 1994).

Headwear

Human hair is known to be a potential carrier of *Staphylococcus aureus*, especially where skin or scalp disease, such as eczema and psoriasis, are present. Keeping the hair clean and tidy should be a prerequisite for all operating room personnel. The helmet total exhaust system is well known for elective joint replacement surgery but traditional headgear is considered necessary only for the 'scrub' team. Effective ventilation is thought to counteract any bacterial shedding, and wearing of traditional headgear by non-scrub staff is considered unnecessary (Humphreys et al 1991a).

Footwear

The constant movement of staff and equipment, including beds, is likely to contribute to contamination of the operating room floor. A correlation between the organisms on the floor and wound infection has not been established. Operating-theatre-restricted footwear remains an important part of operating room protocol and is generally worn for its antistatic and antislip properties, rather than as an infection control measure. Regular cleaning of footwear is desirable to remove splashes of blood and body fluid occurring during surgery.

Overshoes are often worn to cover outdoor footwear when entering an operating room or to cover theatre footwear when leaving the operating suite. The value of these overshoes in reducing the incidence of wound infections has not been established and Humphreys et al (1991b) found no significant increase in the operating room floor colony counts when overshoes were not worn. Apart from the expense (£3 680 000 was spent on overshoes in 1988), there is evidence that contamination of hands occurs when overshoes are put on or removed (Carter 1990). Plastic overshoes also tend to tear (Jones & Jakeways 1988), which defeats the purpose for which they are worn.

With the increase in day surgery units, the use of overshoes for patients could increase. Weightman & Banfield (1994) suggest designated footwear instead of overshoes for patients and visitors.

SAFE MANAGEMENT OF EXCRETIONS AND SECRETIONS

Disposal of urine, faeces and other body fluids

The main outlet for urine and faeces is a machine that sluices, washes and disinfects the urinal or the pan. The machine is connected to the sewage discharge system of the building. Alternatively, a disposable container, either a urinal or a bedpan shell, is disposed of into a macerating machine that converts the container and its content into a pulp, which is subsequently discharged as above.

The washer–disinfector should maintain a minimum of 80°C for a 3-min contact time or 83°C for 1 min to ensure a safe container (Central Sterilising Club (CSC) 1986).

Macerators have been associated with aerosol contamination of the surrounding area and should be checked. In fact, much of the machinery within healthcare settings is governed by a code of planned maintenance, which the Estates department has a responsibility to fulfil.

Bedpan washers and macerators

Both systems are designed to receive human waste and toilet tissue. Each system has its own followers. The choice is often influenced by user preference and the ease with which the machine can be serviced and maintained. It is difficult to quantify the cost of running or maintaining either machine.

With regard to safe practice, macerators dispose of both receptacle and its contents and, providing the door seal remains intact, will pose few contamination problems. Any contamination will be the result of unwashed hands after handling the bedpan, urinal and vomit bowl or sputum container.

The thermal disinfection in washer–disinfectors is sufficient to destroy the pathogens in human waste. There are reports, however, of residual soil still left on bedpans that have been through the wash/disinfection cycle and hence fail the British Standards Institute's soil test ('Washer disinfectors for medical purposes BS 2745: Part 2') (NHSE 1995a). It is possible that the pathogens within the organic matter in the residual soil are protected from disinfection. Suggestions for effective cleaning of bedpan shells and support frames are given in Box 8.1.

Whatever the system, it is vital that staff do not discard inappropriate waste in these machines because they easily become blocked and an engineer then has the unpleasant task of cleaning out and unblocking the drains.

Suction apparatus

Tracheal suctioning is carried out when patients are unable to clear their own airway. The equipment used can become a reservoir for microorganisms (McCulloch 2000). It is recommended that suction containers are changed daily (Creamer & Smyth 1996) but disposable liners are now available in a variety of sizes, depending upon usage, and can be changed when full. Suction equipment and tubing should be changed when they are no longer required by the patient or when the patient is discharged (CDC 1997).

There are occasions when it is necessary to release the content of a suction bottle into the sluice. Extreme care is needed during this procedure and, because there is a risk of splashes to the face and eyes, eye protection must be available. Any contamination of the face and eyes must be rinsed off using copious amounts of water and the incident reported and recorded.

■ **BOX 8.1   Cleaning bedpan shells and support frames**

The cleaning of support frames or bedpan shells is often neglected because there is no visible contamination of the pan. Microorganisms associated with outbreaks have been cultured from such frames. These frames should be washed and stored dry after each use, especially if the same support frame is to be shared. Disinfection might be required in cases of diarrhoeal disease or an outbreak of gastrointestinal infections. Disinfection is also required if frames have been used by patients with pressure ulcers and so have been colonized and/or infected. Ideally, such circumstances demand dedicated support frames and commodes.

The practice of discharging faecal material into the sluice prior to placing the bedpan into the machine is unsafe and should be discouraged. Constant breakdowns or blockages of machinery are frequently quoted reasons. This would indicate a lack of understanding of appropriate use on the part of the staff and a reluctance on the part of the engineer to respond to constant requests from the clinical staff. This problem can be eradicated if:

• only the faecal matter and minimal toilet paper are discharged in the machine
• the machine is not overloaded.

Manufacturers often offer to educate users in the appropriate use of their product; it is a good idea to take advantage of this training.

SAFE MANAGEMENT OF CLINICAL WASTE

Any waste generated in healthcare settings is classed as clinical waste. The Health Service Advisory Committee document 'Safe disposal of clinical waste' (HSAC 1992) details the advice to be incorporated into local waste management policies. The document incorporates current health and safety legislation, the Health and Safety at Work Act (Health Service Advisory Committee (HSAC) 1974), the management regulations and workplace regulations (HSC 1992a,b), HTM 2065 Healthcare Waste Management Segregation (NHSE 1998), the Environmental Protection Act 1990 (DoE 1990), the Radioactive Substances Act (NHSME 1960), and the Control of Substances Hazardous to Health (COSHH) (amendment) Act 1999 (HSE 1999). The COSHH regulations identify the duties of employers regarding hazardous substances at work to which employees and others may be exposed: clinical waste falls within the scope of these regulations. The COSHH assessment becomes an integral part of the local waste disposal policy in terms of risk identification and management.

A policy for the management of clinical waste

The following items have been suggested for an effective policy on the management of clinical waste (HSAC 1992):

• identification of the categories of clinical waste
• specification of the containers/enclosures to be used

- storage
- transport
- handling before disposal
- training needs (for staff at all levels)
- personal protection
- accidents and incidents (reporting, investigation and follow-up)
- spillages
- final disposal.

Those in the process of developing a local policy are referred to the guidance documents. The discussion here is limited to those issues that form part of the teaching requirement for the infection control nurse (ICN).

Categories of clinical waste

Clinical waste is categorized according to the level of risk to staff. There are five categories of waste, each requiring its own control measures. The categories listed here are as stated in the HSAC (1992) guidance:

- *Group A*: all human tissue, including blood (whether infected or not); animal carcasses and tissue from veterinary centres, hospitals or laboratories as well as all related swabs and dressings; waste materials, where assessment indicates a risk to staff handling them (e.g. from infectious disease cases); soiled surgical dressings, swabs and other soiled waste from treatment areas.
- *Group B*: discarded syringe needles, cartridges, broken glass and any other contaminated disposable sharp instruments or items.
- *Group C*: microbiological cultures and potentially infected waste from pathology departments (laboratory and post-mortem rooms) and from other clinical and research laboratories.
- *Group D*: certain pharmaceutical products and chemical wastes.
- *Group E*: items used to dispose of urine, faeces and other body secretions or excretions assessed as not falling within Group A. This includes used disposable bedpans or bedpan liners, incontinence pads, stoma bags or urine containers.

The guidance suggests that the level of risk of Group E items might be difficult to assess, but that they could be offensive and should, therefore, be treated as clinical waste.

All staff members handle clinical waste, although levels of risks will vary according to the category of waste. They require instruction and training about identifying specific categories of clinical waste.

Methods of disposal

Incineration

The guidance recommends incineration as the preferred method of disposal for *all* clinical waste. If this is not practical, the waste in Groups A and B *must* be incinerated. The incineration can be carried out on site or in a licensed and authorized incinerator.

Disinfection

Although the current guidance states that all wastes in Groups A and B must be incinerated, provided there is full compliance with environmental waste disposal requirements and the relevant health and safety guidelines are met, other technologies can be used to treat elements of Group A and B waste. These alternatives to incineration are designed to reduce the risk of infection in handling and transport (Scottish Centre for Infection and Environmental Health (SCIEH) 1994) and to make the waste non-hazardous for disposal by landfill or municipal incinerators. Many of these alternatives have been tried outside the UK and are included here for your information. The intention of these methods is to achieve disinfection of the item and, as such, they are suitable only for certain types of clinical waste.

Microwaving, autoclaving and other heat treatment systems are already in use in the US, Germany and France. Certain microwave systems are not suitable for treating human tissue or cytotoxic drugs because they include a maceration process.

Other methods of disinfection include pyrolysis (prolonged subjection of waste to intense heat in the absence of oxygen, thus bringing about its chemical disintegration), gas sterilization, exposure to radioactivity, disposal by plasma treatment and chemical sterilization using formaldehyde or ethylene oxide.

Landfill

Landfill is an option for the wastes from the remaining groups (C, D and E). The suitability of the waste for landfill will depend on the level of risk and its offensive nature. The landfill sites have to be licensed to accept clinical waste.

Disposal into the sewer

Small amounts of body fluids or tissue and wastes listed in Group E can be macerated and then discharged into the sewer. This requires approval from the sewerage undertaker or sewerage authority. Advice on whether these items can be discharged into sewers can be sought from the Waste Disposal Authority or (in Scotland) the River Purification Board.

Segregation of waste

All wastes, regardless of the method of disposal, should be segregated into colour-coded containers. The colour coding system in Table 8.1 is strongly recommended by the HSAC (1992).

The supply of appropriate containers and sacks is the responsibility of the Supplies department, with advice from and consultation with the local infection control personnel and Estates department.

The labelling of the containers or sacks is a matter for local discussion. Some establishments prefer labelling so that the source can be identified in case of spillage or injury from an item protruding from the sack.

Staff members at all levels should receive instructions on identification, segregation and personal protection (Box 8.2). The importance of thorough

Table 8.1 Colour-coded system for segregation of waste

Colour of bag/container	Type of waste
Yellow	Clinical waste for incineration only
Yellow with black stripes	Clinical waste which is suitable for landfill disposal
Light blue or transparent with light blue lettering	Waste for autoclaving or equivalent treatment before ultimate disposal
Black	Normal household waste

■ **BOX 8.2   Safety points when handling waste and linen**

* Use the appropriate colour-coded bag
* Do not fill bags more than two-thirds full
* Check whether labelling of bags is indicated
* Fasten the bag securely to prevent spillage
* Prevent contamination of staff or other items of linen by using a water-soluble bag as a liner if seepage (e.g. of body fluids or blood) is likely.

---

handwashing and drying after contact with waste, whatever the category, should be emphasized.

Community disposal

The clinical waste generated in general practitioner (GP) and dental surgeries, health centres and nursing homes is subject to the same regulations as in hospitals. The waste from patients' own homes remains a subject of ongoing dialogue. Many local authorities arrange a separate collection for clinical/infected waste if prior arrangements are made. Yellow bags with black stripes are recommended for this method of disposal. This waste can be sent for incineration or landfill at designated, approved and licensed sites.

Although no formal approval exists, some local authorities allow clinical waste arising from home treatment to be disposed of with household waste. Wrapping the waste either in newspaper or plastic bags should be considered.

MANAGEMENT OF SPILLAGES

Accidental spillage of materials can be a serious hazard to health, according to the circumstances and the nature of the substances involved. Spillages can be chemical or biological; only biological spillages are considered here. All biological specimens/body fluids should be considered potentially infectious. The main aim should be to contain, neutralize and dispose of the material safely.

Sodium hypochlorite should be used to neutralize spillages. This agent is rapidly effective against a wide range of microorganisms, including blood-borne viruses, mycobacteria and bacterial spores. It should be used at a high concentration – 1% or 10 000 p.p.m. of available chlorine – although it can be used at a lower concentration (100–1000 p.p.m. of available chlorine) if the spill is removed and the surface cleaned first.

Sodium hypochlorite is corrosive to metal surfaces and can damage rubber and other materials. It is inactivated by organic material and so needs to be used at high concentrations.

CAUTION: diluting sodium hypochlorite with hot water, or mixing it with urine, could result in a rapid release of chlorine that can irritate the eyes and respiratory mucosa.

Clear soluble phenolics can be used instead of sodium hypochlorite. Many phenolics contain a detergent base that allows them to clean as well as disinfect. When used in concentrations of 0.6–2% they are highly effective against mycobacteria and non-sporing bacteria, but poor against viruses. Phenolics are irritants, taint food and damage plastic surfaces. They are not generally recommended for blood spills (Babb 1996).

Peroxygen, quaternary ammonia compounds and iodophores should be used where chlorine-releasing agents are not practical. They are good cleaning agents and are more user and environmentally friendly than sodium hypochlorite or clear soluble phenolics. However, their activity against mycobacteria, spores and non-enveloped viruses is less good (Babb 1996).

Staff members dealing with spillages should consult their organization's own local policies and procedures and/or seek advice from their infection control personnel.

Inexperienced staff and staff with fresh or open cuts or active dermatitis of the hands and arms should be discouraged from clearing up biological spillages. Box 8.3 describes one method of dealing with spills.

One of the COSHH regulations requires the completion of an environmental spillage form (Box 8.4).

■ BOX 8.3 Dealing with spillages

- If practical, close off the immediate area to avoid others becoming involved or contaminated by the spillage
- If sodium hypochlorite is to be used in a confined area, ensure good ventilation
- Put on a plastic apron, gloves, face protection (if required) and overshoes if the spillage is large
- Solutions used to neutralize the spillage will depend on the nature of the substance and local advice should be sought
- Limit the spread of fluid using absorbent disposable towelling or newspapers. Discard the towels into yellow plastic bags for incineration
- Take care to avoid injury if broken glass is present
- Dispose of sharp items into a sharps container
- After the necessary disinfectant contact period, collect the absorbed spillage and discard into a yellow plastic bag or sharps box (if there is sharp debris)
- Remove and discard disposable protective clothing, together with any other contaminated non-sharp disposable materials. Wash and dry hands.

■ **BOX 8.4 Information required on an environmental spillage form**

- Date of incident
- Time
- Location
- Specific area
- Names of persons involved
- State whether persons were contaminated
- State whether medical advice was sought
- Name of person carrying out the cleaning procedure
- Substance spilled (if known)
- Reason for spillage
- Action taken
- Signature and date.

MANAGEMENT OF USED LINEN

Used linen can be processed on site or in a commercial laundry. Local laundering facilities are often encountered in many community elderly care units and some specialist wards, usually for patients' own clothes. The soiling of clothing is as, if not more, likely in these establishments as in a hospital ward and staff need to remain vigilant to adequate processing of clothes and to their own protection when handling contaminated clothes (see Box 8.1).

The guidance set out in HSG (95) 18 (NHSE 1995b), in the Scottish document NHS MEL (1993) 7 (SCIEH 1993) *Hospital Laundry Arrangements for Used and Infected Linen* and in health circular HC (91) 33 *Decontamination of Equipment, Linen and Other Surfaces Contaminated with Hepatitis B and/or Human Immunodeficiency Virus* (DoH 1991) should form a basis for a laundry policy for all areas. The organization or establishment's Estates department should ensure that locally purchased washing machines have the programming ability to meet the disinfection standards set out in HSG (95) 18 (NHSE 1995b).

Categories of used linen

- *Used (soiled and fouled)*: this category includes all used linen, irrespective of state, on occasion it might be contaminated by body fluid or blood.

- *Infected*: this is linen from patients with or suspected of suffering from enteric fever and other salmonella infections; dysentery (*Shigella* spp.); hepatitis A, hepatitis B and hepatitis C (and carriers); open pulmonary tuberculosis; HIV infection; notifiable diseases and other infections in Hazard Group 3 of the COSHH 1999 *Approved List of Biological Agents*. Hazard Group 3 refers to 'an organism that may cause severe human disease and presents a serious hazard to laboratory workers. It may present a risk of spread to the community but there is usually effective prophylaxis or treatment available' (Advisory Committee on Dangerous Pathogens (ACDP) 1995).

• *Heat-labile*: fabrics likely to be damaged by both the normal heat disinfection process and the high temperature are included in this category. These need to be washed at low temperature (40°C). Chemicals such as sodium hypochlorite (150 p.p.m. available chlorine) can be added to the penultimate rinse provided no soiling, detergents or alkali are present and where there is no likelihood of the chemical damaging the fabric.

Transport of used linen

• *Used (soiled and fouled) linen*: this is placed into a polythene or nylon/polyester bag, which is usually white. Use of a water-soluble bag as a liner is recommended if seepage of body fluids or blood is likely.

• *Infected linen*: this is placed immediately, without sorting, into a water-soluble bag or bag with a water-soluble stitched seam of membrane. The sealed bag is then placed into a colour-coded, usually red, nylon or polyester bag.

• *Heat-labile linen*: this is placed in a locally agreed colour-coded bag.

Disinfection of used linen

• *Used (soiled and fouled) linen*: This receives two wash cycles: a sluice wash is followed by a second thermal disinfection cycle in which the load temperature, i.e. the temperature of the wash water in contact with the load, is maintained at 65°C for 10 min or at 71°C for 3 min.

• *Infected linen*: According to HSG (95) 18 (NHSE 1995b), all infected linen receives the same disinfection process as used linen. The Scottish guidance for hepatitis and acquired immunodeficiency syndrome (AIDS) viruses recommends a washing temperature of 93°C for not less than 10 min (SCIEH 1993). The inner bag is transferred into a designated washer without being opened, followed by the outer bag. Infected linen should not be processed in a batch-continuous washing machine in case of a blockage.

• *Heat-labile linen*: This is washed at a low temperature, i.e. 40°C, and dried at 60°C. The disinfection is achieved by adding sodium hypochlorite to the penultimate rinse, although its use is restricted by the presence of soiling, detergents and alkali in the wash. Sodium hypochlorite is not suitable for fabrics treated for fire retardance.

Survival of organisms in the laundry process

The survival of multiresistant enterococci, especially vancomycin-resistant *Enterococcus faecium* has been reported (Freeman et al 1994). This organism is said to be widespread in the environment (Boyle et al 1993) and has been associated with a number of outbreaks (NHSE 1995b). Freeman et al (1994) found that isolates of vancomycin-resistant *Enterococcus faecium* survived temperatures of 65°C for over 20 min and 75°C for 3 min, and therefore survived the temperatures specified by the DoH in HSG (95) 18 (NHSE 1995b). The inclusion of a hypochlorite in the penultimate rinse is effective, although it can be added only in the absence of soiling, detergent and alkali and if the fabric is not likely to be damaged by chemicals. It is also possible that the organisms persist in the washing machines and continue to contaminate the linen, allowing their reintroduction into the original ward or other hospitals.

The destruction of hepatitis B virus at temperatures specified in the DoH guidance document HSG (95) 18 (NHSE 1995b) has not been established but is stated in the Scottish guidance document NHS MEL (1993) 7 (SCIEH 1993). Kobayashi et al (1984) recommend a minimum temperature of 93°C for hepatitis B but the DoH suggests that the heat inactivation at the temperatures suggested combined with the considerable dilution factor stage should render the linen safe to handle on completion of the wash cycle.

Role of infection control in laundry management

Infection control personnel have a vital role in monitoring the laundering of linen. The same laundry might serve many hospitals and infection control personnel can arrange a rota of visiting the designated laundry to ensure safe laundering. They might even want to share the testing of laundered items to ensure that contamination is not reintroduced on laundered linen.

Domestic linen

Most linen can be washed adequately in domestic washing machines. Special arrangements might be required for contaminated linen from people with infections. Community staff should liaise with infection control and hospital laundry personnel.

REFERENCES

Adams D, Bagg J, Limaye M et al 1992 A clinical evaluation of glove washing and reuse in dental practice. Journal of Hospital Control 20(3):153–162

Advisory Committee on Dangerous Pathogens (ACDP) 1995 Categorisation of pathogens according to hazard and categories of containment, 3rd edn. HMSO, London

Babb JR 1996 Application of disinfectants in hospitals and other health care establishments. Infection Control Journal of South Africa 1(1):4–12

Belkin NL 1994 Gowns: selection on a procedure-driven basis. Infection Control and Hospital Epidemiology 15:713–716

Berger SA, Kramer M, Nagar H, Finkelstein A 1993 Effect of surgical mask position on bacterial contamination of the operative field. Journal of Hospital Infection 23:51–54

Boyle JF, Soiumakis SA, Rendo A 1993 Epidemiological analysis and genotypic characterization of nosocomial outbreak of vancomycin-resistant enterococci. Journal of Clinical Microbiology 31:1280–1285

Brehler R 1996 Contact urticaria caused by latex-free nitrile glove. Contact Dermatitis, p 34, 296

British Medical Association (BMA) 1989 Code of practice for sterilization of instruments and control of cross infection. BMA Publications, London

British Standards Institution (BSI) 1994a Medical gloves for single use. Part 1: specification for freedom from holes (BS-EN 455-1). BSI, London

British Standards Institution (BSI) 1994b Medical gloves for single use. Part 2: specification for physical properties (BS-EN 455-2). BSI, London

British Standards Institution (BSI) 1994c Medical gloves for single use. Part 3: requirements and testing for biological evaluation (BS-EN 455-3). BSI, London

Burke FJT, Wilson NHF, Cheug SW 1995 Factors associated with the skin irritation of hands experienced by dental practitioners. Contact Dermatitis 32:35–38

Carter R 1990 Ritual and risk. Nursing Times 86(13):63–64

Centers for Disease Control (CDC) 1988 Universal precautions for prevention of transmission of human immunodeficiency virus, hepatitis B virus and other bloodborne pathogens in health care settings. Morbidity and Mortality Weekly Report 37:24

Centers for Disease Control (CDC) 1997 Guidelines for prevention of nosocomial pneumonia. Morbidity and Mortality Weekly Report 46 no. RR1, CDC, Atlanta

Central Sterilising Club (CSC) 1986 Washer disinfection machines. Working Party Report no. 1. Hospital Infection Research Laboratory, Birmingham

Charnley J 1979 Low friction arthroplasty of the hip. Springer-Verlag, Berlin

Cole RP, Gault DT 1989 Glove perforation during plastic surgery. British Journal of Plastic Surgery 42:481–483

Creamer E, Smyth EG 1996 Suction: reducing infection risks. Journal of Hospital Infection 34(1):1–9

De-Groot Kosolchar J, Jones JM 1989 Permeability of latex and vinyl gloves to water and blood. American Journal of Infection Control 17:196–201

Department of the Environment (DoE) 1990 Environmental Protection Act (1990) Waste management: the duty of care, a code of practice. HMSO, London

Department of Health (DoH) 1991 Decontamination of equipment, linen or other surfaces contaminated with hepatitis B or human immunodeficiency virus (HC(91)33). HMSO, London

Department of Health (DoH) 1998a The Interdepartmental Working Group on Tuberculosis. The prevention and control of tuberculosis in the United Kingdom: UK guidance on the prevention and control of transmission of: 1. HIV-related tuberculosis; 2. drug-resistant, including multiple drug-resistant, tuberculosis. DoH, The Scottish Office, The Welsh Office, London

Department of Health (DoH) 1998b Expert Advisory Group on AIDS and the Advisory Group on Hepatitis. Guidance for clinical health care workers: protection against infection with blood-borne viruses. DoH, London

Department of Health (DoH) 2001 The EPIC Project: developing national evidence-based guidelines for preventing healthcare associated infections. Journal of Hospital Infection 47(suppl):S1–S82

Doebbeling BN, Pfaller MA, Housten AK, Wenzel RP 1988 Removal of nosocomial pathogens from contaminated gloves: implications for glove reuse and handwashing. Annals of Internal Medicine 109:394–398

Duguid JP 1946 The size and duration of air carriage of respiratory droplets and droplet nuclei. Journal of Hygiene (Cambridge) 44:471–479

Duguid JP, Wallace AT 1948 Air infection with dust liberated from clothing. Lancet ii:845–849

Eckersley JRT, Williams DM 1990 Glove punctures in an orthopaedic trauma unit. British Journal of Accident Surgery 2:177–178

Fogg D 1989 Bacterial barrier of latex and vinyl gloves. AORN Journal 49:1101–1105

Freeman R, Kerans AM, Lightfoot NF 1994 Heat resistance of enterococci. Lancet 344:64–65

Gerhardt GG 1989 Results of microbiological investigations on the permeability of procedure and surgical gloves. Zentralblatt fur Hygiene 188:336–342

Haglund U, Junghams K 1997 Glove powder – the hazards which demand a ban. European Journal of Surgery. Scandinavian University press, Sweden

Health and Safety Commission (HSC) 1992a Workplace (health, safety and welfare) regulations 1992. Approved code of practice. HMSO, London

Health and Safety Commission (HSC) 1992b Management of Health and Safety at Work Act Regulations 1992. Approved Code of Practice. HMSO, London

Health and Safety Executive (HSE) 1992 Personal protective equipment at work regulations: guidance on regulations. HMSO, London

Health and Safety Executive (HSE) 1999 Control of substances hazardous to health (COSHH) (Amendment) Act 1999. Approved codes of practice. HSE Books, London

Health Service Advisory Committee (HSAC) 1974 Health and Safety at Work Act (1974). HMSO, London

Health Service Advisory Committee (HSAC) 1992 Safe disposal of clinical waste. HMSO, London

Humphreys H et al 1991a The effect of surgical theatre head-gear on air bacterial counts. Journal of Hospital Infection 19:175–180

Humphreys H et al 1991b Theatre over-shoes do not reduce operating theatre floor bacterial count. Journal of Hospital Infection 17:117–123

Infection Control Nurses Association (ICNA) 1999 Glove usage guidelines. ICNA, Bathgate, UK

Jones M, Jaheways M 1988 Over-estimating overshoes. Nursing Times 84(41): 66–71

Kobayashi H, Tsuzuki M, Koshimizu K et al 1984 Susceptibility of hepatitis B virus to disinfectants or heat. Journal of Clinical Microbiology 20(2):214–216

Korniewicz DM, Laughon B, Cyr W et al 1990 Leakage of virus through used vinyl and latex examination gloves. Journal of Clinical Microbiology 28:787–788

Korniewicz DM, Kirwin M, Cresci K et al 1994 Barrier protection with examination gloves: double vs. single. American Journal of Infection Control 22:12–15

Lars P, Naver S, Gottrup F 2000 Incidence of glove perforations in gastrointestinal surgery and the protective effect of double gloves: a prospective, randomized controlled study. European Journal of Surgery 166:1–3

McCulloch J 2000 Infection control: science, management and practice. Whurr Publishers, London

Medical Devices Agency (MDA) 1996 Latex sensitisation in the health care setting – the use of latex gloves (DB(96)01). HMSO, London

Medical Devices Agency (MDA) 1998 Latex medical gloves (surgeons' and examination) powdered latex medical gloves (surgeons' and examination) (SN(98)25). HMSO, London

Mitchell NJ, Hunt S 1991 Surgical face masks in modern operating theatres – a costly and unnecessary ritual? Journal of Hospital Infection 18:239–242

National Health Service Executive (NHSE) 1995a Management policy on washer–disinfectors (30/80 HTM2030). NHS Estates, London

National Health Service Executive (NHSE) 1995b Hospital laundry arrangements for used and infected linen (HSG(95)18). DoH, London

National Health Service Executive (NHSE) 1998 Healthcare waste management segregation (HTM 2065). HMSO, London

National Health Service Management Executive (NHSME) 1960 Radioactive Substances Act. NHME Estates, London

Olsen RJ, Lynch P, Coyle MB Examination gloves as barriers to hand contamination in clinical practice. Journal of the American Medical Association 270(3):350–353

Ormerod LP 2000 BTS guidelines: control and prevention of tuberculosis in the United Kingdom: code of practice 2000. Joint Tuberculosis Committee of the British Thoracic Society. Thorax 55:887–901

Orr NW 1981 Is a mask necessary in the operating theatre? Annals of the Royal College of Surgery of England 63:390–392

Orr NW, Bailey S 1992 Masks in surgery. Annals of the Royal College of Surgery of England 20:57

Parker LJ 2000 Biogel reveal: a puncture indication system from Regent Medical. British Journal of Nursing 9(17):1182–1185

Richmond PW, McCabe M, Davies JP, Thomas DM 1992 Perforation of gloves in an accident and emergency department. British Medical Journal (Clinical Research edn) 304:879–880

Romney MG 2001 Surgical face masks in the operating theatre: re-examining the evidence. Journal of Hospital Infection 47:251–256

Scottish Centre for Infection and Environmental Health (SCIEH) 1993 Hospital laundry arrangements for used and infected linen (NHS MEL(1993)7). SCIEH, Glasgow

Scottish Centre for Infection and Environmental Health (SCIEH) 1994 Management of clinical waste and heat treatment processes. An advisory paper for Scotland (NHS MEL(1994)88). SCIEH, Glasgow

Smock M, Shiel M 1990 The role of surgeon and procedure gloves in infection control. Nursing Standard 4(7):24–26

Tunevall TG 1991 Postoperative wound infections and surgical face masks: a controlled study. World Journal of Surgery 15:383–388

Tunevall TG, Jörbrck H 1992 Influence of wearing masks on the density of airborne bacteria in the vicinity of the surgical wound. European Journal of Surgery 158:263–266

Ward V, Wilson J, Taylor L et al 1997 Preventing hospital-acquired infection: clinical guidelines. PHLS, London

Weightman NC, Banfield KR 1994 Protective overshoes are unnecessary in a day surgery unit. Journal of Hospital Infection 28:1–3

Whyte W 1988 The role of clothing and drapes in the operating room. Journal of Hospital Infection 11(suppl C):2–17

Yassin MS, Lierl MB, Fischer TJ 1994 Latex allergy in hospital employees. Annals of Allergy 72(3):245–249

Means of transmission

9

■ CONTENTS

SUMMARY

This chapter examines methods used by microbes to transfer from their place of reservoir to susceptible individuals, and the actions required to curtail their spread.

INTRODUCTION

The skin is the largest organ in the body and protects and isolates the body from the outside world. It presents an effective mechanical barrier to the penetration of the underlying structures by harmful microorganisms. Microorganisms, or skin flora, live on skin surfaces and produce substances known to have antimicrobial properties. The presence of skin flora is also thought to prevent or slow down colonization by other exogenous microorganisms (Mims et al 1993).

Both Gram-positive and Gram-negative microorganisms are known to exist on the skin and can be found at any site on the body, including the perineum and the genital tract (Noble 1993). Up to 50% of the population are thought to carry *Staphylococcus aureus* in their anterior nares (Williams et al 1960). These organisms are responsible for a significant number of hospital-acquired wound and skin infections.

There is the potential for the transference of organisms from the nose to the hands, and from the hands to a vulnerable site on a susceptible patient. The skin flora or resident organisms rarely cause disease in a healthy host, but they are opportunistic, and create problems when they are found on or in a vulnerable host.

Microorganisms that are transferred from one patient to another, called transient organisms, are the main cause of cross-infection in clinical settings. This is because:

- the human body is familiar with and able to cope only with its own organisms
- the patient is compromised by the illness that has resulted in their hospital admission as well as by the treatment received.

The 1994 prevalence survey (Emmerson et al 1996) showed that 9.6% of patients with hospital-acquired infection were suffering from skin infections. Infections of the skin are a result of:

- a breach in the integrity of intact skin creating a portal of entry
- systemic infections manifesting on the skin
- skin damage due to toxin from organisms, for example toxic shock syndrome, scarlet fever or necrotizing fasciitis.

Dispersal of microorganisms from these patients, as well as from the normal skin flora, has implications for procedures such as bed making and aseptic techniques such as wound dressings.

Colonization

The patient's skin flora can alter either as a result of antibiotic therapy or by colonization with hospital organisms carried on the hands of staff (Barrett-Connor 1978, Bennett & Brachman 1979). The skin and mucous membranes of older and debilitated people are more likely to become colonized with Gram-negative bacteria (Johanson 1969), and the hands of paraplegic patients have also been found to have been colonized with Gram-negative organisms (Chin & Davies 1978). This can result in the colonized patient becoming infected or in the organisms being transmitted to other susceptible patients by direct or indirect contact.

Hospital patients develop infection through the skin because:

- they received a traumatic injury before entering a hospital, and/or
- the integrity of the skin is compromised through diagnostic or therapeutic procedures, such as surgical incisions, aspirations, biopsies, injections, cannulation, debridement etc. (Axnic & Yarborough 1984).

HANDWASHING

Many factors contribute to the development of a hospital-acquired infection; patient to patient cross-colonization and/or infection can occur by many routes (Fig. 9.1) making it difficult to establish a link between any one variable. Hospitals today admit severely ill patients who require frequent

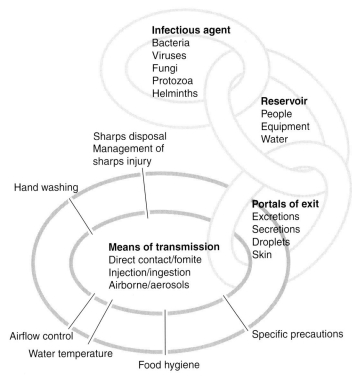

Figure 9.1 Breaking the chain of infection: means of transmission.

invasive procedures and devices, with an increasing risk of transmission of pathogenic organisms between them.

The relationship between the hands of healthcare workers and the spread of microorganisms among patients has been known since the nineteenth century (Marc LaForce 1993). A simple but effective means of protecting patients from hospital-acquired infection is handwashing. It is universally considered to be the most basic but vital infection control measure, but it is also one of the most neglected of practices (DoH 2001, ICNA 1999, Larson & Killian 1982).

Hands as the vector

The evidence to support the link between handwashing and contact transmission of infection was first established by Oliver Wendell Holmes in the US (1843) and in Europe by Ignaz Semmelweis (1861). They both showed a drop in the rate of puerperal sepsis and its associated mortality when doctors washed their hands between examining women during childbirth. Other evidence to support the link between hands and cross-infection can be said to be indirect, on the basis that organisms that were causing infections in patients were also recovered from the hands of the carers. Wolinsky et al (1960) confirmed the role of unwashed hands in the transmission of *Staphylococcus aureus* in a newborn nursery. Casewell & Phillips (1977) recovered an endemic strain of *Klebsiella* species from the skin of patients and from nurses' hands in an intensive therapy unit, establishing an association between hand-washing and the termination of the epidemic. Other studies have shown contamination of hands by, and its relationship to, hospital-acquired infections by Gram-negative organisms (Guenthner et al 1987, Knittle et al 1975). Viable hepatitis A virus (HAV) has been found on the hands of health personnel, who might play a part in the transmission of this virus (Mbithi et al 1992).

Cross-transmission of organisms is not always easy to detect. Patients can be discharged home, transferred to other wards or perhaps colonized rather than infected. Colonized patients act as undetected sources of cross-infection to others.

Cross-infections are confirmed in the laboratory by a variety of identification methods, such as phage typing, pyocin typing, serotyping and modern molecular methods. Schaberg and colleagues (1980) demonstrated, using these typing methods, that approximately 15% of endemic infection in hospitals occur in clusters, suggesting that cross-infection has taken place. Because such extensive examination of infections is expensive, time-consuming and impractical, many cases of cross-infection go undetected.

Organisms do survive and multiply on human hands, with a potential to infect others or the self. Reybrouck (1983) found that *Staphylococcus aureus* could be isolated from the hands of between 25% and 65% of nurses in a general hospital. Many studies have dealt with the level of contamination of hands during care procedures. Gram-negative bacilli are thought to contaminate between 20% and 30% of healthcare personnel generally, reaching up to 80% in personnel working in intensive care and burns units (Knittle et al 1975).

A number of experimental studies suggest an easy acquisition and spread of organisms. In clinical situations, Casewell & Phillips (1977) found that even undertaking specific clean nursing procedures resulted in contamination of nurses' hands with 100–1000 klebsiellae on each hand. Sanderson & Weissler (1992) studied contamination of nurses' hands by coliforms in the spinal injuries unit and general surgical wards. The activities included:

- bed-making
- handling patients and their clothing, wash cloths, bowls and towels
- handling used linen
- sluice room activities
- changing urinary catheters and drainage bags
- touching curtains and bedside furniture
- medicine rounds.

Bacterial contamination without apparent soiling of the hands has been shown during contact with patients. Dirty activities such as dealing with body secretions and excretions result in much heavier contamination of the hands, even when gloves are worn (Noone et al 1983). Handwashing results in a significant reduction in the carriage of potential pathogens, as well as in a reduction in the spread of infections (Daschner et al 1982, Larson 1988, Larson et al 1988).

Mortality from bacteraemia and septicaemia and pneumonia in hospital-ized patients remains high. The major route of transmission of infection in these patients is thought to be the hands of hospital personnel (Bauer et al 1990, Casewell & Phillips 1977, Peacock et al 1988). Organisms require a mode of transport, and hands are by far the most convenient vehicle.

Principles of handwashing

The purpose of handwashing is to remove dirt and/or to reduce the level of organisms present on the hands. Organisms found on the skin might be transient or resident (Shanson 1999). The resident bacteria live permanently in the openings of the hair follicles and the sebaceous glands. They rarely cause problems in a healthy host and, indeed, protect the skin against col-onization by transient organisms. The transient organisms are found on the surface of the skin or beneath the horny layer of superficial cells known as the stratum corneum. This layer is essentially made up of bacteria deposited from outside sources. In the vast majority of cases, a healthy body is able to defend itself against transient organisms, the majority of which are removed by the mechanical action of handwashing or the chemical action of hand decontamination.

Choosing a handwashing agent

The choice of handwashing agent, the duration of the wash and the tech-nique used (Box 9.1) depend on the procedure to be undertaken and the susceptibility of the patient. Box 9.2 shows the handwashing schedule that is recommended by most experts. The type of handwash is divided into:

- routine handwash
- surgical handwash.

Routine handwash

This is the most common form of handwashing practised in both the home and institutional setting. The aim is to remove all transient organisms. Blowing the nose, using the toilet, handling soiled nappies and cleaning toilets are some of the personal actions that result in significant hand con-tamination. In hospital, practices that involve direct contact with patients and used equipment often produce high levels of contamination. These organisms are easily removed by washing the hands with soap and running water, and applying friction for 10–15 s (Fig. 9.2). The most important element in effective handwashing is mechanical friction (Ayliffe et al 1978).

In most care settings handwashing with liquid soap and water is adequate. Staff are more likely to use a solution that is pleasant and does not harm the skin. Emollients are now standard additions to the majority of detergent products. Liquid soap dispensers with disposable cartridges reduce the risk of contamination compared to refillable containers. They should be wall mounted and preferably operated by the elbow, wrist or foot (Ayliffe et al 1978). The use of aqueous antiseptic solutions will reduce transient and

■ BOX 9.1   Handwashing technique

- Complete coverage of the hands with the handwashing agent is vital. Taylor (1978) showed that parts of the thumbs, backs of fingers, backs of hands and underneath the fingernails are frequently missed.
- Wetting the hands before applying the handwashing agent facilitates complete coverage and will reduce the drying effect on the skin.
- Debris collected under the fingernails can result in a high microbial count inside gloved hands and should be removed. A gentle 'brushing' or use of a nail stick will avoid damage and subsequent colonization of the subungual area.
- Short nails are desirable because the majority of organisms are found under or around the fingernails (McGinley et al 1988).
- False fingernails are a host to potential pathogens, including yeasts, and should be avoided by healthcare workers (Anon 1999, Moolenaar et al 2000).
- The bacterial counts are higher under and around rings (Hoffman et al 1985) but bacteria can be removed effectively by manipulating rings during handwashing (Jacobson et al 1985). Wearing of jewellery in clinical settings should be limited to a wedding ring (Salisbury et al 1997).
- Sufficient contact time with the antiseptic agent is essential to achieve adequate antisepsis (Reybrouck 1986). This is dependent upon the agent being used.
- Thorough rinsing and drying of hands is important to prevent skin irritation.
- Disposable paper towels are more effective in further reducing the flora than cloth towels (Ansari et al 1991). Cloth towels are rarely used in patient care areas but might be preferred in general practice, dental surgeries and patients' own homes.
- The use of cloth towels, if unavoidable, needs to be strictly controlled. Damp cloth towels will become contaminated and should be dried between use. They should be changed at least daily and laundered appropriately.
- The use of hot air dryers should be discouraged in patient care areas. An increase of more than 500% in the bacterial count was demonstrated with hot air dryers (Knight et al 1993, Redway et al 1994). An increase of bacterial contamination in the local environment was also noted. People in the study rarely used hot air dryers for long enough to ensure more than 55–65% dryness; drying was often completed by wiping hands on the clothes. Hot air dryers also tend to be noisy, which discourages their use during the night.
- Hand lotions are advisable to prevent skin dryness, but can become contaminated. Single-use cartridge dispensers or pump-action bottles should be used. Compatibility is required between hand lotions and handwashing agents when making a choice.
- Handwashing agents can also become contaminated. Bars of soap should be maintained dry, refilling of liquid soap containers and antiseptic agents should not occur. Disposable cartridges are the current choice.

resident organism levels and will achieve hand antisepsis. This is important when patients' vulnerability predisposes them to infection from resident organisms. Newborn infants, intensive care patients and severely immuno-compromised patients all fall into this category.

■ **BOX 9.2   Handwashing schedule**

Thorough handwashing must be carried out:
- Before:
  - performing invasive procedures
  - caring for susceptible patients
  - preparing or handling food
  - any other activity where a risk of transmitting infection is anticipated
  - starting work and leaving work areas (visiting the canteen, end of shift)
  - wearing sterile gloves
  - leaving source isolation
- Before and after:
  - touching wounds and dressings of any type
  - administering medication
  - touching urethral catheters and intravenous lines
  - emptying urine drainage bags
- Between:
  - significant or prolonged contact with different patients, particularly in high-risk areas such as the intensive therapy unit (ITU), special care baby unit (SCBU) and the burns unit
  - any situation that involves direct patient contact, for example bathing, assisting to move and toileting
- After:
  - situations likely to cause microbial contamination (contact with blood and body fluids, secretions or excretions)
  - touching sources likely to be contaminated with clinically significant microorganisms (urine measuring devices, suction bottles, specimen collection pots)
  - caring for patients infected or colonized with important organisms where there is a risk of serious cross-infection (methicillin-resistant *Staphylococcus aureus* (MRSA), gentamycin-resistant *Klebsiella pneumonia*, *E. coli* 0157, *Clostridium difficile*, rotavirus and respiratory syncytial virus (RSV))
  - personal contamination (using the toilet, blowing or wiping the nose, etc.)
  - removing gloves
  - bed-making
  - handling contaminated laundry and waste.

Surgical handwash

During surgery, the skin is breached, allowing organisms direct and easy access to internal tissues and organs. Many surgical procedures are lengthy and a large proportion of surgical gloves will be perforated at the end of the operation (Paulssen et al 1988). Antiseptics that provide both immediate and prolonged antibacterial activity are the agent of choice in these situations. A surgical handwash requires not only the removal of transient organisms but also the reduction of residential organisms to a minimum level. Although soap, water and friction are effective in removing transient

Hands should be wet first; take one squeeze of liquid soap from the dispenser. Wash as shown using five strokes on each movement and a total washing time of at least 10 seconds.

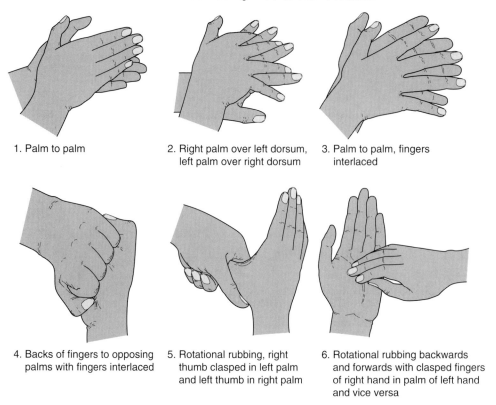

1. Palm to palm

2. Right palm over left dorsum, left palm over right dorsum

3. Palm to palm, fingers interlaced

4. Backs of fingers to opposing palms with fingers interlaced

5. Rotational rubbing, right thumb clasped in left palm and left thumb in right palm

6. Rotational rubbing backwards and forwards with clasped fingers of right hand in palm of left hand and vice versa

After washing, hands should be thoroughly rinsed to avoid irritation.

Figure 9.2 Standard handwashing technique.

organisms there is a possibility of an increase in the level of resident organisms following a social handwash. This is thought to be as a result of increased shedding of the desquamating epithelium that contains these organisms. These resident organisms can be pathogenic if given the opportunity to invade a patient. An antimicrobial wash is needed to kill or inhibit the resident organisms and reduce the numbers further (Lilly & Lowbury 1978, Lilly et al 1979, Reybrouck 1986).

A further advantage of using an antiseptic agent is the persistent antibacterial activity of the residue on the skin following handwashing. Such antibacterial action is desirable when frequent handwashing is difficult, as during prolonged surgical procedures.

Handwashing agents

Some of the commonly used antiseptic agents include chlorhexidine gluconate, iodophors, triclosan and hexachlorophane. Antiseptics kill or inhibit microorganisms and reduce their level further by their residual effect, but this becomes inactivated by contact with organic material. The detergent base in antiseptic washes also allows for the physical removal of any contamination. The level of activity against different microorganisms varies with each agent. Another influencing factor in choosing an agent is acceptance by the user as skin sensitivity is a problem area for many health-care workers.

Chlorhexidine gluconate

This is a broad-spectrum antiseptic effective against Gram-positive bacteria but has little activity against Gram-negative bacteria, fungi, viruses or tubercle bacilli (Ayliffe et al 1984). Its residual effect remains active on the skin for several hours making it an ideal surgical scrub. It is available as a washing agent in 4% concentration in a detergent base or as a combination with alcohol for skin antisepsis and handrub.

Iodophors

Iodophors are broad-spectrum agents. They have good activity against Gram-positive and Gram-negative organisms, tubercle bacilli, fungi and viruses. They have little residual activity and are neutralized in the presence of organic matter. Iodophors contain iodine and a carrier such as povidone and can be harsh on the skin.

Triclosan

This has achieved popularity as an effective agent against MRSA. The persistent residual activity of triclosan on the skin makes its use as a bathing agent ideal for patients colonized with MRSA.

Hexachlorophane

This is a bacteriostatic agent for Gram-positive organisms but has little activity against Gram-negative bacteria, fungi, viruses or tubercle bacilli.

Alcohols

Alcohols in the form of handrubs and handgels are relatively safe on the skin and have good activity against most microorganisms except spores. Reduction in microbial counts is rapid and substantial. The application of alcohol is as effective in surgical scrubs as in hand antisepsis. The length of time the alcohol is in contact with hands has to be increased for surgical scrubs (Larson et al 1990). Despite an absence of residual activity in alcohols, the bacterial count has been shown to drop for several hours after gloving (Lilly et al 1979). This makes the use of alcohols for surgical scrubs economic and effective.

   Although not inactivated by small amounts of blood, alcohols are not considered to be good cleaning agents. They should not be used on hands that are physically soiled. Hands that have been contaminated with body fluids must be washed with soap and water before applying an alcohol handrub.

Isopropyl alcohol at 70% concentration with either chlorhexidine or triclosan is commonly used. An alternative is a combination of alcohols. An emollient is added to counteract the drying effect of the alcohol. For alcohol to be effective and to prevent skin irritation, it must be allowed to evaporate completely.

Ethical considerations of non-compliance

Handwashing is universally considered to be the most basic but vital infection control measure, but it is also one of the most neglected areas of practice (Bryan 1986). Studies have shown less-than-required compliance with handwashing by both medical and nursing staff (Albert & Condie 1981, Larson & Killian 1982). Periodic high-profile campaigns might prove effective in reminding staff but motivation has been shown to decrease with time (Williams & Buckles 1988). An important and powerful force is the patient and their relatives. Wenzel & Pfaller (1991) achieved a high compliance rate by advising high-risk patients to request handwashing of all healthcare workers entering their room. Jarvis (1994) made the following observation:

> If health care workers cannot be educated to comply, perhaps we should tell patients about the importance of handwashing: how many doctors and nurses would ignore a patient's request that they wash their hands first?

A recent study in the US, replicated in the UK, encouraged patients to give cards to staff asking them to wash their hands. As a consequence, an increased compliance to handwashing policies was observed (McGuckin et al 2001). An educational hospital-wide programme introduced into a Geneva hospital improved compliance and a reduction in MRSA transmission rates (Pittet et al 2000).

The new guidelines for hand hygiene from the Centers for Disease Control (CDC), due for publication in 2002, are considering recommending the replacement of soap and water with alcohol rubs. The shift towards recommending waterless agents is based on improper handwashing techniques and low compliance to policies. Times recommended for the decontamination of hands in protocols of 15, 30 or 60s bear no resemblance to what actually happens in practice. Eleven studies referenced in the draft guidelines evaluated that the average duration of handwashing by healthcare workers ranges from 7 to 10s. Consequently, alcohol handrubs are recommended (Pugliese et al 2001) because they:

- take less time to reduce microbial loads than other agents
- provide better access because sinks and water are not used
- are less irritating to hands than soap and water.

Observing clinical practice, the wearing of latex gloves appears to be the norm for the majority of nursing procedures. As such, the risk of physical soiling of the hands is minimal. Therefore an increase in the use of alcohol handrubs might be acceptable.

SPECIFIC PRECAUTIONS

Universal precautions

The concept of universal precautions was introduced in the US in the mid-1980s to minimize the occupational risk of blood-borne viral infections in healthcare workers (CDC 1987). The guidelines were drawn up largely in response to the human immunodeficiency virus (HIV), especially following reports of hospital personnel becoming infected with HIV through needle-stick injuries and skin contamination with patients' blood. The main assumption underlying the advent of universal precautions was that many patients with blood-borne infections are not recognized and therefore precautions should be applied to all patients, regardless of their presumed status (CDC 1987). In 1988 the guidelines were updated to include prevention of exposure to blood, body fluids visibly contaminated with blood, and semen and vaginal secretions. Although the risk of transmission was unknown from cerebrospinal, amniotic, peritoneal, pericardial, pleural and synovial fluids, these were included. The guidelines did not include faeces, urine, nasal secretions, sputum, sweat, tears, or vomit unless they contained visible blood. The 1988 guidelines also emphasized immunization against hepatitis B virus (HBV) (CDC 1988).

Body substance isolation

Universal precautions are intended to apply only to fluids that might transmit HIV and certain other blood-borne pathogens. In body substance isolation, barrier precautions are recommended for contact with all body excretions and secretions. These include, in addition to blood and blood-stained fluids, faeces, urine, saliva, sputum, wound drainage and vomit from all patients, regardless of their infection status (Lynch et al 1987, 1990). The rationale underlying these guidelines is that all the above can potentially contain infectious agents. The emphasis is on the use of gloves when handling these body substances. The main advice is to:

- put on clean gloves just before contact with mucous membrane or non-intact skin
- wear clean gloves when contact with moist substance is anticipated
- use a face mask when entering the room of patients with infections transmitted via the airborne route
- be immunized against certain infections likely to be transmitted via the airborne route, for example measles, mumps, rubella and varicella.

The value of universal precautions/body substance isolation

According to Gerberding et al (1995) universal precautions and/or body substance isolation 'avoid discrimination against certain patients based on their HIV serostatus or the presence of risk factors for HIV infection' and will, hopefully, prevent transmission of infection from patient to staff, as well as from an infected staff member to a patient. With regard to

---

■ **BOX 9.3** **Universal precautions**

- Apply good basic hygiene practices with regular handwashing
- Cover existing wounds or skin lesions with waterproof dressings
- Avoid invasive procedures if suffering from chronic skin lesions on hands
- Avoid contamination of person by use of appropriate clothing
- Protect mucous membranes of eyes, mouth and nose from blood splashes and blood-stained fluids
- Prevent puncture wounds, cuts and abrasions in the presence of blood/blood-stained body fluids
- Avoid sharps usage wherever possible
- Institute safe procedures for handling and disposal of needles and other sharps
- Institute approved procedures for sterilization and disinfection of instruments and equipment
- Clear up spillages of blood and other body fluid promptly and disinfect surfaces
- Institute a procedure for safe disposal of contaminated waste.

HIV, the main hazard to healthcare workers is percutaneous exposure to HIV-infected blood. Heptonstall et al (1993) have documented 118 cases of occupationally acquired HIV world-wide, four of which occurred in the UK. Anecdotal evidence, however, would suggest that the majority of healthcare workers associate universal precautions with the wearing of protective clothing for blood and body fluid contact. Prevention of percutaneous injuries, safe disposal of needles and other sharp instruments and appropriate disinfection/sterilization of reusable equipment used in performing invasive procedures are rarely included.

The value of universal precautions or body substance isolation in preventing transmission of HIV has not been established. The jury is still out on whether either, both or a combination of these measures result in lower rates of other nosocomial infections. Most organizations advocate the use of universal precautions for all body fluids. The important message, however, is the assessment and management of risks associated with each patient care activity. Education and auditing staff awareness of hazards and practice remain pivotal in protecting both patients and staff.

In the UK, the Advisory Group on Hepatitis (UK Health Departments 1993), under the aegis of the Advisory Committee on Dangerous Pathogens (ACDP 1990) has recommended similar guidelines (Box 9.3).

Policies and guidelines

The Infection Control Standards Working Party (ICSWP) document *Standards in Infection Control in Hospitals* (ICSWP 1993) depicts the areas and procedures that policies should cover. It also includes a comprehensive list of reference material governing each policy. It is vital that infection control policies are written by the infection control personnel in consultation with the relevant users of the policy, to guide and protect healthcare personnel. All managers and practitioners have a responsibility to ensure that policies are read, understood and complied with.

In January 2001, the DoH published the first national evidence-based guidelines for infection control (DoH 2001). These guidelines are systematically developed broad statements (principles) of good practice that can be used to develop local protocols and policies. The type and grade of supporting evidence is linked explicitly to each recommendation. The document states that 'all recommendations are endorsed equally and none is regarded as optional' (DoH 2001).

PATIENT PRACTICES

A number of practices are common to all patient care areas irrespective of specialty; these practices are designed to manage risks and protect patients and staff. Healthcare workers will be in a position to manage risks and provide 'informed care' if they understand the factors that contribute to both intrinsic and extrinsic risks.

Bed-making

Williams et al (1960) showed that bacteria accumulate in large numbers in patients' bedding. Organisms in patients' bedding can be from their faecal flora, skin or from an infected site. Sanderson and Alshafi (1995) isolated organisms from both top and bottom sheets of patients with a urinary tract infection caused by the same organisms. Organisms included *Enterobacter cloacae, Escherichia coli, Klebsiella pneumoniae, Enterococcus faecalis, Candida tropicalis* and group B streptococci. It is suggested that organisms on bedding could contaminate the hands of patients and staff and be distributed into the environment of the ward by particles of lint.

Bed-making has been known to result in the dissemination of microorganisms into the air (Litsky 1971, Noble 1962, Noble & Davies 1965, Shooter et al 1958). Noble (1962) found air counts of *Staphylococcus aureus* of more than 50 particles per cubic foot during bed-making. These organisms will eventually settle on horizontal surfaces until they become airborne again or are lifted on hands. Box 9.4 outlines good bed-making practice.

■ **BOX 9.4   Bed-making**

- Strip the bed by folding each item of bedding separately and avoid 'scooping'. Scooping involves close contact with staff's own clothing, resulting in contamination. The bedlinen is more likely to fall on the floor than separated sheets or blankets.
- Bedding must not touch the floor. Organisms on the floor could be transferred on to the bedding.
- Avoid shaking of bedclothes because this causes dissemination of large amounts of organisms into the surrounding environment.
- Take the linen skip to the bed to avoid 'hugging' bedclothes when transporting them to the skip.
- Plastic aprons should be worn if there is likely to be close physical contact with the patient.

Bed-bathing

A survey by Greaves (1985) showed that there were more bacteria on a patient's skin after a bed-bath than before. The reasons for this include:

- not changing the water often enough
- insufficient rinsing of patients' washcloths
- not cleaning washbowls after use.

Many organisms are picked up by the washcloth from the patient's body and transferred into the water. These eventually create a 'soup' of bacteria, which are then transported on the cloth to various other parts of the body. The organisms will continue to survive, and possibly multiply, unless the washcloth is rinsed thoroughly under running hot water. The storage of the cloth should allow for it to dry between each use. Washcloths must never be wrapped around soap in a wash bag and the soap should not be stored in a wet soap dish.

Inappropriately cleaned washbowls have resulted in transmission of *Klebsiella* pneumonia in a number of surgical patients (Joynson 1978). Thorough washing with detergent and water followed by drying should be routine practice with individual washbowls advisable.

SHARPS DISPOSAL

Use and disposal of sharps

Many procedures in healthcare settings are invasive and require the use of devices that can penetrate the human body. Healthcare workers have always been aware of the potential hazards of using such instruments but the seriousness of the risk became evident when the first case of needlestick injury related to HIV was documented (Anon 1984). Sharps injury with inoculation of blood and other potentially infectious body fluids has been identified as the most important mechanism for transmitting hepatitis B and HIV to healthcare workers. Whereas evaluation and refinement of invasive devices and instruments continues (Anon 1993), every effort should be made to reduce the risk of sharps injuries (Box 9.5). All work with sharp instruments should be careful, attentive and unhurried. Special care should be taken when using needles and scalpels, when handling sharp instruments after procedures, when cleaning used instruments and when disposing of used needles and other sharps (British Medical Association (BMA) 1990).

Sharps containers – BSI specifications

Sharps containers should comply with British Standard 7320 or its equivalent. Sharps containers must (HSAC 1992, SCIEH 1994):

- be puncture-resistant and leak-proof, even if they topple over or are dropped
- be capable of being handled and moved while in use with minimal danger of the content spilling or falling out
- be provided with a handle(s) that is not part of any closure device; the position of the handle must not interfere with the normal use of the container

> ■ **Box 9.5   Safety precautions in dealing with sharps**
>
> - Avoid recapping, bending, breaking or otherwise manipulating used needles.
> - If removal of the needle from the syringe is unavoidable, forceps should be used, or the needle should be approached carefully along the barrel of the syringe, using a gloved hand. Alternatively, sharps boxes with needle-removing facilities should be used. However, extreme vigilance is required to prevent injuries and contamination.
> - Used needles and other disposable sharps should be discarded in the sharps containers provided (DoH 1987).
> - The sharps containers should conform to the British Standards Institution specification set out in BS 7320 (BSI 1990) and the United Nations Standard (UN 3291).
> - The container must not be over-filled and items should be carefully dropped in, not pushed down.

- have an aperture that, in normal use, will inhibit removal of the contents but will ensure that it is possible to place items intended for disposal into the sharps container using one hand, without contaminating the outside of the container
- have a closure device attached for sealing when the container is three-quarters full or ready for disposal
- have a horizontal line to indicate when the container is three-quarters full, and be marked with the words 'Warning – do not fill above the line'
- be made of material that can be incinerated
- be yellow
- be clearly marked with the words 'Danger', 'Contaminated Sharps Only', 'Destroy by incineration' or 'To be incinerated'.

FOOD HYGIENE

Catering and food hygiene

Safe food is necessary to avoid widespread illness due to infectious diseases, and food handlers are integral to the process of providing safe food. Individual food handlers have legal obligations to avoid contaminating food (Painter 1995). The term 'food handlers' applies to a wide range of healthcare staff, from the professional producers in the catering department to anyone who delivers, serves or otherwise handles unwrapped food (DoH 1992). A healthcare worker making a slice of toast for a patient or opening a carton of milk is classed as a food handler. All food handlers are liable for any adverse incidents that occur in association with food preparation or consumption on healthcare premises.

Whether the care establishment uses a conventional or cook–chill or cook–freeze catering system, the main responsibility for the prevention of the introduction of infection into the food premises rests with catering managers. The catering manager is supported by local environmental health officers and the organization's infection control personnel.

The Food Safety (General) Regulations (DoH 1995a) are concerned with consumer protection and form the basis of practice in catering establishments. Safe catering practice incorporates the structure of the food premises, food hygiene and personal hygiene. It also includes the temperature control during receipt, storage, processing and distribution of food as laid down in the Food Safety (Temperature Control) Regulations (DoH 1995b): the food has to be kept at either $<8°C$ or $>63°C$. In cases of cook–chill and cook–freeze catering, $<3°C$ is recommended during both transport and storage (DoH 1989).

The *Food Safety (General Food Hygiene) Regulations* (DoH 1995a) are supported by the new *Controls Assurance Standard: Catering and Food Hygiene* (NHSE 2001). This places a requirement on the NHS organizations to comply with current food safety legislation.

Food poisoning outbreaks in healthcare settings have highlighted the risks of contamination of food in catering. The most common causes are listed by Barrie (1996) as:

- preparing food too long in advance
- storing food at ambient temperatures
- cooling food too slowly before placing it in a refrigerator
- not reheating food to temperatures at which food poisoning bacteria can be destroyed
- using contaminated food
- undercooking meat, meat products and poultry
- not thawing frozen poultry and meat for long enough
- cross-contamination between raw and cooked food
- keeping hot food below 63°C
- infected food handlers.

The effects of food poisoning range from mild gastrointestinal symptoms to significant illness and death (Joseph & Palmer 1989). Protection of patients from food-borne illness has attained a very high profile since the major outbreak of salmonella food poisoning at Stanley Royd Hospital (DHSS 1986), which resulted in 19 deaths. The Committee of Inquiry on the Stanley Royd Hospital outbreak (DHSS 1986) state that:

> *The solution to all problems of avoiding contamination of food lies in:*
>
> - *proper hygiene*
> - *proper cooking*
> - *proper handling*
> - *proper storage of food.*

The Expert Working Group Guidance document entitled *Food Handlers: Fitness to Work* (DoH 1995c) suggests that the:

> *Management in the food industry must minimise the risk of food becoming contaminated by:*
>
> - *training and/or instructing, and supervising staff in the safe handling of food*
> - *ensuring employees have a working understanding of the principles of hygiene*

- *advising staff of their obligation to report to management any infectious or potentially infectious conditions*
- *excluding infectious or potentially infectious food handlers as specifically required by UK food hygiene legislation in accordance with the guidance*
- *liaising with enforcement authorities as appropriate*
- *ensuring that others, such as maintenance engineers, who may come in contact with food or food surfaces do not cause contamination and*
- *providing clean hygienic working environment.*

Food handlers

The Food Safety (General Food Hygiene) Regulations (DoH 1995a) specify mandatory training for food handlers. The catering manager or supervisors should assess the risks associated with food handlers' activities. The section on employee health in Chapter 3 discusses issues in relation to infections in food handlers.

Ward kitchens and ward-based food handlers

Some elementary training and a safe code of practice should apply to healthcare workers at a ward level. The food is served by both the nursing and domestic staff, who should understand the importance of serving meals within 15 min of reheating (DoH 1989), discarding delayed meals, and the drawbacks of reheating food in microwave ovens (Barrie 1996).

The responsibility for ward kitchen hygiene, including disposal of waste, rests predominantly with the domestic staff. Nurses, however, are constant frequenters of ward kitchens and handle refrigerators, dishwashers, microwave ovens, ice-making machines, and so on. They can easily contaminate surfaces and equipment with inadequately washed hands following contact with patients, especially those with gastrointestinal infections, as well as maternity, paediatric, elderly and psychiatric patients in whom faecal soiling is likely (Abbot et al 1960, Cruickshank 1984, Palmer & Rowe 1983).

Ward dishwashers and manual washing-up

The importance of a high standard of washing-up has been recognized. Both methods are practised in ward kitchens. Manual washing-up requires two sinks to ensure thorough rinsing of crockery and cutlery. However, the water temperature might be inconsistent and the standard of washing-up will vary. Dishwashers are more reliable, as well as more practical. Commercial dishwashers that achieve a thermal disinfection at 82°C are preferred (DHSS 1976). Most dishwashers operate on an automatic soap-feeding system. The cleaning schedule for ward kitchens should incorporate daily removal of food residue and thorough cleaning of dishwashers. The ward dishwashers should be part of the planned maintenance programme of the organization. Cowan et al (1995) state that 'provision of hygiene crockery and cutlery should form an integral part of any Code of Good Practice' and as such should be incorporated into infection control environmental audit.

Microwave ovens

Microwave ovens are a regular feature in many ward kitchens. Microwave ovens are open to misuse: reheating of delayed meals or food brought in by patients' visitors. Microwave ovens heat food unevenly and should never be used to heat food for neutropenic patients (Lund et al 1989, Knutson et al 1987). According to Barrie (1996) only 1000 W commercial microwave ovens should be allowed in wards. If used, the heated food should be tested with a temperature probe to ensure a temperature of 75°C or piping hot. Whether used for patients' meals or staff food, the use of microwave ovens should be rigidly controlled and they should be maintained and cleaned regularly.

Inspection of food premises

The day-to-day inspection of kitchens and food handling areas rests with the hospital staff involved in food management. A more structured and official inspection is recommended by the Department of Health (DHSS 1986). The inspection should be carried out twice a year by hospital management, the catering manager, the infection control personnel, a member of the estates department and, possibly, the consultant in communicable diseases control (CCDC). The environmental health officers carry out their inspection according to the Food Safety Act (1990) Code of Practice No. 8: Food Hygiene Inspections (DoH 1990). Full reports of these inspections are submitted to the hospital's Chief Executive and the Infection Control Committee.

Rehabilitation, milk kitchens, diet kitchens

Some patients are encouraged to cook as part of their rehabilitation programme, or as members of the team in a community home. In some instances, the guidance or the policy on food hygiene might have to be modified. Healthcare staff associated with these activities need to be aware of their own responsibilities and obtain advice as necessary.

The preparation of milk feeds should be carried out in dedicated milk kitchens if possible. Milk is an ideal growth medium for many pathogenic bacteria. Contamination of milk feeds can occur as a result of inadequate disinfection of feeding bottles, teats, mixing or dispensing equipment or from the hands of staff. Warming the feed in a contaminated sink or container can also result in the contamination of the feed.

Commercially prepared presterilized infant feeds are now used. Where local feed preparation continues, staff should receive training on:

- techniques of feed preparation to include thorough cleaning of equipment
- personal hygiene, especially handwashing
- placing of feed in the refrigerator (at 4°C) within 30 min
- discarding unsterilized milk after 24 h
- thorough cleaning and drying of containers used to warm the feed
- thorough cleaning of reusable bottles and teats to remove feed residue

- the correct strength of disinfectant, if local disinfection practised:
  - hypochlorite 125 p.p.m. available chlorine is recommended (Babb 1996)
  - the solution should be mixed freshly each day; the date and time of mixing should be charted
  - removal of air bubbles and total immersion of teats and bottles for 1 h
  - careful removal of bottles and teats following disinfection; they should be checked for integrity before use.

Kitchens where specialist diets are prepared require a higher level of awareness of hygiene regulations and practice. All specialist kitchens should be included in routine inspections.

ENVIRONMENTAL CONTROLS

Operating rooms

The majority of postoperative infections in wounds, other than clean wounds, appear to be from endogenous sources, that is, from the patient's own flora. The operating room environment can influence some surgical wound infection and this suggests that a degree of environmental control is necessary (Holton & Ridgeway 1993).

Ventilation

The operating room ventilation serves a dual purpose of preventing infection of the patient's wound and providing a comfortable atmosphere for the surgical team to work in. The primary source of bacteria in the operating room is the people. Microbial contamination in the form of skin scales is generated through the physical activities of staff members. The concentration of bacteria has been found to be proportional to activity and numbers of people in the room (Hambraeus & Laurell 1980, Lidwell et al 1967).

Although most people disperse bacteria of low pathogenicity, approximately 10% of men and 1% of women also disperse *Staphylococcus aureus*, which is associated with wound infections from exogenous sources. It is generally accepted that microorganisms in the air of operating rooms are associated with infections in prosthetic joint surgery (Lidwell et al 1983). The air movement in operating rooms is designed to curtail the transfer of bacteria from less clean to clean areas and to reduce the airborne bacterial contamination. Only a small number of bacteria are required to produce deep infections in orthopaedic surgery. Here, an ultra-clean air system that allows a further reduction of airborne contamination is generally used.

Tuberculosis: isolation room requirements

Guidance for the management of patients suspected or confirmed with pulmonary tuberculosis suggests that, based on UK data, aerosol transmission can normally be prevented by isolation of patients in a single room.

Such isolation is preferably combined with measures to stop airflow to other patient areas using negative pressure ventilation.

Because of the known possibility of transmission of infection from and to HIV-infected patients and the seriousness of multidrug-resistant tuberculosis, additional precautions for patients in these categories should be considered on a case by case basis (DoH 1996).

A national survey undertaken to assess if practices were consistent with the new guidance found that only 35% of Trusts had access to negative pressure facilities for the isolation of infectious patients (Wiggam & Hayward 2000).

REFERENCES

Abbott JO, Hepner ED, Clifford C 1960 Salmonella infections in hospital. A report from the Public Health Laboratory Service Salmonella Subcommittee. Journal of Hospital Infection 1:307–314

Advisory Committee on Dangerous Pathogens (ACDP) 1990 HIV – the causative agent of AIDS and related conditions, 2nd revision of guidelines. HMSO, London

Albert RK, Condie F 1981 Handwashing patterns in medical intensive care units. New England Journal of Medicine 304:1465–1466

Anon 1984 Needlestick transmission of HTLV-III from a patient infected in Africa. Lancet ii:1376–1377

Anon 1993 Needle safety update. Hospital Infection Control 20:49–57

Anon 1999 Reviews Minerva. British Medical Journal 319:1080

Ansari SA, Springthorpe VS, Sattar SA et al 1991 Comparison of cloth, paper and warm air drying in eliminating viruses and bacteria from washed hands. American Journal of Infection Control 19:243–249

Axnic KJ, Yarborough M 1984 Infection control: an integrated approach. CV Mosby, St Louis

Ayliffe GAJ, Babb JR, Quoraishi AH 1978 A test for hygienic hand disinfection. Journal of Clinical Pathology 31:923–928

Ayliffe GAJ, Coates D, Hoffman PN 1984 Chemical disinfection in hospitals. PHLS, London

Babb JR 1996 Application of disinfectants in hospitals and other health care establishments. Infection Control Journal of South Africa 1(1):4–12

Barrett-Connor B 1978 Epidemiology for infection control nurses. CV Mosby, St Louis

Barrie D 1996 The provision of food and catering services in hospital. Journal of Hospital Infection 33:13–33

Bauer TM, Ofner E, Just HM, Daschner FD 1990 An epidemiological study assessing the relative importance of airborne and direct contact transmission of microorganisms in a medical intensive care unit. Journal of Hospital Infection 15:301–310

Bennett JV, Brachman PS 1979 Hospital infections. Little Brown, Boston, MA

British Medical Association (BMA) 1990 A code of practice for the safe use and disposal of sharps. BMA Publications, London

British Standards Institution (BSI) 1990 Specification for sharps containers. BS 7320, HCC/34. BSI, London

Bryan CS 1986 Of soap and Semmelweis. Infection Control 7(9):445–447

Casewell M, Phillips I 1977 Hands as a route of transmission of *Klebsiella* species. British Medical Journal ii:1315–1317

Centers for Disease Control (CDC) 1987 Recommendations for prevention of HIV transmission in health-care settings. Morbidity and Mortality Weekly Report 36(suppl 2S):S1–S18

Centers for Disease Control (CDC) 1988 Update: universal precautions for prevention of transmission of human immunodeficiency virus, hepatitis B virus, and other blood-borne pathogens in health care settings. Morbidity and Mortality Weekly Report 37:337–384, 387–388

Chin P, Davies DG 1978 Hand flora. Journal of Hygiene 77:93–96

Cowan ME, Allen J, Pilkington F 1995 Small dishwashers for hospital ward kitchens. Journal of Hospital Infection 29:227–231

Cruickshank JG 1984 The investigation of salmonella outbreaks in hospitals. Journal of Hospital Infection 5:241–242

Daschner FD, Frey P, Wolff G et al 1982 Nosocomial infections in intensive care wards: a multicentre prospective study. Intensive Care Medicine 8:5–9

Department of Health (DoH) 1987 Used sharps disposal. Safety Information Bulletin SIB(87)31. DoH, London

Department of Health (DoH) 1989 Guidelines on cook–chill and cook–freeze catering systems. HMSO, London

Department of Health (DoH) 1990 Food Safety Act 1990. HMSO, London

Department of Health (DoH) 1992 Management of food services and food hygiene in the National Health Service (HSG(92)34). HMSO, London

Department of Health (DoH) 1995a Food safety (general food hygiene) regulations. Food hygiene (general) regulations. HMSO, London

Department of Health (DoH) 1995b Food Safety 1995 (Temperature Control) Regulations 1958. Food Hygiene (Amendment) Regulations. HMSO, London

Department of Health (DoH) 1995c Food handlers: fitness to work. Guidance for food businesses, enforcement officers and health professionals. HMSO, London

Department of Health (DoH) 1996 The Interdepartmental Working Group on Tuberculosis. The prevention and control of tuberculosis in the United Kingdom: recommendations for the prevention and control of tuberculosis at a local level. DoH, Wetherby

Department of Health (DoH) 2001 The EPIC Project: developing national evidence based guidelines for preventing healthcare associated infections. Journal of Hospital Infection 47(suppl):S1–S82

Department of Health and Social Security (DHSS) 1976 Dishwashing in hospital wards. Domestic Services Management Advice Note No. 2. HMSO, London

Department of Health and Social Security (DHSS) 1986 The report of the Committee of Inquiry into the outbreak of food poisoning at Stanley Royd Hospital. HMSO, London

Emmerson AM, Enstone JE, Griffin M et al 1996 The second prevalence survey of infection in hospitals – overview of the results. Journal of Hospital Infection 32:175–190

Gerberding JL, Lewis FR, Schecter WP 1995 Are universal precautions realistic? Special Clinics of North America 75(6):1091–1105

Greaves A 1985 'We'll freshen you up dear ... '. Nursing Times 81(10)(suppl):3–6

Guenthner SH, Owen Hendley J, Wenzel RP 1987 Gram-negative bacilli as nontransient flora on hands of hospital personnel. Journal of Clinical Microbiology 25:488–490

Hambraeus A, Laurell G 1980 Protection of the patient in the operating suite. Journal of Hospital Infection 1:15–30

Health Service Advisory Committee 1992 Safe disposal of clinical waste. HMSO, London

Heptonstall J, Gill ON, Porter K et al 1993 Health care workers and HIV: surveillance of occupationally acquired infection in the United Kingdom. CDR Review (3)11/PHLS, London

Hoffman PN, Cooke EM, McCarville MR, Emmerson AM 1985 Microorganisms isolated from skin under wedding rings worn by hospital staff. British Journal of Medicine 290:206–207

Holmes OW 1843/1936 The contagiousness of puerperal fever. Reprinted (1936). In: Medical classics. Williams & Wilkins, Baltimore, MD, vol 1, 211–243

Holton J, Ridgeway GL 1993 Commissioning operating theatres. Journal of Hospital Infection 23:153–160

Infection Control Nurses Association (ICNA) 1999 Guidelines for hand hygiene. ICNA, Edinburgh

Infection Control Standards Working Party (ICSWP) 1993 Standards in infection control in hospitals. PHLS, London

Jacobson G, Thiele JE, McCune JH, Farrel LD 1985 Handwashing: ring wearing and number of microorganisms. Nursing Research 31:186–188

Jarvis WR 1994 Handwashing – the Semmelweis lesson forgotten? Lancet 344(12):1311–1312

Johanson WG 1969 Changing pharyngeal bacteria in hospital patients. New England Journal of Medicine 28:1137–1140

Joseph CA, Palmer SR 1989 Outbreaks of salmonella infection in hospitals in England and Wales 1978–1987. British Medical Journal 298:1161–1164

Joynson DHM 1978 Bowls and bacteria. Journal of Hygiene (Cambridge) 80:423–425

Knight B, Evans C, Barrass S, McHardy B 1993 Hand drying: a survey of efficiency and hygiene. The Applied Ecology Research Group, University of Westminster, London

Knittle MA, Eitzman DV, Baer H 1975 Role of hand contamination of personnel in the epidemiology of Gram-negative nosocomial infections. Journal of Paediatrics 86:433–437

Knutson KM, Martin EH, Wagner WK 1987 Microwave heating of food. Food Science Technology 20:101–110

Larson E 1988 A causal link between handwashing and risk of infection? Examination of evidence. Infection Control 9:28–36

Larson E, Killian M 1982 Factors influencing handwashing behaviour of patient care personnel. American Journal of Infection Control 10:93–99

Larson EL, Oram MT, Hedrick E 1988 Nosocomial infection rates as an indicator of quality. Medical Care 26(7):676–684

Larson E, Butz AM, Gullette DL, Laughton BA 1990 Alcohol for surgical scrubbing? Infection Control and Hospital Epidemiology 11:139–140

Lidwell OM et al 1967 Comparison of three ventilation systems in an operating theatre. Journal of Hygiene (Cambridge) 65:193–205

Lidwell OM et al 1983 Airborne contamination of wounds in joint replacement operations: the relation to sepsis rates. Journal of Hospital Infection 4:111–113

Lilly HA, Lowbury EJL 1978 Transient skin flora. Journal of Clinical Pathology 31:919–922

Lilly HA, Lowbury FJL, Wilkins MD, Zaggy A 1979 Delayed antimicrobial effects of skin disinfection by alcohol. Journal of Hygiene (London) 82:497–500

Litsky BY 1971 Germs make trouble when nurses make beds. Modern Nursing Homes 27(5):52–56

Lund BM, Knox MR, Cole MB 1989 Destruction of *Listeria monocytogenes* during microwave cooking. Lancet i:218

Lynch P, Jackson MM, Cummings MJ, Stamm E 1987 Rethinking the role of isolation practices in the prevention of nosocomial infections. Annals of Internal Medicine 107:243–246

Lynch P, Cummings MJ, Roberts PL et al 1990 Implementing and evaluating a system of generic infection precautions: body substance isolation. American Journal of Infection Control 18:1–12

Marc LaForce F 1993 The control of infections in hospitals: 1750 to 1950. In: Wenzel RP (ed) Prevention and control of nosocomial infections, 2nd edn. Williams & Wilkins, Baltimore, MD

Mbithi JN, Springthorpe S, Boulet JR, Sattar SA 1992 Survival of hepatitis A virus on human hands and its transfer on contact with animate and inanimate surfaces. Journal of Clinical Microbiology 30:757–763

McGinley KJ, Larson EL, Leyden JJ 1988 Composition and density of microflora in the subungual space of the hand. Journal of Clinical Microbiology 26:950–953

McGuckin M, Waterman R, Storr J, Bowler ICJW 2001 Evaluation of a patient-empowering hand hygiene programme in the UK. Journal of Hospital Infection 48(3):222–227

Mims CA, Playfair JHL, Roitt IM et al 1993 Medical microbiology. Mosby Year Book Europe, London

Moolenaar RL, Crutcher JM, San Joaquin VH et al 2000 A prolonged outbreak of *Pseudomonas aeruginosa* in a neonatal intensive care unit: did staff fingernails play a role in disease transmission? Infection Control and Hospital Epidemiology 21(2):80–85

National Health Service Executive (NHSE) 2001 Controls assurance standard: catering and food hygiene. NHSE, London

Noble WC 1962 The dispersal of staphylococci in hospitals. Journal of Clinical Pathology 15:552–558

Noble WC (ed) 1993 The skin microflora and microbial skin disease. Cambridge University Press, Cambridge

Noble WC, Davis RR 1965 Studies on the dispersal of staphylococci. Journal of Clinical Pathology 10:16–19

Noone MR, Pitt TL, Bedder M et al 1983 *Pseudomonas aeruginosa* colonisation in an intensive therapy unit: role of cross infection and host factors. British Medical Journal 286:341–344

Painter MJ 1995 Chairman's forward to food handlers: fitness to work. DoH, London

Palmer SR, Rowe B 1983 Investigation of outbreaks of *Salmonella* in hospitals. British Medical Journal 287:291–293

Paulssen J, Eidem T, Kristiansen R 1988 Perforations in surgeons' gloves. Journal of Hospital Infection 11:82–85

Peacock JE, Marsik FJ, Wenzel RP 1988 Methicillin-resistant *Staphylococcus aureus*: introduction and spread within a hospital. Annals of Internal Medicine 93:526–532

Pittet D et al 2000 Effectiveness of a hospital-wide programme to improve hand hygiene. Lancet 356:1307–1312

Pugliese G, Favero MS 2001 Medical news: alcohol rubs. CDC's new hand-hygiene guidelines. Infection Control and Hospital Epidemiology 22(1):56–57

Redway K, Knights B, Bozoky Z et al 1994 Hand drying: bacterial types associated with different hand drying methods and with hot air dryers. The Applied Ecology Research Group, University of Westminster, London

Reybrouck G 1983 Role of hands in the spread of nosocomial infections. 1. Journal of Hospital Infection 4:103–110

Reybrouck G 1986 Handwashing and hand disinfection. Journal of Hospital Infection 8:5–23

Salisbury DM, Hutfilz P, Treen LM et al 1997 The effect of rings on microbial load of health care workers' hands. American Journal of Infection Control 25:24–27

Sanderson PJ, Weissler S 1992 Recovery of coliforms from the hands of nurses and patients: activities leading to contamination. Journal of Hospital Infection 21:85–93

Sanderson PJ, Alshafi KM 1995 Environmental contamination by organisms causing urinary-tract infection. Journal of Hospital Infection 29:301–303

Schaberg DR, Haley RW, Highsmith AK et al 1980 Nosocomial bacteriuria: a prospective study of case clustering and antimicrobial resistance. Annals of Internal Medicine 93:420–425

Scottish Centre for Infection and Environmental Health (SCIEH) 1994 Management of clinical waste and heat treatment processes. An advisory paper for Scotland (NHS MEL(1994)88). SCIEH, Glasgow

Semmelweis I 1861 The aetiology, the concept, and the prophylaxis of childbed fever. Hartlenben's Verlag-Expedition, Pest, CA

Shanson DC 1999 Microbiology in clinical practice, 3rd edn. Butterworth Heinemann, Oxford

Shooter RA, Smith MA, Griffiths JD 1958 Spread of staphylococci in surgical wards. British Medical Journal 1:607–613

Taylor L 1978 An evaluation of handwashing techniques 1. Nursing Times 74:54–55

UK Health Departments 1993 Protecting health care workers and patients from hepatitis B. Recommendations of the Advisory Group on Hepatitis. HMSO, London

Wenzel RP, Pfaller MA 1991 Handwashing: efficacy versus acceptance. A brief essay. Journal of Hospital Infection 18(suppl B):65–68

Wiggam SL, Hayward SL 2000 Hospitals in England are failing to follow guidance for tuberculosis infection control – results of a national survey. Journal of Hospital Infection 46:257–262

Williams E, Buckles A 1988 A lack of motivation. Nursing Times/Journal of Infection Control Nursing 84(22):63–64

Williams R, Blowers R, Garrod LP, Shooter R 1960 Hospital infection. Lloyd Luke, London

Wolinsky E, Lipsitz PJ, Mortimer EA et al 1960 Transmission of staphylococci between newborns: direct versus indirect transmission. Lancet ii:620–622

Portals of entry

10

■ CONTENTS

SUMMARY

This chapter considers how microbes enter the susceptible host and the actions necessary to prevent this happening.

INTRODUCTION

Many care professionals' work activities and procedures carry a risk of infection, either to patients or to the practitioners themselves. The essence of safe practice is 'knowing' the consequences of each action or inaction. Patient care activities, based on knowledge, can be described as 'informed' care.

The introduction to infection control starts with the understanding of the principles of practice, that is, what, when and how actions are to be taken and where these principles can be applied.

Understanding the principles that govern each action is the first stage in becoming a safe practitioner and providing quality care. According to Larson et al (1988) 'there is a core of practices that are within the control of carers and that modify the patient's risk of developing infection'. Choosing to ignore the application of certain basic steps that should be the principle underlying each practice can predispose the patient to the risk of acquiring an infection. A failure to carry out safe practice knowingly can be interpreted as a desire to harm those under care. Quality care is assured when the healthcare worker is able to make explicit the hazard associated with each practice.

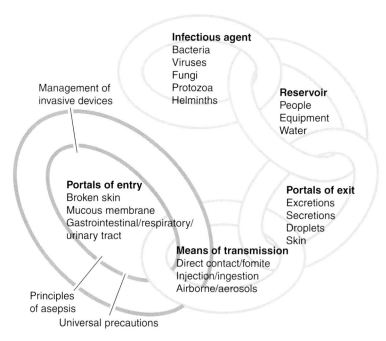

Figure 10.1 Breaking the chain of infection: portals of entry.

PRINCIPLES OF ASEPSIS

Adherence to the principles of asepsis suggests that every effort has been made to:

- guarantee the safety of the equipment used (correct decontamination processes)
- reduce the level of microbial contamination of the site requiring manipulation (antisepsis)
- ensure that no microorganisms are introduced (asepsis).

Antisepsis is the reduction of the number of microorganisms already present on the body site prior to a procedure. An alcohol-based antiseptic such as chlorhexidine or povidone–iodine is generally used to reduce the skin flora before surgery. Wound cleansing during ward dressing procedures is recommended only if it is dirty, when lotions such as sterile water or normal saline are sufficient.

Asepsis suggests a procedure designed to prevent any introduction of microorganisms to the site and is achieved by a non-touch technique and use of sterile gloves.

SURGICAL WOUND INFECTIONS

For a postoperative patient, the ideal outcome is the cure of the condition, primary healing and an uneventful recovery. Surgical wound complications result in human suffering, extended hospital stay and treatment that

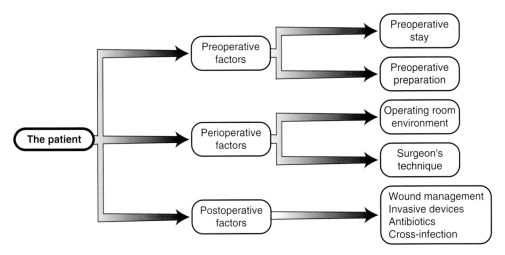

Figure 10.2 External factors responsible for surgical wound and other infections.

consume scarce resources and lead to patients' loss of income and productivity (Cruse 1992, Plowman et al 2000).

Surgical wound infections accounted for 18.9% of hospital-acquired infections in the 1980 prevalence survey (Meers et al 1981) and 10.7% in 1993–94 (Emmerson et al 1996). Early discharge and day surgery could account for the lower figure in the latter survey. Many infections develop following patients' discharge. Postdischarge infection rates have been found to range from 21 to 84% (Law et al 1990). The implications of earlier discharge and day surgery have not yet been assessed, but could be substantial.

The length of inpatient stay increases significantly in patients with surgical wound infections. The average length of stay is said to range from 5 days to 20.5 days (Bremmelgaard et al 1989). Mishriki and colleagues (1992) identified an extra 480 days in a surgical wound survey of 1242 consecutive patients where 83 became infected. Most factors associated with the development of surgical wound infections are outside the control of nurses (Fig. 10.2).

Classification of surgical wounds

The risk of infection in surgical wounds is dependent upon the contamination that occurs at the time of surgery and the ability of the body to resist that contamination. Wounds are categorized according to the level of contamination:

- Clean wounds: operations in which a viscus is not opened. This category also includes a non-traumatic, uninfected wound where no inflammation is encountered and where no break in technique has occurred
- Clean–contaminated wounds: a viscus is entered but without spillage of contents. Also included in this category are non-traumatic wounds where a minor break-in technique has occurred
- Contaminated wounds: a viscus is entered and gross spillage occurs or a fresh traumatic wound from a relatively clean source results in the

patient being admitted via Accident and Emergency (A&E). Acute non-purulent inflammation might also be encountered
• Dirty wounds: old traumatic wounds from a dirty source, with delayed treatment, devitalized tissue, clinical infection, faecal contamination or foreign body (Altmeier 1979, Ayliffe & Lowbury 1982, National Research Council of Medical Sciences (NRC) 1964).

Preoperative factors

A direct link between the length of preoperative stay and succeeding wound infections has been well established (Table 10.1). Two possible explanations are that:

1. patients requiring an extended preoperative stay are likely to be debilitated, or present with a coexisting illness
2. preoperative stay results in lowering a patient's resistance or increased pathogenic skin contamination (Mishriki et al 1992).

There is a strong association between preoperative shaving and wound infection (Table 10.2). Studies have shown a wound infection rate of 5.6% in shaved patients as opposed to 1% in those not shaved or using depilatory cream.

Dry, and sometimes clumsy, razor shaving damages the deeper layers of skin, causing bleeding or wound exudates that act as a medium for bacterial growth. Abrasions and damage to the dermal layer from shaving remain a tradition. The reasons for shaving are often purely aesthetic, or to allow easy changes of postoperative wound dressings. If hair removal is unavoidable, shaving should be completed *immediately* before surgery to prevent bacterial multiplication in the serum oozing from the damaged skin.

Table 10.1 Relation between number of preoperative days and likelihood of infection (Cruse 1992)

Number of days	Percentage of wounds infected
1	1.1
7	2.1
14 or more	3.4

Table 10.2 Relationship between shaving and wound infection rate in clean surgery (Cruse 1992)

Shaving	Percentage of infection
Razor shaving (2 hours preoperative)	2.3
Hair clipped	1.7
Neither shaving nor clipping	0.9

Perioperative factors

The majority of postoperative infections in wounds, other than clean wounds, appear to be from endogenous sources, that is, from the patient's own flora. Environmental control is necessary within the operating room to reduce the risk of wound infection, as the primary source of bacteria in the operating room is the people. Microbial contamination is generated through the physical activities of the staff. The concentration of bacteria has been found to be proportional to activity and numbers of people (HIS Working Party 2001).

Sterility of instruments

Sterility is a process that kills all microorganisms. Sterilization is necessary if the instrument penetrates intact skin or mucous membranes, enters sterile body cavities or is in contact with a breach in the skin or mucous membrane. Efficient sterile services departments serve most operating rooms. It is necessary for all staff to check the integrity of sterile packages.

Processing of some heat-labile items, for example, endoscopes, is often carried out by theatre personnel and it is imperative that they are appropriately trained before taking on such an important responsibility.

Duration of surgery

A report on the incidence of wound infection in England and Wales (Public Health Laboratory Service (PHLS) 1960) identified a direct link between the length of the operation and the infection rate. This was further supported in a report by the National Research Council (NRC 1964). Cruse (1992) provides the following explanations:

- bacterial contamination increases with time
- the tissues in the operative area are damaged by drying and retractors
- a longer operation is usually associated with increased use of sutures and electrocoagulation, which reduces the local resistance of the wound
- longer procedures are more likely to be associated with blood loss and shock, thereby reducing the general resistance of the patient.

Use of sutures and drains

The number of microorganisms required to produce infection is lowered substantially in the presence of sutures, clips and staples (Edlich et al 1973). Wound drains are useful in reducing dead space and preventing collection of blood, exudates or other body fluid (haematoma) that could act as a culture medium. Drains can be an entry point for bacteria down to the tip of the (open) drain or, in cases of closed drains, introduce a foreign body reaction and increase the risk of infection.

Skill of the surgeon

A very significant association has been identified between the skill of the operator and the wound infection rate (Cruse & Foord 1980). Wounds are said to heal without complication when there is gentle handling of tissue, careful haemostasis, adequate blood supply, removal of devitalized tissue, absolute reduction of dead space and wound closure without tension.

Drapes

Body drapes

These are used to create a barrier between the wound site and the patient's own skin bacteria and to keep the patient warm. A 'bacterial strike-through' has been shown to occur with cotton drapes (Beck & Collette 1952). Cruse (1992) suggests a layer of sterile plastic on the thigh under cotton drapes. This inexpensive draping has been shown to be as effective as expensive disposable drapes.

Incision drapes

These comprise a thin plastic adhesive film placed over the skin at the site of operation and incised through. Studies have shown little benefit of these drapes (Lilly et al 1970, Raahave 1976). In fact, Cruse (1992) quotes a 1.5% infection rate in clean surgery using cotton drapes that increased to 2.3% when plastic adhesive drapes were used in addition. French et al (1976) have shown a reduction in the level of bacterial contamination when plastic drapes were used. Plastic drapes have not been shown to significantly reduce the frequency of wound sepsis (Cruse & Foord 1980, Maxwell et al 1969, Paskin & Lerner 1969).

Wound edge drapes

These are used to drape the wound edge. The main source of bacteria entering the wound is thought to be at or close to the wound (Whyte 1988). Wound edge drapes are thought to prevent bacteria at the edge of the skin from getting into the wound (Raahave 1976).

Postoperative factors

Infections in a surgical unit are not limited to wound infections; virtually any body system can be affected. Consideration of postoperative factors should include practices and treatments that could result in an adverse outcome.

Wound dressing material

Wounds can readily acquire bacteria and need to be covered. The protection provided by the traditional dressings such as dry gauze and Gamgee is limited in the presence of wound exudates. Modern dressings, such as hydrogel and hydrocolloids, provide a moist environment that improves wound epithelialization and granulation. They are impermeable to bacteria but allow moisture vapour to escape and retain heat and the antimicrobial effect of wound exudates. Polymer films, used as primary adhesive transparent dressings, also maintain the moist environment and wound exudates and are equally effective.

Aseptic technique

Almost all clinical areas will boast their own individual wound dressing technique. There is little scientific basis for these procedures. The intention of the dresser is to keep the bacterial contamination low. The level of air-borne bacterial contamination of the immediate surroundings during wound dressing is considerably lower with hydrocolloid dressings than with conventional absorbent cotton wool or gauze (Lawrence 1994). Irrespective of the type of dressing used, the question should always be asked 'Is it necessary?'

Antibiotics

The role of antibiotics as both prophylaxis and therapy in surgical patients in minimizing morbidity and mortality is well established. The development of resistance by many bacteria has generated different and serious problems for both patients and the clinical environment.

Cross-infection

Cross-contamination and infection of wounds occur periodically. The infection control team (ICT) constantly monitors surveillance of alert organisms and alert conditions.

Infection rates in clean operations are likely to become one measure of effectiveness of an infection control programme in surgery (DoH 2001a). If surgical wound infections are to become a benchmark for successful infection control practice, then nurses need to be involved in the effectiveness debate by making a positive and 'informed' contribution.

MANAGEMENT OF INVASIVE DEVICES

Infection prevention in relation to the genitourinary system

The genitourinary tract is the most common site of infection both in hospitals and the wider community. Urinary catheterization is an essential component of patient care. It is estimated that, in a district general hospital (DGH) up to 2500 patients are catheterized over a 12-month period (Mulhall et al 1988). Patients with long-term catheters make up approximately 4% of the community nursing caseload and up to 28% of those in residential care (Getliffe 1990, Ouslander 1987, Roe & Brocklehurst 1987).

Urethral catheterization is associated with many complications, the most important being urinary tract infection (UTI); 86% of UTIs are said to be associated with instrumentation, usually catheterization (Roe et al 1986, Slade & Gillespie 1985). The 1994 prevalence survey (Emmerson et al 1996) found 23.2% of hospital-acquired infections to be those of the urinary tract. Other complications include significant bacteriuria (Mulhall et al 1988), septic complications with significant patient mortality (Murphy et al 1983), urethral strictures, pressure necrosis, encrustation, blockage, bypassing and spasm (Blandy 1980, Kennedy & Brocklehurst 1982, Roe & Brocklehurst 1987). There is also a potential for creating a reservoir for multiple-resistant organisms, and this has implications both for the patient and for the organization. Highly toxic and expensive antibiotic therapies have to be used because the resistance of the organisms reduces the choice.

National evidence-based guidelines include guidance for preventing infections associated with the insertion and maintenance of short-term indwelling urethral catheters in acute care (DoH 2001b). They cover issues of:

- assessing the need for catheterization
- selection of catheter type
- aseptic catheter insertion
- catheter maintenance.

Reasons why catheterized patients develop infection

Falkiner (1993) lists the following reasons why catheterized patients develop UTIs:

- a catheter is a foreign body
- the catheter interferes with the normal process of urine excretion and continual flushing effect
- the catheterized bladder becomes a continuous culture apparatus
- the reservoir of urine in the bladder (approximately 20 ml) is continually reinoculated with urethral and other organisms
- formation of biofilms on the surface of catheters that have been in place for a period of time. Biofilms interfere with effective antibiotic therapy or antiseptic washouts.

The above complications would suggest that catheterization should only take place if absolutely essential. Slade & Gillespie (1985) provide the following possible indications for catheterization:

- relief of acute or chronic retention due to anatomical or physiological obstruction
- care for debilitated patients with urinary incontinence
- for complex preoperative drainage to facilitate transurethral surgery
- postoperative drainage
- paralysis and spinal injury
- bladder irrigation
- measurement of urinary output and urodynamic investigations or diagnostic purposes
- administration of cytotoxic drugs.

Slade & Gillespie (1985) have also defined what constitutes short-, medium- and long-term catheterization:

- short-term: 1–7 days, for example, for perioperative care
- medium-term: 7–28 days, for example, for postoperative catheterization for elderly orthopaedic patients
- long-term: 28 days or more.

Urinary catheterization – the system

This incorporates the catheter, drainage bag and the method of drainage. 'Closed' systems of drainage and Foley-type balloon catheters are widely used.

The catheter material

The material can be plastic, latex, Teflon-coated, hydrogel-coated latex, siliconized latex or silicone:

- plastic catheters are used for 'non-indwelling' catheterization
- latex catheters have been linked to urethral stricture formation and are not suitable for use as indwelling catheters (Belfield 1988, Blandy 1980, Burkitt et al 1986)
- hydrogel or silicone-elastomer-coated latex or silicone catheters are less susceptible to encrustation (Talja 1990) and less prone to bacterial adherence (Roberts 1993)
- silicone catheters are less irritating to the urethra but are prone to bacterial adherence (Roberts 1993, Talja 1990).

Catheter size

A narrow gauge catheter is less likely than a larger gauge catheter to cause urethral irritation. Larger catheters cause expansion of the urethra as it retreats from the source of irritation (Falkiner 1993). Bypassing and leakage of urine around the catheter can occur (Kennedy & Brocklehurst 1982, Roe 1987). Small-dimension catheters are advised:

- 12–14 Ch for females and 14–16 Ch for males
- 18 Ch if urine is concentrated or cloudy
- 18–20 Ch for long-term catheterization
- 22 Ch in the presence of blood and debris (Falkiner 1993).

The ideal lengths to avoid loops and kinks are:

- females – 25 cm
- males – 40 cm.

Balloon size

With continuous drainage, the catheterized bladder is in a permanent state of collapse. As such, it is likely to come in contact with the balloon or catheter tip, a risk that is greater with a larger balloon than a smaller one. Balloons in 10 ml and 30 ml sizes are widely available. 30 ml balloons are used in chronically catheterized women with weak pelvic muscles or applied to the prostatic bed to stop postoperative bleeding in men (Falkiner 1993).

Balloons must be filled with sterile water
Air will cause the balloon to float and tap water and saline can block the inflation channel with crystals or debris, making deflation difficult (Falkiner 1993).

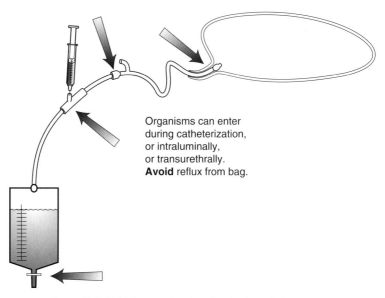

Organisms can enter
during catheterization,
or intraluminally,
or transurethrally.
Avoid reflux from bag.

Figure 10.3 Multiple entry sites in a closed urinary drainage system.

Drainage bag

Urine enters a bag through a non-return valve and is emptied through a tap at the bottom of the bag. A rubber sleeve is fitted to the bag tubing to facilitate specimen collection. The urine specimen is extracted through the rubber sleeve (although this can pose a risk of needlestick injury; alternatives are now marketed).

Closed drainage system

The closed drainage system has been available since 1928 and used routinely since the 1950s (Parker 1999).

Portals of entry

Figure 10.3 shows the potential entry points for microorganisms into a closed urinary drainage system (Garibaldi 1993, Garibaldi et al 1980, Kunin & McCormack 1966, Maizels & Schaeffer 1980, Thornton & Andriole 1970). Box 10.1 suggests how to prevent transmission of bacteria by these routes.

Intermittent self-catheterization by patients

Intermittent self-catheterization is a safe and effective way of managing patients with retention or incontinence due to neuropathic or hypotonic bladder (Hunt et al 1996). It entails insertion of a catheter into the bladder, draining out all the urine and removing the catheter. The technique can be mastered by children as young as 4 years old and adults in their 80s (Anderson & Grant 1991, Hunt & Oakshott 1993, Whitelaw et al 1987), as well as by people with spinal cord injuries, multiple sclerosis and physical

■ BOX 10.1   Urinary catheterization

Millions of patients are catheterized in a variety of care settings; always consider the alternatives before catheterizing a patient.

Preparation of the genital area

The distal urethra and the area surrounding the genitalia are normally colonized by skin and faecal flora. Thorough cleaning with an antiseptic solution is necessary prior to insertion.

A strict code of asepsis

A break in the aseptic technique can lead to the introduction of organisms into the urinary system, and can also contaminate the drainage system.

Trauma

- A lack of expertise or a large-bore catheter can result in meatal and urethral damage, leading to further colonization with hospital flora
- Use of anaesthetic gel before catheterizing women helps dilate the urethra allowing easy passage of the catheter and reducing the risk of trauma (de Courcy-Ireland 1993).

Inadequate light

Inadequate lighting, especially when catheterizing women, can result in the catheter inadvertently touching the surrounding area or being placed in the vagina (if this happens, the catheter must be discarded and the gloves changed).

Maintenance of the integrity of the drainage system

- Continuous movement of an unanchored catheter can cause sphincter damage, irritation of the urethra and also introduce organisms from the external meatus into the urinary system
- Other complications include frequent breaks in the drainage system and lack of unobstructed urine flow
- Urine specimens should be obtained from the sampling port and not by opening the catheter–drainage-tube connection.

The emptying procedure

- The bag should be emptied when it contains 500 ml urine or every 8 h, unless the patient's condition demands otherwise
- Emptying the catheter bag has been identified as creating an entry port for ascending infection (Pick 1990). Strict observance of handwashing is necessary before and after the procedure. Gloves should be worn when emptying the bag and removed on completing the procedure and hands washed. Each bag should be emptied separately as required, and not as part of a ward routine. The tap must be closed securely and wiped with a tissue to prevent environmental contamination
- The receptacle used should be heat disinfected in a bedpan washer or washed in hot water and detergent, dried and stored inverted. The use of a disposable urinal is acceptable.

■ **BOX 10.1** *(continued)*

Meatal care

Faeces, exudates or encrustation can collect around the meatal–catheter junction and become a focus for microorganisms. The site should be washed with soap and water and dried once daily and as necessary.

Duration of catheterization

There is a direct link between the duration of catheterization and increased risk of infection. Catheters should be removed as soon as possible. The risk of infection in suprapubic and intermittent catheterization is lower than in urethral catheterization (Warren 1995).

Bladder irrigation

Bladder irrigation is carried out to remove excessive blood and clots following bladder surgery or catheter blockage in long-term catheterized patients. There is little evidence to suggest that antiseptic irrigations are beneficial and Falkiner (1993) recommends sterile saline for this purpose.

Drainage bag changes

Catheter bags should be changed in case of damage or leakage, the accumulation of sediment or when the bag becomes odorous (Checko et al 1991).

Placement of drainage bags

Catheter bags should be attached to a catheter bag holder and placed below the patient's bladder. They should never be placed on the floor.

Patient education

Education of patients about their catheters has been shown to have a significant effect on patients' knowledge and acceptance (Roe 1987, 1993).

---

disabilities (Hill & Davies 1988, Hunt et al 1984, Hunt & Whittaker 1990, Lapides et al 1976, Robinson et al 1985, Webb et al 1990). Hunt et al (1996) provide the following positive effects of intermittent catheterization:

- the bladder can empty completely and under the patient's control
- residual urine is eliminated, so reducing symptomatic urinary infections
- urinary drainage is ensured, so preventing or improving dilatation of the upper urinary tract.

A clean rather than aseptic technique is advocated. A clean procedure with minimal time of the catheter in the bladder and drinking more than 2 litres of fluid a day is recommended (McSweeney 1989).

A number of studies have advocated the drinking of cranberry juice for the prevention of UTI. It is suggested that cranberry juice provides an alternative approach for prevention of UTI that could result in decreased use of antimicrobials (Kontiokari et al 2001).

Infection prevention in relation to the vascular system

Numerous comprehensive papers have been written on this subject (Elliott 1993, Goodinson 1990a,b,c, Hamilton 1993, Haynes 1989, Henderson 1995, Johnson 1994, Keenlyside 1992, Livesley 1993, Oldman 1991, Rotstein et al 1995, Wilkinson 1991, 1996, Wilson 1994).

Intravenous therapy is an important adjunct to the total management of many patients. It is used both in the hospital and community setting to:

- administer i.v. solutions, medication, blood products, total parenteral nutrition (TPN)
- monitor critically ill patients
- obtain blood specimens.

Intravenous therapy is extremely common. A multicentre study undertaken by Nystrom et al (1983) found that of 10 616 surgical patients investigated, 63% had an intravenous device inserted while in hospital. Wilkinson (1996) estimated that between 18 and 80% of general hospital admissions have some form of i.v. therapy, and approximately 200 000 central venous catheters (CVCs) are used annually in the UK in 1993 (Elliott 1993).

Complications of intravenous devices

The complications include thrombophlebitis and chemical phlebitis, extravasation (tissuing), localized infections, bacteraemia and septicaemia.

Thrombophlebitis

Thrombophlebitis is defined as 'an acute inflammation of a vein receiving fluids and is characterized by erythema, pain, swelling and development of a palpable venous cord (cording)' (Lodge & Brennan 1987). It occurs in 75% of all hospitalized patients receiving intravenous therapy. The inflammation response is said to correlate with the amount of bacterial adherence to the cannula. Thrombophlebitis can be reduced by attention to asepsis during insertion.

Chemical phlebitis

High or low acid pH, osmolality of infusate, cannula composition and intravenous medication as well as particulate matter can all predispose to chemical phlebitis (Goodinson 1990c, Lodge & Brennan 1987).

Extravasation (tissuing)

Extravasation is thought to be related to the nature and volume of fluids used as well as the gauge of the cannula. The aetiology of extravasation is said to be either:

- vasoconstriction due to the irritation of the endothelium by the infusate, which restricts the flow and results in a rise in intraluminal pressure
- a rupture of the vein wall or accidental removal of the cannula tip from the vein (Hecker et al 1984, Lodge & Brennan 1987).

Localized infections

Localized infections are associated with erythema, oedema, purulent exudates and tenderness during manipulation. There might be tenderness at the site, especially during catheter manipulation. Erythema, oedema and cellulites along the subcutaneous tract of a tunnelled device can also be encountered (Elliott 1993).

Bacteraemia

In 1991, 4000 cases of line-associated bacteraemia were reported (Elliott 1993).

Septicaemia

Between 0.2 and 8% of patients receiving an intravenous infusion develop septicaemia (Shanson 1999). Intravenous catheter-related sepsis has been reported to range from 0 to 15% (Elliott 1993). It causes significant morbidity and mortality.

Risk factors

Henderson (1995) has suggested the following risk factors associated with the development of vascular related complications.

- Patient related:
  - age (<1 year old, >60 years old)
  - alterations in host defences:
    - loss of skin integrity
    - diminished granulocyte function
    - immunosuppression and immunodeficiency
  - severity of underlying illness
  - presence of distant infection
- Hospital related:
  - catheter material
  - catheter type and function
  - location of catheter
  - type of placement (percutaneous versus cut-down)
  - duration of placement
  - emergency versus elective placement
  - skill of the operator
  - alteration of microflora surrounding insertion site.

Henderson (1995) states that each entry into the intravenous delivery system, be it for phlebotomy, drug administration or any other purpose, increases the risk of bacterial contamination of the system. It has been shown conclusively that repeated entry into the system is linked with catheter-associated infection.

Product-related risk factors

Many plastics are thrombogenic because of their chemical composition or their biophysical surface properties (Goodinson 1990a, Tebbs et al 1994):

- organisms are less likely to adhere to smooth than to irregular surfaces
- steel needles cause less thrombophlebitis than Teflon or silicone

- steel needles are associated with extravasation and infiltration
- antibiotic (teicoplanin)-coated central venous catheters have been found to be effective against Gram-positive and Gram-negative bacteria, although there is a potential for antibiotic resistance with these catheters
- Hickman and Broviac catheters are made of silicon elastomer. The tissue grows into the Dacron cuff, securing the catheter and preventing bacteria from skin migrating into the wound (Wilson 1994).

Catheter design

Any size of cannula can cause mechanical irritation, endothelial shearing and venospasm. But the longer and larger the cannula the greater the trauma so:

- use the smallest cannula possible
- use the thinnest possible needle
- remember that there is a higher rate of infection with triple lumen catheters than with single lumen catheters.

Access of organisms into the vein

Extraluminal and intraluminal (on the external or internal surface of the catheter)

- Skin organisms enter the insertion wound, attach to the external surface of the catheter and colonize the distal tip of the catheter
- Organisms colonizing the catheter hub can be introduced intraluminally when using a luer lock
- Colonization of the internal surface of the catheter is greater when it is used for longer periods.

Haematogenous seeding (distant infection)

Microorganisms from other sites of infection in the patient's body are transferred by the blood flow to the catheter.

Contaminated infusate resulting in bacteraemia

Intrinsic contamination of infusate is uncommon but occurs when:

- the manufacturing is faulty
- transport and storage are poor
- the use of the equipment is inappropriate.

Extrinsic contamination can occur when:

- there is poor adherence to policy
- there is poor aseptic technique
- drugs are added or inserted into the cannula
- fluid or administration sets are changed
- blood and blood products are administered.

Boxes 10.2 to 10.5 contain guidance on total intravascular therapy management.

■ **BOX 10.2** Intravenous therapy

Site
- Siting over mobile joints can lead to a risk of phlebitis and extravasation
- Catheters placed in the groin or elsewhere in the lower extremities are associated with an increased risk of infection (Henderson 1995).

Shaving
Microscopic damage from skin shaving can result in increased microbial colonization and infection (Wilson 1994).

Asepsis
Skin flora, especially *Staphylococcus epidermidis*, remains the major source of organisms in intravenous-related sepsis. Duggan et al (1985) found that 7 of 52 septicaemias (including one death) were caused by *Staphylococcus epidermidis*. The organisms can be introduced into the vein from the patient's own flora and also from the hands of the person siting the device. Before performing a cannulation:

- Ensure thorough washing of hands, either by soap and water or an alcohol handrub
- Carry out adequate preparation of the insertion site. For central venous catheters (CVCs), chlorhexidine in alcohol is recommended as the most effective antiseptic (DoH 2001b). For peripheral cannulation, alcoholic-based chlorhexidine or povodine–iodine is recommended for skin cleansing (Elliott & Faroqui 1995, Maki et al 1991), although alcohol-impregnated swabs are frequently used. The solution must be allowed to dry before siting the cannula. The components of the intravascular device, including the boot and hubs, should be observed for signs of damage, particularly from alcohol (Elliott & Faroqui 1995)
- Avoid contamination of the catheter tip during insertion.

Anchoring the catheter
Anchoring the catheter prevents trauma to the vein and reduces the risk of mechanical phlebitis. It also prevents migration of skin organisms into the wound, which can be aided by catheter movement.

Always use sterile tape or occlusive dressing and sterile scissors. Contaminated tape has been implicated in device-related infections (Bauer & Densen 1979, Oldman 1991).

Dressings
Transparent or gauze dressings can be used (Infection Control Nurses Association (ICNA) 2001). The advantages of transparent dressings are that they:

- secure the catheter
- allow for continuous inspection
- protect the site from contamination by other wounds
- allow patients to bathe or to shower
- can be left on for the lifetime of the catheter.

■ **BOX 10.2** (*continued*)

However, increased microbial colonization of the insertion site has been associated with their use. This results in localized and systemic infections, probably due to the accumulation of moisture under the dressing encouraging microbial overgrowth.

Gauze dressings reduce the risk of infection but require frequent changes and make it difficult to observe the site.

In-line filters

The role of in-line filters in the prevention of infection has yet to be established (ICNA 2001). According to guidelines (HICPAC 2001) their use is not supported by the research for infection control purposes. The main points of entry for microorganisms are the skin, insertion site and the catheter hub. In-line filters are used when administering i.v. drugs of high molecular size to reduce the risk of phlebitis and accidental air administration into the circulatory system (Falchuk et al 1985).

The advantages of in-line filters are that they:

- prevent passage of air and particulate matter in fluids and drugs
- can be used safely for 96 hours
- save costs and nursing time because the giving sets are changed every 96 hours.

  Their disadvantages are that:

- they cannot be used for blood, blood products, lipids or on Swan–Ganz catheters
- a combination of intravenous fats and other parenteral nutrition fluids limits their use in parenteral nutrition.

Frequency of dressing changes

- Manipulation of any part of the intravenous delivery system can result in contamination
- Advice on the frequency of dressing changes varies from daily to every other day to three times a week or longer
- It might be prudent to change only when the dressing fails, unless observation or condition indicates otherwise.

Handling of administration equipment

Lines frequently accessed to administer drugs and other additives are more likely to be contaminated (Maki et al 1987).

Infusion fluid is easily contaminated when:

- drugs are added or inserted into the cannula
- fluids and administration sets are changed.

Preventive measures

Skin scales adhere by electrostatic charge to plastic tubing, allowing organisms to enter the system when infusion fluids are changed (Newsome 1985).

■ **BOX 10.2** (*continued*)

Hands must be decontaminated using alcohol handrub to reduce the risk of contamination:

- wash hands before accessing lines
- do not allow intravenous line connections to touch non-sterile surfaces
- handle sterile connections with sterile gloves
- practise antiseptic cleaning of the cannula hub and stopcock before manipulation
- practise strict asepsis when introducing additives
- administer drugs through a latex membrane.

Administration sets – changing frequencies

Changing of administration sets every 24 h has been advocated by the DoH since 1972. However, many studies have demonstrated a 72-h interval between changes to be entirely safe practice (ICNA 2001, Jakobsen et al 1986, Josephson et al 1985, Maki et al 1987). For certain products (e.g. blood, blood products or lipid emulsions), which pose a greater risk of bacterial growth, the set should be changed more frequently, at least every 24 h (Jarvis & Highsmith 1984).

Duration of catheter placement

The risk of infection increases with the length of time the device remains in place. It is therefore advisable to remove a peripheral catheter every 48 to 72 h. Leaving a catheter in place for longer than 72 h significantly increases the risk of infection (Maki & Ringer 1987, Maki et al 1973, Rhame et al 1979).

Emergency versus elective insertion

Catheters inserted during an emergency are at a high risk for infection as there might be a break in aseptic technique during insertion (Henderson 1995). Catheters sited in an emergency should be resited as soon as practical.

Subcutaneous fluid administration

Administration of fluids via the subcutaneous route (also known as hypodermoclysis) is a means of managing dehydration, especially in the elderly. Commonly used in the 1940s it fell out of favour with the increased use of intravenous fluid administration (Hughes 1989). Its use is advocated for the elderly, terminally ill and others and is recommended for those unable to have intravenous fluids (Eugene & Berger 1981, Fainsinger et al 1994, Martin et al 1996).

The cannula should be sited in loose subcutaneous tissue where the needle will not be jostled (Noble-Adams 1995). Insertion should be under aseptic techniques and the site changed every 24 h (Wood 1994).

■ BOX 10.3   Central venous catheters

The skin insertion wound is a major source of contamination of central venous catheters (CVCs) (Egebo et al 1996). Multiple lumen CVCs are associated
with higher catheter-related bloodstream infections (CR-BSI) than single-lumen
CVCs. This increased risk could be associated with increased trauma at insertion
and increased manipulation of the multiple ports postinsertion (Farkas 1993,
Hilton et al 1988).

Site
The infection rate has been shown to be higher for the internal jugular site than
for the subclavian (Pinilla 1983).

Organisms commonly associated with CVC-related infections
Most skin colonizing Gram-positive organisms, such as *Staphylococcus aureus* and
Staphylococcus epidermidis, are associated with CVC-related infections. Gram-neg-
ative organisms, such as *Escherichia coli*, *Pseudomonas* species and *Klebsiella* species,
Serratia and fungi like *Candida*, are found especially in total parenteral nutrition.

Asepsis
Many epidemics of device-associated bacteraemia have been linked to hospital
staff carrying the epidemic strain of bacteria on their hands (Henderson 1995).
For this reason, insertion of CVCs should be regarded as a surgical procedure
similar to placement of prosthetic devices:

- use an antiseptic handwash
- wear sterile gloves
- apply skin antiseptic liberally, and allow it to dry. Chlorhexidine is the
  recommended agent of choice (DoH 2001b).

Duration
The replacement of CVCs is a controversial issue. Some researchers consider
duration of cannulation to be an infection risk and advocate change between 3
and 7 days, while others report little evidence of increased risk. National guidelines (DoH 2001b) recommend the following:

- Do not routinely replace non-tunnelled CVCs as a method to prevent
  catheter-related infection
- Use guide-wire-assisted catheter exchange to replace a malfunctioning
  catheter or to exchange an existing catheter if there is no evidence of
  infection at the catheter site or proven CR-BSI
- If CR-infection is suspected, but there is no evidence of infection at the
  catheter site, remove the existing catheter and insert a new catheter over a
  guide wire: if tests reveal CR-infection, the newly inserted catheter should
  be removed and, if still required, a new catheter inserted at a different site
- Do not use guide-wire-assisted catheter exchange for patients with
  CR-infection. If continued vascular access is required, remove the implicated
  catheter and replace it with another catheter at a different insertion site.

■ BOX 10.4 Total parenteral nutrition

This form of vascular therapy differs from the i.v. or central methods because:

- Parenteral infusion through peripheral infusion lines is associated with lower risk of infection and is recommended for short-term nutritional support (Hansell 1989).
- Total parenteral catheters remain in place much longer than other types of catheter and are more likely to become contaminated
- The composition of the infusate supports the growth of different microorganisms, that is, *Candida* species.
- There is an increased risk of thrombosis because of the hypertonicity of the solution. Thrombosis may result in infection.
- Patients receiving total parenteral nutrition are often suffering from severe illnesses such as neoplasm, trauma, diseases causing bowel inflammation, and so on, and are at risk from bacteraemia. The seeding of the catheter here is high.

Siting
This is as for central venous catheter placement.

Management
- The parenteral catheter should not be used for administering drugs or taking blood
- The manipulation of the catheter must be carried out using strict asepsis
- Taps or stopcocks should not be attached to the administration set
- The infusate and the giving set should be changed every 24 h using strict asepsis.

Peripheral inserted central catheters
- Single- or double-lumen central venous access devices are available in sizes ranging from 2 to 6 French gauge. These are considered suitable for total parenteral nutrition, cytotoxic chemotherapy, certain antibiotics and vesicant fluid (Brown 1989, Goodwin & Carlson 1993).
- A peripherally inserted cannula should be considered for patients requiring parenteral therapy for 5 days or more (Kyle & Myers 1989).

Stopcocks and caps

These are frequently manipulated for the administration of drugs, i.v. fluids and blood sampling. They are entry sites for microorganisms and the risk of infection cannot be ignored.

Needleless i.v. systems

These allow for the connection of syringes to i.v. catheters without the use of needles. Their introduction is primarily to prevent the risk of needlestick injury. If used correctly as instructed by manufacturers, and following strict

■ **BOX 10.5   Dialysis**

Dialysis, mainly used to treat uraemic patients, might be short or long term. Continuous ambulatory peritoneal dialysis (CAPD) is prone to both insertion site infection and peritonitis. Common skin organisms can contaminate the catheter or the alteration in the skin flora of CAPD patients can lead to peritoneal contamination with enteric pathogens. Contamination of the dialysate delivery system during bag exchanges can also lead to pathogens entering the peritoneal cavity (Levison & Bush 1995). A strict code of asepsis during catheter insertion, management of the wound and bag exchanges is paramount.

asepsis for the cleaning of ports before and after use, there should be no increased risk of infection (ICNA 2001).

Infection prevention in relation to the respiratory system

Both upper and lower respiratory tract infection are found in healthcare settings. Infections of the lower respiratory tract, especially pneumonia, carry a high mortality rate. Lower respiratory tract infections (LRTI) accounted for 22.9% of hospital-acquired infections in the 1994 Prevalence Survey (Emmerson et al 1996). Hospital-acquired chest infections can be found in any aspect of patient care but are more commonly associated with:

• intubation
• intensive care units
• antibiotics
• surgery
• chronic lung disease
• advanced age
• immunosuppression (Pennington 1995).

Endotracheal intubation for short-duration surgery or for long-term mechanical ventilation for respiratory failure is associated with a high level of hospital-acquired pneumonia (Shanson 1999). Tracheostomy is often performed on patients receiving long-term respiratory aid and it increases the risk of LRTI, especially pneumonia (Cross & Roup 1981).

Endotracheal tubes can cause irritation and injury of the respiratory mucosa, predisposing the area to colonization with potential pathogens. Endotracheal tubes bypass the natural infiltration system of the nose and the mucociliary clearance system of the airways.

Patients requiring mechanical ventilation are often critically ill with many underlying problems (such as chronic obstructive pulmonary disease, immunosuppressive diseases or diabetes). Any of the risk factors discussed earlier could be present. These patients are treated with numerous antimicrobials that can lead to pneumonia as a consequence of selection for more resistant organisms. Respiratory therapy equipment also becomes a source of bacterial contamination.

Box 10.6 outlines the principles of good respiratory therapy management.

■ BOX 10.6   Respiratory therapy management

- Segregate colonized and infected patients from other patients
- Strict hand hygiene both before and after contact with susceptible patients and equipment
- Prevention of contamination of respiratory therapy equipment. This includes:
    - face masks
    - nasal cannulae
    - tubing, for example, oral, endotracheal
    - ventilation and anaesthetic tubing
    - humidifiers
    - rebreathing bags
    - oxygen tents
    - aerosol-producing equipment, for example, nebulizers
- Consider single-use items when possible. Reusable items must be decontaminated after use, between patients and/or at time intervals every 24–48 h
- Do not routinely change ventilator circuits more frequently than every 48 h (Centers for Disease Control (CDC) 1997)
- Use of high-efficiency bacterial filters to prevent contamination of the spirometer and machinery is recommended. High-efficiency bacterial filters that provide heat/moisture exchange, instead of hot water bath humidifiers, are preferred. If hot water bath humidification is used, only sterile fluids should be used. Do not 'top up' the solution; discard the remnant of fluids before replenishing
- A specialist department should disinfect laryngoscope blades. Autoclave sterilization is the recommended method (Centers for Disease Control (CDC) 1997)
- Mini-nebulizers must be washed, dried and wiped thoroughly after each use. These are for single patient use only
- Use a plastic apron and gloves when handling secretions from infected patients
- Use of masks and protective eyewear is recommended if contamination of the face is likely during cough-inducing procedures.

Respiratory equipment as a major reservoir and source of organisms

The organisms contaminating respiratory equipment invariably originate from the ventilated patient. Most critically ill patients become colonized with Gram-negative organisms within a matter of days following admission (Pennington 1995). Humidifiers, nebulizers and disposable respiratory tubings have all been found to be contaminated.

Laryngoscope blades have been associated with *Pseudomonas aeruginosa* pneumonia and septicaemia in patients in a paediatric cardiac intensive care unit (Foweraker 1995). Laryngoscope blades were also identified as a source of *P. aeruginosa* contamination in another special care baby unit (Neal et al 1995). Dried secretions were found on the blades around the bulb, as well as in the lateral groove.

Pulmonary function test apparatus has been associated with cross-infection with tuberculosis (Hazaleus et al 1981). Nasogastric tubes have also been associated with hospital-acquired pneumonia (Veazey 1981).

Respiratory syncytial virus (RSV), which is commonly associated with bronchiolitis, frequently causes pneumonia in infants and children. Hospital-acquired RSV infections have been documented (Hall 1983) as has been the spread of hospital-acquired *Haemophilus influenzae* (Howard 1991). *Pseudomonas cepacia*, frequently found in cystic fibrosis and immunosuppressed patients, is known to be associated with slowly declining lung function. Some cystic fibrosis patients succumb to an accelerated and fatal deterioration in pulmonary function with fever, necrotizing pneumonia and septicaemia with this organism (Lancet 1992). *Pseudomonas cepacia* has also been cultured from the environmental surfaces and respiratory equipment.

CDC guidelines for the prevention of nosocomial pneumonia (CDC 1997) give the following examples of semi-critical items used on the respiratory tract. They state that if the items are directly or indirectly in contact with mucous membranes of the respiratory tract, they should be sterilized or put through high-level disinfection before reuse. Items include:

- anaesthesia device or equipment including:
  - facemask or tracheal tube
  - inspiratory and expiratory tubing
  - Y-piece
  - reservoir bag
  - humidifier
- breathing circuits of mechanical ventilators
- bronchoscopes and their accessories (biopsy forceps and specimen brushes are critical items and are sterilized before reuse)
- endotracheal and endobronchial tubes
- laryngoscope blades
- mouthpieces and tubing of pulmonary-function testing equipment
- nebulizers and their reservoirs
- oral and nasal airways
- probes of CO_2 analysers, air-pressure monitors
- resuscitation bags
- stylets
- suction catheters
- temperature sensors.

With the increased emphasis on decontamination of reuseable equipment, respiratory and anaesthetic equipment are now being considered and included in infection control policies (King & Cooke 2001).

Infection prevention in relation to the gastrointestinal system

A wide variety of pathogens is responsible for gastrointestinal infections. These include bacteria, viruses and parasites and can be confined to the upper small bowel producing non-inflammatory infection, or might produce inflammatory infection in the colon. Some enteric pathogens cause systemic infections. Commonly known as diarrhoeal disease, the symptoms of infectious gastroenteritis include nausea and/or vomiting, abdominal discomfort, cramp or pain, and fever. Diarrhoea might be accompanied by pus or blood. Gastroenteritis can affect any age of patient and can be very debilitating. The pathogens can be acquired by the faecal–oral route, that is, from faecally contaminated food, fluid or fingers. In food-associated infections, the food:

1. acts as a vehicle for the organisms as in food-borne illness
2. provides optimum conditions for bacteria to multiply and/or produce toxins as in food poisoning. *Staphylococcus aureus* in contaminated food can produce a toxin that resists destruction during food preparation. The ingested toxin can produce illness within hours of consumption.

Organisms responsible for common gastrointestinal diseases include (CDR Review 1995):

* *Bacillus* species
* *Campylobacter* species, *Clostridium perfringens, Cryptosporidium* species
* *Escherichia coli* verotoxin producing and enteropathogenic
* *Giardia* species
* Hepatitis A virus
* *Salmonella* (excluding typhoid and paratyphoid), *Shigella* species, *Staphylococcus aureus*
* Gastroenteritis viruses – rotavirus, small round-structured viruses.

Another well established cause of diarrhoeal disease in care settings is antibiotics. Antibiotics disrupt the normal gut flora, leading to recolonization of the gut. The usual anaerobes are replaced with an organism such as *Staphylococcus aureus* or *Candida*. Many broad-spectrum antibiotics inhibit the normal flora, allowing the organism *Clostridium difficile* to multiply. The toxin produced by *Clostridium difficile* produces severe diarrhoea, requiring treatment. Cross-infection amongst patients receiving antibiotic therapy is common. Outbreaks of gastrointestinal infections affecting patients and staff in care settings are well recognized. The main aim during such outbreaks is to identify the pattern of the disease and curtail its spread. The movement of staff and patients between wards and within the affected area creates an ideal environment for the spread of infection.

Enteral feeds

Contamination of enteral feeds occurs during preparation, dilution and decanting of feeds and the assembling and subsequent handling of the feeding system (Anderton 1995). Bacterial contamination of enteral feeds is thought to cause diarrhoea, pneumonia and septicaemia (Freedland et al 1989, Levy et al 1989, Navajas et al 1992, Thurn et al 1990, Veazey 1981).

Prepackaged, sterile, ready-to-use feeds have to an extent eliminated some of these risks. Safe handling of parenteral and enteral feeds is included in the guidance document of the 'Parenteral and enteral group of the British Diabetic Association' (Anderton 2000) and in a clinical review by Anderton (1995).

REFERENCES

Altmeier WA 1979 Surgical infections: incisional infections. Little Brown, Boston, MA, p 287–306

Anderson JB, Grant JBF 1991 Postoperative retention of urine: a prospective urodynamic study. British Medical Journal 302:894–896

Anderton A 1995 Reducing bacterial contamination in enteral tube feeding. Clinical review. British Journal of Nursing 4(7):368–376

Anderton A 2000 Microbial contamination of enteral tube feeds: how can we reduce the risk? The Parenteral and Enteral Nutrition Group of the British Dietetic Association. Nutricia Clinical Care Ltd, Wiltshire

Ayliffe GAJ, Lowbury EJL 1982 Hospital acquired infection: principles and prevention. Wright, Bristol

Bauer E, Densen PL 1979 Infections from contaminated elastoplast. New England Journal of Medicine 300(7):370

Beck WC, Collette TS 1952 False faith in the surgeon's gown and drape. American Journal of Surgery 83:125–126

Belfield PW 1988 Urinary catheters. British Journal of Medicine 296:836–837

Blandy JP 1988 Urethral stricture. Postgraduate Medical Journal 56:383–418

Bremmelgaard A, Raahave D, Beier-Holgersen R et al 1989 Computer-aided surveillance of surgical infections and identification of risk factors. Journal of Hospital Infection 13:1–3

Brown J 1989 Peripherally inserted central catheters – use in home care. Journal of Intravenous Nursing 12(2):144–147

Burkitt DS, Barwell NJ, Wilson AGM 1986 Urethral catheter strictures. Lancet i:688–689

Centers for Disease Control (CDC) 1997 Guidelines for prevention of nosocomial pneumonia. Morbidity and Mortality Weekly Report 46(RR-1):1–79

Checko PJ, Hierholzer WJ, Pearson DA 1991 Recommendations for urinary catheter and drainage bag changes. American Journal of Infection Control 19:255–256

Communicable Disease Report (CDR) Review 1995 The prevention of human transmission of gastrointestinal infections, infestations, and bacterial intoxications. PHLS, London

Cross AS, Roup B 1981 Role of respiratory assistance devices in endemic nosocomial pneumonia. American Journal of Medicine 70:681

Cruse PJE 1992 Classification of operations and audit of infection. In: Taylor EW (ed) Infection in surgical practice. Oxford University Press, Oxford

Cruse PJE, Foord R 1980 The epidemiology of wound infection; a ten year prospective study of 62 939 wounds. Surgical Clinics of North America 60:27–40 de Courcy-Ireland K 1993 An issue of sensitivity: use of analgesic gel in catheterizing women. Professional Nurse 8(11):738–742

Department of Health (DoH) 2001a Performance indicators for the NHS, draft document. HMSO, London

Department of Health (DoH) 2001b The EPIC project: developing national evidence-based guidelines for preventing healthcare associated infections. Journal of Hospital Infection 47(suppl):S1–S82

Duggan JM, Oldfield GS, Ghosh HK 1985 Septicaemia as a hospital hazard. Journal of Hospital Infection 6:406–412

Egebo K, Toft P, Jacobsen CJ 1996 Contamination of central venous catheters. The skin insertion wound is a major source of contamination. Journal of Hospital Infection 32:99–104

Eldlich RF, Panek PH, Rodehaever GT et al 1973 Physical and chemical configuration of sutures in the development of surgical infection. Annals of Surgery 117:679

Elliott TSJ 1993 Line-associated bacteraemia's. Communicable Disease Report 33(7):R91–R95

Elliott TSJ, Faroqui MH 1995 Letter. Journal of Hospital Infection 31(1):77–78

Emmerson AM, Enstone JE, Griffin M et al 1996 The second prevalence survey of infection in hospitals – overview of the results. Journal of Hospital Infection 32:175–190

Eugene Y, Berger MD 1981 Nutrient by hypodemodysis. Journal of the American Geriatrics Society 32(3):199–202

Fainsinger RL et al 1994 The use of hypodemodysis for rehydration in terminally ill cancer patients. Journal of Pain and Symptom Management 9(5):298–302

Falchuk KH, Peterson L, McNeil BJ 1985 Microparticulate-induced phlebitis. Its prevention by in-line filtration. New England Journal of Medicine 312(2):778–782

Falkiner FR 1993 The insertion and management of indwelling urethral catheters – minimising the risk of infection. Journal of Hospital Infection 25:79–90

Farkas JC, Lui N, Bleriot JP et al 1993 Single versus triple lumen central catheter related sepsis: a prospective randomised study in a critically ill population. American Journal of Medicine 3:277–282

Foweraker JE 1995 The laryngoscope as a potential source of cross-infection (letter). Journal of Hospital Infection 29:315–316

Freedland CP, Roller RD, Wolfe BM, Flynn NM 1989 Microbial contamination of continuous drip feedings. Journal of Parenteral and Enteral Nutrition 13:18–22

French MLV, Eitzen HE, Ritter MA 1976 The plastic surgical adhesive drape: an evaluation of its efficiency as a microbial barrier. Annals of Surgery 184:46–50

Garibaldi RA 1993 Hospital acquired urinary tract infections. In: Wenzel RP (ed) Prevention and control of nosocomial infections, 2nd edn. Williams & Wilkins, Baltimore, MD, p 600–613

Garibaldi RA, Burke JP, Britt Miller WA, Smith CB 1980 Meatal colonization and catheter-associated bacteriuria. New England Journal of Medicine 303:316–318

Getliffe KA 1990 Catheter blockage in community patients. Nursing Standard 5:33–36

Goodinson SM 1990a The risk of IV therapy. Professional Nurse 5(5):235–238

Goodinson SM 1990b Reducing risk of infection in IV therapy. Professional Nurse 5(11):572–575

Goodinson SM 1990c Complications of peripheral venous cannulation. Professional Nurse 6(3):175–177

Goodwin M, Carlson I 1993 The peripherally inserted catheter – a retrospective look at three years of insertion. Journal of Intravenous Nursing 13(5):297–305

Hall CB 1983 The nosocomial spread of respiratory syncytial viral infections. Annual Review of Medicine 34:311–319

Hamilton H 1993 Care improves while costs reduce. Professional Nurse 8(9):592–596

Hansell DT 1989 Intravenous nutrition: the central or peripheral route? Intravenous Therapy and Clinical Monitoring July:184–190

Haynes S 1989 Infusion phlebitis and extravasation. Professional Nurse 5(3):160–161

Hazaleus RE, Cole J, Berdichewsky M 1981 Tuberculin skin test conversion from exposure to contaminated pulmonary function testing apparatus. Respiratory Care 26:53–55

Hecker J, Fisk G, Lewis G 1984 Phlebitis and extravasation with intravenous infusions. Medical Journal of Australia 140:658–660

Henderson DK 1995 Bacteraemia due to percutaneous intravascular devices. In: Mandell GL, Dolin R, Bennett JE (eds) Principles and practice of infectious diseases, 4th edn. Churchill Livingstone, New York

Hill VB, Davies WE 1988 A swing to intermittent clean self-catheterization as a preferred mode of management for the dextrous spinal cord patient. Paraplegia 26:405–412

Hilton ET, Haslett M, Borenstein V et al 1988 Central catheter infection: single versus triple lumen catheters. American Journal of Medicine 8(4):7–72

Hospital Infection Control Practices Advisory Committee 2001 Draft guideline for the prevention of intravascular catheter-related infections. Available: http://www.cdc.gov/nicdod/hip

Hospital Infection Society (HIS) 2001 Working Party. Infection control and operating theatres. Draft document. Available: http://www.his.org.uk

Howard AJ 1991 Nosocomial spread of Haemophilus influenzae. Journal of Hospital Infection 19:1–3

Hughes JD 1989 Hypodermoclysis. Australian Journal of Hospital Pharmacy 19(3):182–183

Hunt GM, Oakshott P 1993 Self-catheterization: worth a trial. Geriatric Medicine 23:17–18

Hunt GM, Whittaker RH 1990 A new device for self catheterization in wheelchair-bound women. British Journal of Urology 66:162–163

Hunt GM, Oakshott P, Whittaker RH 1996 Intermittent catheterization: simple, safe and effective but underused. British Medical Journal 312:103–107

Hunt GM, Whittaker RH, Doyle PT 1984 Intermittent self-catheterization in adults. British Medical Journal 289:467–468

Infection Control Nurses Association (ICNA) 2001 Guidelines for preventing intravascular catheter-related infection. ICNA, London

Jarvis WR, Highsmith AK 1984 Bacterial growth and endotoxin production in lipid emulsion. Journal of Clinical Microbiology 19(1):17–20

Jakobsen CJ, Grabe N, Nielsen E et al 1986 Contamination of intravenous infusion systems – the effect of changing administration sets. Journal of Hospital Infection 8:217–223

Johnson S 1994 A time and money saver? Cost comparison of IV therapy with and without Pall 96 filters. Professional Nurse 10(2):94–96

Josephson A, Gombert ME, Sierra MF et al 1985 The relationship between intravenous fluid contamination and the frequency of tubing replacement. Infection Control 6:367–370

Keenlyside D 1992 Every detail counts – infection control in IV therapy. Professional Nurse 7(4):226–232

Kennedy AP, Brocklehurst JC 1982 The nursing management of patients with long-term indwelling catheters. Journal of Advanced Nursing 7:411–417

King TA, Cooke RPD 2001 Developing an infection control policy for anaesthetic equipment. Journal of Hospital Infection 47(4):257–261

Kontiokari T, Sundqvist K, Nuutinen M et al 2001 Randomised trial of cranberry–loganberry juice and *Lactobacillus* GG drink for the prevention of urinary tract infections in women. British Medical Journal 322:1–5

Kunin CM, McCormack RC 1966 Prevention of catheter induced urinary tract infections by sterile closed drainage. New England Journal of Medicine 274:1155–1161

Kyle K, Myers J 1989 Peripherally inserted central catheters – development of a hospital-based programme. Journal of Intravenous Nursing 13(5):287–290

Lancet 1992 *Pseudomonas cepacia* – more than harmless commensal? (Editorial). Lancet 339:1385–1386

Lapides J, Diokno AC, Gould FR, Lowe BS 1976 Further observations on self-catheterization. Journal of Urology 116:169–171

Larson EL, Oram MT, Hedrick E 1988 Nosocomial infection rates as an indicator of quality. Medical Care 26(7):676–684

Law DJW, Mishriki SF, Jeffery PJ 1990 The importance of surveillance after discharge from hospital in the diagnosis of postoperative wound infection. Annals of the Royal College of Surgeons (England) 72:207–209

Lawrence JC 1994 Dressings and wound infection. American Journal of Wound Infection 167(suppl 1A):21S–24S

Levison ME, Bush LM 1995 Peritonitis and other abdominal infections. In: Mandell GL, Bennett JE, Dolin R (eds) Principles and practice of infectious diseases, 4th edn. Churchill Livingstone, New York

Levy J, Van Laethem Y, Verhaegen G et al 1989 Contaminated enteral nutrition solutions as a cause of nosocomial bloodstream infection: a study using plasmid fingerprinting. Journal of Parenteral and Enteral Nutrition 13:228–234

Lilly HA, London PS, Lowbury EJL, Porter MF 1970 Effects of adhesive drapes on contamination of operation wounds. Lancet i:431–432

Livesley J 1993 Securing methods for peripheral cannulae. Nursing Standard 7(31):31–34

Lodge JPA, Brennan TG 1987 Insertion technique, the key to avoiding infusion phlebitis: a prospective clinical trial. British Journal of Clinical Practice 41(7):816–818

Maki D, Ringer M 1987 Evaluation of dressing regimens for prevention of infection with peripheral vascular intravenous catheters: gauze, a transparent polyurethane dressing, and an iodophor-transparent dressing. Journal of the American Medical Association 258:2396–2403

Maki D, Goldman D, Rhame F 1973 Infection control in intravenous therapy. Annals of Internal Medicine 79:867–887

Maki D, Botticelli J, LeRoy M et al 1987 Prospective study of replacing administration sets for intravenous therapy at 48 vs 72 hour intervals. 72 hours is safe and cost effective. Journal of the American Medical Association 258:1777–1781

Maki DG, Alvarado CJ, Ringer MA 1991 A prospective randomized trial of povidone–iodine, alcohol and chlorhexidine for the prevention of infection with central venous and arterial catheters. Lancet 338:339–343

Maizels M, Schaeffer AJ 1980 Decreased incidence of bacteriuria associated with peroxide instillation of hydrogen peroxide into the urethral catheter drainage bag. Journal of Urology 123:841–845

Martin S, Corrado O, Alldred A 1996 Guidelines for the administration of subcutaneous fluids. United Leeds Teaching Hospital NHS Trust, Leeds

Maxwell NJ, Ford CR, Peterson DE, Richards RC 1969 Abdominal wound infections and plastic drape protectors. American Journal of Surgery 118:844–848

McSweeney P 1989 Self-catheterization – a solution for some incontinent people. Professional Nurse 4(8):399–401

Meers P, Ayliffe GAJ, Emmerson A et al 1981 Report on the national survey of infection in hospitals. Journal of Hospital Infection 2(suppl):1–51

Mishriki SF, Jeffery PJ, Law DJW 1992 Wound infection: the surgeon's responsibility. Journal of Wound Care 1(2):32–36

Mulhall AB, Chapman RG, Crow RA 1988 Bacteriuria during indwelling urethral catheterization. Journal of Infection 11:253–262

Murphy DM, Falkiner FR, Carr M et al 1983 Septicaemia after transurethral prostatectomy. Journal of Urology xxii:133–135

National Research Council of Medical Sciences (NRC) 1964 Postoperative wound infections. The influence of ultraviolet irradiation of the operating room and various other factors. Annals of Surgery 160(suppl 2):1–192

Navajas MFC, Chacon DJ, Solvas JFG, Vargas RG 1992 Bacterial contamination of enteral feeds as a possible risk of nosocomial infection. Journal of Hospital Infection 26:111–120

Neal TJ, Hughes CR, Rothburn MM, Shaw NJ 1995 The neonatal laryngoscope as a potential source of cross-infection (Letter). Journal of Hospital Infection 30:315

Newsome SW 1985 Infection control in intensive care: problems with vascular access. Care of the Critically Ill 1(2):15–16

Noble-Adams R 1995 Dehydration: subcutaenous fluid administration. British Journal of Nursing 4(9):488–494

Nystrom B, Olesen-Larsen S, Dankert J et al 1983 Bacteraemia in surgical patients with intravenous devices: a European multi-centre incidence study. Journal of Hospital Infection 4:338–349

Oldman P 1991 A sticky situation: microbiological study of adhesive tape used to secure IV cannulae. Professional Nurse 6(5):265–269

Ouslander JG 1987 Complications of chronic indwelling urinary catheters among male nursing home patients: a prospective study. Journal of Urology 138:1191–1195

Parker LJ 2000 Applying the principles of infection control to wound care. British Journal of Nursing 9(7):394–404

Paskin DL, Lerner HJ 1969 A prospective study of wound infections. American Surgeon 35:627–629

Pennington JE 1995 Nosocomial respiratory infections. In: Mandell GL, Bennett JE, Dolin R (eds) Principles and practice of infectious diseases, 4th edn. Churchill Livingstone, New York

Pick D 1990 Standards of excellence. Nursing 4(24):17–18

Pinilla JC 1983 Study of the incidence of intravascular catheter infection and associated septicaemia in critically ill patients. Critical Care Medicine 11(1):21–25

Plowman R, Graves N, Griffin M et al 1999 The socio-economic burden of hospital-acquired infection. PHLS/London School of Tropical Medicine and Hygiene, London

Public Health Laboratory Service (PHLS) 1960 Incidence of surgical wound infection in England and Wales. Lancet ii:659–663

Raahave D 1976 Effects of plastic skin and wound drapes on the density of bacteria in operation wounds. British Journal of Surgery 63:936–940

Rhame F, Maki D, Bennett J 1979 Intravenous cannula-related infections. In: Bennett J, Brachman P (eds) Hospital infections. Little Brown, Boston, MD

Roberts JA 1993 Adherence to urethral catheters by bacteria causing nosocomial infections. Urology 41(4):338–342

Robinson R, Cockram M, Strode M 1985 Severe handicap in spina bifida: no bar to intermittent self-catheterization. Archives of Diseases of Childhood 60:760–766

Roe BH 1987 Catheter care and patient teaching. PhD Thesis. University of Manchester, Manchester

Roe BH 1993 Catheter-associated urinary tract infections: a review. Journal of Clinical Nursing 2:197–203

Roe BH, Brocklehurst JC 1987 Study of patients with indwelling catheters. Journal of Advanced Nursing 12(6):713–718

Roe BH, Chapman RG, Crow R 1986 A study of the procedure for catheter care recommended by district health authorities and schools of nursing. Nursing Practice Research Unit, University of Surrey, Guildford

Rotstein C, Brock L, Roberts RS 1995 The incidence of first Hickman catheter related infection and predictors of catheter removal in cancer patients. Infection Control and Hospital Epidemiology 16(8):451–458

Shanson DC 1999 Microbiology in clinical practice, 3rd edn. Butterworth Heinemann, Oxford

Slade N, Gillespie WA 1985 The urinary tract and the catheter. Infection and other problems. John Wiley, Chichester

Talja M 1990 Comparision of urethral reaction to full silicone, hydrogel-coated and siliconized latex catheters. British Journal of Urology 66(6):652–657

Tebbs SE, Sawyer A, Elliott TSJ 1994 Influence of surface morphology on in-vitro bacterial adherence to central venous catheters. British Journal of Anaesthesiology 72:587–591

Thornton GF, Andriole VT 1970 Bacteriuria during indwelling catheter drainage. Journal of the American Medical Association 214:339–342

Thurn J, Crossley K, Gerdis A et al 1990 Enteral hyperalimentation as a source of nosocomial infection. Journal of Hospital Infection 15:203–217

Veazey JM Jr 1981 Hospital-acquired pneumonia. In: Wenzel RP (ed) Handbook of hospital acquired infections. CRC Press, Florida

Warren JW 1995 Nosocomial urinary tract infection. In: Mandell GI, Bennett JE, Dolin R (eds) Principles and practice of infectious diseases, 4th edn. Churchill Livingstone, New York

Webb RJ, Lawson AL, Neal DE 1990 Clean intermittent self catheterization in 172 adults. British Journal of Urology 65:20–23

Whitelaw S, Hammonds JC, Tregellas R 1987 Clean intermittent self catheterization in the elderly. British Journal of Urology 60:125–127

Whyte W 1988 The role of clothing and drapes in the operating room. Journal of Hospital Infection 11(suppl C):2–17

Wilkinson R 1991 The challenge of intravenous therapy. Nursing Standard 5(28):24–27

Wilkinson R 1996 Nurses' concerns about IV therapy and devices. Nursing Standard 10(3):35–37

Wilson J 1994 Preventing infection during IV therapy. Professional Nurse March: 388–392

Wood PC 1994 Hypodormoclysis guidelines. North Shae Hospital, Auckland, New Zealand

Susceptible hosts

CONTENTS

SUMMARY

This chapter discusses the factors that contribute to an individual's susceptibility to acquiring infection and the steps taken to minimize risks.

INTRODUCTION

In infectious diseases, the final outcome can depend as much, if not more, on the susceptibility of the person as on factors relating to the microorganism itself (Ayliffe 1986). Donowitz (1987) has listed a number of factors that increase the host susceptibility, these include (Fig. 11.1):

- Age: very young children and people over the age of 65 years
- An underlying disease such as diabetes, blood and respiratory disorders and cardiopulmonary disease
- The therapy for disease, for example, chemotherapy used to suppress the bone marrow in patients with leukaemia, lymphoma and those

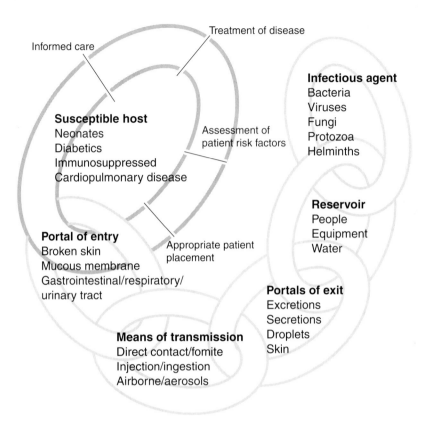

Figure 11.1 Breaking the chain of infection: susceptible hosts.

undergoing bone marrow or organ transplant; steroids and cancer-cell-suppressing (cytotoxic) drugs, which can result in interference with the host defences and in depression of immunity. Steroids are known to increase the risk of infection
- Treatments and procedures carried out whilst in hospital, especially invasive techniques such as surgery, urinary catheterization and intravenous therapy.

ASSESSMENT OF PATIENT RISK FACTORS

Infection risks are identified as host related (intrinsic) or as a result of pre-scribed therapeutic treatment procedures related to medical and nursing care (extrinsic).

Extremes of age

Children aged 1 year and under and people aged 65 years and over are at an increased risk of infection.

The newborn, normal weight infant relies on maternal antibodies for protection against infection for a period of 3–6 months, until its immune system is fully developed. Premature delivery and low birth weight add significantly to the infant's susceptibility.

Elderly people suffer changes in their cell-mediated and humoral immunity that can lead to poor healing ability (Saltzman & Peterson 1987) as well as poor cough reflex and poor circulation (Ben-Yehuda & Weksler 1992). Poor nutrition is also common in the elderly. They often suffer from chronic illnesses that are associated with infection and are often on immunosuppressive drugs (Crossley & Peterson 1995).

Studies have shown not only an increase in wound infection rate with advancing age, but that age influences infection rate independently of other factors (Cruse & Foord 1980, Davidson et al 1971, Farber & Wenzel 1980, Leigh 1981, Mishriki et al 1990, 1992, NRC 1964).

Nutrition and build

Both obese and emaciated individuals are susceptible to complications.

Obese people often lack many elements required for healing. The blood supply to fatty tissue is poor, so the tissue heals more slowly. There is also an increased risk of contamination of a wound during surgery for people with surplus fat, because the procedure can take longer. Obese people may not have a balanced diet containing essential nutrients, hence they might be as malnourished as underweight and emaciated individuals. Postoperative wound and chest infections are high in obese people (Choban et al 1995).

Malnutrition impairs host defences by weakening the immune response. The metabolic reserves are decreased and the integrity of the epithelial surfaces is affected in emaciated and malnourished people. Reduction in infections, including surgical wound infections, has been shown to be commensurate with improved nutrition (Hamilton 1982).

Breach in the integrity of skin

Trauma, surgical wounds, venous and pressure ulcers and stab wounds such as a cannula through the skin are examples of a transgression of the first line of defence. Apart from creating a portal of entry for microorganisms, lesions and wounds are susceptible to colonization with pathogenic microbes, including antibiotic-resistant organisms of significant concern.

Trauma

Trauma results in a break in the integrity of skin. Traumatized skin and mucosal surfaces become contaminated during injury and allow pathogens to bypass the first line defences (Fiore et al 1995). Trauma often results in devitalized soft tissues, which provides an ideal environment for pathogens to multiply. Invasive devices and wound drains, often necessary in traumatized patients, create a portal of entry for these organisms. Multiple trauma cases are nursed in intensive care units where further colonization of injured surfaces and devices with hospital flora is almost inevitable.

Pregnancy

Cellular immunity declines in pregnancy. The maternal immune response is defective during pregnancy in order that fetal tissue is not rejected.

Physiological changes in the bladder and ureters during pregnancy predispose pregnant women to urinary tract infection (Patterson & Andriole 1995). Certain persistent infections such as cytomegalovirus and herpes simplex virus can be reactivated, placing infants at risk of contracting secondary infections during pregnancy or during passage through the infected maternal tract (Hirsch 1995, Ho 1995).

The pH and the vaginal flora change during pregnancy and colonization or infection with organisms such as *Trichomonas vaginalis* or haemolytic group B streptococci are common.

Premature rupture of the membrane, instrumental delivery and retained products of conception are predisposing factors in the infection of damaged and vulnerable tissue following delivery or abortion.

Substance, drug and alcohol abuse

Substance abuse, of either drugs or alcohol, has been associated with infections. Often, alcoholism, malnutrition and exposure to cold go together, predisposing to infection (Musher 1995). Drug abuse, especially intravenous drug abuse, predisposes the users to a multitude of infections, mainly through puncture wounds. Immunological abnormalities can exist in drug abusers. The puncture wounds provide an access point for organisms and have been known to be abnormally colonized with *Staphylococcus aureus* (Levine & Sobel 1995).

Smoking

Tobacco-related complications such as coronary heart disease, chronic obstructive pulmonary disease (COPD) and atherosclerotic peripheral vascular disease increase the smoker's risk of infection (Nagachinta et al 1987). Cigarette smoking is considered to be the most important factor in chronic bronchitis. Many cigarette smokers suffer from respiratory disorders, such as COPD, which is often accompanied by complications such as chest infection. Long-term steroid therapy, often a treatment in many chronic conditions, reduces the body's defences further (Reynolds 1995).

Drug therapy as a risk factor

Conditions like leukaemia and lymphoma are treated with radiotherapy and/or chemotherapy to suppress abnormal cell production. Unfortunately, the cytotoxic nature of the treatment results in the destruction of normal cells. It also leaves the patient highly susceptible to infectious agents.

Patients suffering from malignant tumours are exposed to similar treatments with subsequent immunosuppression. In a small study of septicaemia, Duggan et al (1985) established that immunosuppressive drugs significantly worsen the prognosis compared with immunosuppressive disease. In the study, all three patients who died as a result of septicaemia were taking immunosuppressive drugs but did not have immunosuppressive disease, whereas five patients who had immunosuppressive disease but were not taking immunosuppressive drugs survived. Steroids are usually given in the form of long-term corticosteroid therapy for many chronic conditions.

They interfere with the body's natural ability to defend itself against infection (Reynolds 1995).

Antimicrobials are known to be associated with increased risk of infection, especially pneumonia. This is thought to be due to the selection of more resistant bacteria during treatment of the initial infection.

Resistance to antimicrobials is becoming a major problem in many countries. Serious infections, once easily treated with antibiotics, are becoming untreatable. The emergence of methicillin-resistant *Staphylococcus aureus* (MRSA) and resistance to vancomycin in *Staphylococcus aureus* and enterococci has created difficulties for treatment (Edmond et al 1996). Further complications include antibiotic-associated diarrhoea and *Clostridium difficile*-associated colitis (Fekety 1995). Hospital-acquired *Clostridium difficile* diarrhoea in the UK increased sixfold between 1990 and 1993 (Riley 1994). Patients with *Clostridium difficile*-associated diarrhoea have a significantly longer stay in hospital (Macgowan et al 1995).

Resistance by bacteria to antimicrobials generates problems that can be serious for patients as well as the clinical environment. Mehtar (1992) has summarized these as follows:

- The antibiotics required to treat multiple-resistant bacteria are usually more potent, costly and require the parenteral route of administration
- The morbidity, and occasionally mortality, is increased with multiresistant bacteria, particularly those involved in hospital-acquired infections
- The hospital environment becomes colonized with resistant bacteria and the spread of these bacteria is further increased via clinical and non-clinical equipment
- Hospital stay is prolonged and occasionally further surgical intervention is required.

Vulnerable children

Children with conditions predisposing them to immune defects, children receiving transplants and those requiring invasive device treatments pose a challenge for the staff. The infection control principles discussed previously should form a basis of each care practice.

INFECTION PREVENTION IN DIFFERENT CARE SETTINGS

Trauma patients

Traumatized patients are at an increased risk of infection because:

- The first line of defence, skin or mucosal surfaces, is bypassed, allowing contamination a direct entry point.
- The devitalized and ischaemic injured tissue becomes colonized with microbes that gain access to vulnerable sites via surgical drains, intravenous lines, urinary catheters and endotracheal tubes.

- Multiple trauma patients invariably require intensive care. These patients quickly become colonized with hospital-acquired pathogens.
- Traumatized, ill patients might require tracheostomy, are immobilized, develop bedsores and require constant manipulation of invasive devices.
- Impaired mobility, pH changes, fasting and antibiotic therapy in critically injured patients often lead to a loss of protective colonization provided by normal gut flora (Fiore et al 1995).

Intensive care and special care baby units

The severity of the illness, extensive nature of drug and invasive therapy, the frequent manipulation of the body and the number of devices used make patients – whether adult, neonate or paediatric – highly susceptible to hospital-acquired infections. The risks associated with host, treatments, procedures and practices have been identified elsewhere in the chain of infection. Although the principles governing practice points can be readily applied, the intensity and the degree of manipulation of invasive devices, and of these severely ill patients, demand a strict and high level of infection control practice.

Medical and elderly care wards

Patients admitted to these wards can be highly vulnerable to infection because of their advanced age and many underlying conditions. Many patients are admitted with lower respiratory tract infections or exacerbation of their airways, which can predispose them to superimposed chest infections. Many patients can develop antibiotic-associated complications, which require careful infection control measures.

Immunosuppressed patients are often nursed in a single room of a medical ward. Immunocompromised patients are vulnerable to infections from opportunist organisms, that is, those organisms that rarely cause problems in an immunocompetent person. So they can be vulnerable to their own endogenous organisms. Box 11.1 highlights some points to consider when working with elderly and immunocompromised patients.

Obstetric units

Maternal infection is associated with the delivery process, whether it is vaginal or caesarean:

- In vaginal delivery, an association was found between the number of vaginal examinations and post-caesarean febril morbidity and wound infection rates (Nice et al 1996). Multiple vaginal examinations can introduce vaginal and intestinal organisms into the uterus, and should be kept to a minimum.
- Ruptured membranes increase the risk of infection, requiring the need for an antiseptic handwash and the wearing of sterile gloves.
- Tissue trauma and laceration of the vaginal wall is often a feature of vaginal delivery and provides entry for organisms present in the vagina.

- Microorganisms can be introduced during manual removal of the placenta.
- Episiotomy allows entry for organisms present around the perineum.

■ **BOX 11.1   Points to consider**

- Urinary catheters and vascular devices, including a cannula without infusion, should remain in place for the shortest possible period.
- Nebulizers and inhalers should be washed after each use and wiped with alcohol-impregnated swabs.
- A solution of sodium bicarbonate (in warm tap water) helps to remove the mucus from suction catheters.
- Oxygen masks can become contaminated with sputum from patients. These should be washed and dried thoroughly after each use. They are single-patient items and should not be used for more than one patient.
- Staff members and visitors with infections should be excluded from caring for and visiting immunosuppressed patients.
- Scrupulous handwashing before contact with immunosuppressed patients is vital.
- Immunosuppressed patients may be vulnerable to certain foods, especially uncooked foods.

Caesarean section

The wound infection rate following caesarean section has been placed between 1 and 9% (Creighton et al 1991). Risk factors for the development of postoperative wound infections after caesarean sections have been described by Webster (1988) and Rehu & Nilsson (1990) to include:

- obesity
- socioeconomic status
- length of operation
- skill of operator
- use of drains
- previous post-caesarean section infection and type of incision (horizontal versus vertical).

Women undergoing a caesarean section are catheterized prior to the surgery. The procedure for this varies, from the catheter being inserted immediately before surgery and either being left to drain on a sterile pad and removed at the end of the surgery or being removed immediately after emptying the bladder before surgery (Leigh et al 1990). Occasionally, indwelling catheters are inserted and left for 1 or 2 days. Parrot et al (1989) found a urinary tract infection rate of 14.5%, whereas Wrightson (1996) reported a rate of 33% when catheters were left in for 24 to 48h postsurgery. Both the management and duration of urinary catheterization can require a closer examination.

Many women develop mastitis after delivery. Nipples often crack and allow colonization or infection with *Staphylococcus aureus*. Abscess formation in breasts due to engorgement and milk stasis can occur (Jensen et al 1991).

Postdelivery care

The basic hygiene education of women should include care of the perineal area, especially after passing urine or defaecation. Women may also need guidance on the care of breasts and nipples. They need to report immediately to the midwife any redness, tenderness and cracked or split nipples.

Paediatric patients

Paediatric wards are often a mixture of non-immune and infected children. Infections of children include childhood diseases such as varicella-zoster (chickenpox), mumps, pertussis (whooping cough), measles, rubella, viral and bacterial gastrointestinal infections and other viral infections, such as respiratory syncytial virus (RSV), hepatitis A and herpes. Box 11.2 outlines some of the problems that face nursing staff on paediatric wards.

■ **BOX 11.2   Problems that may be found on paediatric wards**

- Maintaining basic hygiene and barrier precautions can be difficult
- Environmental surfaces and objects such as toys are easily contaminated and are likely to be shared with other patients
- Physical contact with paediatric patients is often closer than with adult patients
- Parents and members of the family who are often involved closely in the care might not understand the necessary hygiene and barrier procedures
- Visitors and siblings might visit whilst carrying or suffering from transmissible diseases
- Parents of infected children can pose a risk to other non-immune children by visiting them.

It could be useful to produce an information leaflet describing the importance of:

- Not visiting a child if suffering from infections
- Proper handwashing practices before and after contact with the child, nappies, bedding, environment, and so on
- Not visiting other children on the ward or sharing sweets and toys with other children
- Not allowing visiting siblings to play with other patients on the ward.

Parents and visitors will also need instructions on the way the child's infection could spread and the precautions needed to stop that spread.

Child day centres

Infectious diseases occur frequently in child day centres. This is a result of the relatively low state of immunity of children, the degree of close contact between the children and attendants and the difficulties in maintaining a high standard of hygiene. Infections acquired in the nursery can spread to staff, family members and the community. Environmental hygiene is important because playpens, highchairs and nappy changing areas can easily become contaminated.

Schools

Schools are vulnerable to outbreaks of infection. These outbreaks can disrupt the daily routine and require costly control measures. Close physical contact in classrooms and in the playgrounds provides an ideal environment for cross-transmission of microorganisms between children. Some infectious diseases remain difficult to control. Chickenpox can be transmitted during the final phase of its incubation period before there are visible indications of the disease. Gastrointestinal infections spread because the affected children do not report their condition to the school staff and many can be infected before the problem is recognized.

Once the spread of an infection is known, the school staff must report it to, and obtain advice from the Community Infection Control Nurse (CICN) or the Environmental Health Officer (EHO). Some basic steps can be introduced immediately if a problem is suspected:

- Prompt removal from school of children with symptoms
- High standard of environmental hygiene for cleaning toilets, door handles, sink taps, etc.
- Strict and supervised handwashing of children after visiting the toilet and before meals.

Many EHOs find poor handwashing facilities on inspection of schools. Often only cold water is supplied, with no soap or towels.

Severely disabled children are attended by specially qualified assistants. The children might be doubly incontinent and possibly require intermittent catheterization. CICNs can provide infection control advice and support to staff working with these children.

Mental health settings

Large old buildings that once housed mental health and learning disability patients are now rare. Patients in the acute stages of illness are often nursed in dedicated wards of general hospitals and non-acute patients remain in small community homes and units. The community units might be purpose built or adapted from a residential home. Whatever the environment, the infection control management can pose a number of problems.

The nature of the illness and behaviour of many patients demand increased awareness and a very high level of infection control standards. The policies and guidelines, as well as health and safety guidelines, DoH directives, legislation, and the removal of Crown Immunity, are relevant in these establishments. The importance of safe food handling was highlighted by the Stanley Royd Report (DHSS 1986).

Nursing and residential homes

Residents in long-term care facilities, such as nursing and residential homes, often have bacterial infections that can be transmitted directly between patients or indirectly on the hands of staff or via contaminated equipment. Infections of the urinary and lower respiratory tracts, decubitus, venous and arterial ulcers and skin can pose a major problem. Diarrhoeal diseases, especially viral, can spread with extreme ease in long-term care facilities. Infected residents are treated with multiple courses of antimicrobials or require hospitalization. This process selects strains more resistant to antibiotics (John & Ribner 1991). These resistant strains are then likely to disperse in the environment. Three major reasons why antibiotic resistance is a particular problem are:

1. Antibiotics used empirically in long-term facility residents infected with resistant bacteria can lack specific antimicrobial activity
2. Transfer of these residents to acute care centres inadvertently jeopardizes the receiving institution by introducing a new set of antibiotic-resistant genes into a different patient population
3. Infection control measures necessary to detect or to limit endemic, resistant pathogens fall outside the standard practice of most long-term care facilities.

Resistant microbes, especially MRSA, create anxiety amongst staff in these settings. The DoH leaflet entitled *MRSA – What Nursing and Residential Homes Need to Know* (DoH 1996) provides sound basic advice for homes caring for colonized residents. The DoH has also circulated infection control guidelines specifically aimed at residential and nursing homes (Public Health Medicine Environment Group (PHMEG) 1996). Workers who have no care background and who might have received very little training in basic infection control practice often staff long-term care facilities, especially residential homes.

General practice and dental surgeries

Increasingly, general practice surgeries offer treatments and services once performed only in hospitals. Such procedures include:

- gastrointestinal endoscopies
- minor surgery
- cervical smears
- family planning clinics
- blood glucose and cholesterol monitoring services.

Practice nurses perform a range of procedures, including:

- immunizations
- venepuncture
- auriscope examination
- cervical smears
- assisting with minor surgical procedures (Atkin et al 1993).

Various surveys have established inadequate and varied decontamination methods practised by practice nurses (Farrow et al 1988, Morgan et al 1990). Many GPs did not clean or disinfect earpieces of auriscopes between patients (Overend et al 1992). Another survey of GPs in England and Wales identified a significant lack of understanding about the risks associated with resheathing used needles, risks of cross-infection and methods of decontamination (Foy et al 1990).

Infection control in dentistry received prominence when the transmission of human immunodeficiency virus (HIV) by a Florida dentist to six patients was reported (Ciesielski et al 1992, Hillis & Huelsenback 1994). Infections like hepatitis B virus (HBV) and herpes simplex have also been transmitted in dental practices (Scully et al 1990). Comprehensive infection control procedures for dental practices are produced by the British Dental Association (BDA 1991, Glenwright & Martin 1993). However, compliance with infection control procedures has been found to be inadequate (Porter et al 1996, Scully & Mortimer 1994, Scully et al 1992, 1993). Compliance with protective wear remains an individual responsibility but infection control nurses (ICNs) might have the opportunity to provide training and support to staff responsible for appropriate decontamination of instruments.

Patients' own homes

Increasingly, patients with debilitating illness requiring specialist treatment and invasive devices are being cared for in their own homes. Preparation of such patients will have started whilst still in hospital. The community staff often work in constrained environmental circumstances, depending upon the individual home of the patient. Sanitation could be a problem, with community staff having to carry supplies of paper towels, soap or alcohol handrub to facilitate hand hygiene.

The organisms found in the home might be different from and not so virulent as those in hospitals. But clinical practices need to be underpinned by basic hygiene and infection control principles. Family members and anyone associated with the care of the patient need a basic knowledge of safe practice. They also require a basic understanding of routes of transmission of the microorganisms likely to be met and the methods of care of medical devices and procedures to stop their spread must remain the cornerstone of practice.

UNDERLYING CONDITIONS AND DISEASES

Diabetes

Cardiovascular disorders are more common in people with diabetes than in the general population. There could also be accompanying degenerative changes in blood vessels and decreased nutrition to cells, which can affect the natural healing process (Jarrett 1985). Arterial and venous leg ulcers are common in diabetic patients. These ulcers are colonized with organisms that frequently lead to infections of ulcers or other wounds in diabetic patients. Often, a minor trauma in patients with diabetic neuropathy and arterial vascular insufficiency leads to cellulitis, soft tissue necrosis or osteomyelitis with a draining sinus requiring surgical interventions. Colonization and infections are common in these wounds (Swartz 1995). Organisms are readily available for transmission to another susceptible site on the body. The risk of hospital-acquired infection is increased in diabetic patients (Stamm et al 1997).

Respiratory disorders

The respiratory tract contains an impressive array of defence mechanisms. The filtration 'tree' of the upper airway and tracheobronchial tree trap the invading microorganisms, which are transported away from the lungs by cilia and expelled by coughing. The bronchial secretions also contain anti-microbial substances such as lysozyme (Tramont & Hoover 1995).

Conditions likely to obstruct the smooth passage of air through the lungs are:

• chronic bronchitis
• emphysema
• asthma
• bronchiectasis
• cystic fibrosis.

Patients with chronic obstructive pulmonary disease are likely to encounter the following problems:

• impaired coughing mechanism
• increased secretions
• ischaemia
• susceptibility to colonization of the lower respiratory tract with Gram-negative organisms.

Certain procedures are known to bypass the natural defences in the respiratory tract, such as:

• intubation
• mechanical respiratory aids
• tracheostomy.

Finally, cigarette smoke is also known to interfere with the effectiveness of the natural defences in the respiratory tract (Tramont & Hoover 1995).

Blood disorders

Blood disorders range from anaemia to leukaemia, lymphoma, myeloma, agranulocytosis and thrombocytopenia.

In most instances of blood disorder there is a degree of anaemia. Anaemic patients could have poor nutrition, as well as poor skin conditions predisposing them to pressure ulcers and infection.

Leukaemia is characterized by an abnormal proliferation of immature white cells that tend to interfere with bone marrow function leading to the production of fewer normal blood cells. The resulting anaemia, leucopenia or thrombocytopenia increases the patient's vulnerability to infections from agents that are normally considered to be of low pathogenicity.

Lymphoma is characterized by an abnormal structure of cells in lymph nodes. Many symptoms associated with lymphoma create a favourable medium for development of infection.

A partial or complete absence of neutrophils in agranulocytosis makes the patient extremely susceptible to serious infection.

When platelet disorders occur, there is interference in the number or the function of platelets that affects the coagulation process. The tendency to bleed easily leads to anaemia and associated complications. Duke (1994) provides a comprehensive literature on various blood disorders.

INFORMED CARE

The delivery of care should be based on understanding the factors that predispose patients and sometimes staff to the risk of infection. The actions then required to minimize such risks can be taken.

Evaluating practices and questioning risk management, risk factors and quality assurance

The process of care, irrespective of the discipline, centres on assessment of patients, planning and implementing care and evaluating the outcome. The purpose of the assessment is to plan care to meet the patients' requirements, be they dietary, degree of hands-on care, risk of falls, pressure ulcers or infections. The quality of the assessment will depend on the level of knowledge and understanding of the practitioner of what to 'look for'. The nursing process suggests that the needs of patients are assessed on the basis of their admitting condition and their history. Infection risks can be included in the initial and ongoing assessment (Fig. 11.2). Infection risks in patients are constantly changing based on the treatment and procedures. The care plan needs to reflect these ever changing risk factors.

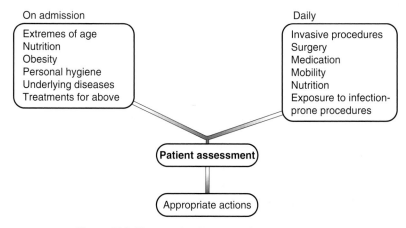

Figure 11.2 Theoretical underpinning of patient assessment.

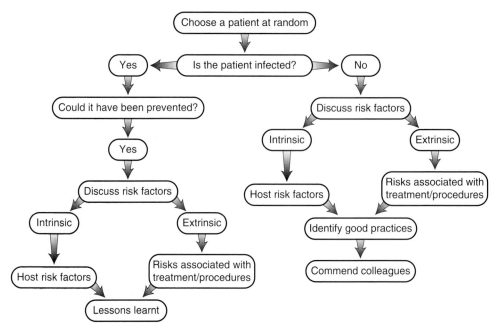

Figure 11.3 Questioning infection and evaluating care against risk factors.

The importance of nursing assessment of infection risks was advocated by Webster & Bowell (1986) and Bowell (1990, 1992):

- There should be a formal assessment of intrinsic and extrinsic patient risk factors documented in medical and nursing notes
- Review dates appropriate to individual risk factors should be documented
- The documented infection control care plan and its evaluation should reflect the individual patient's changing risk factors.

Most infections, whatever their origin, will, on investigation, reveal predisposing factors. Both inherent and treatment-related risk factors require identification and appropriate management so that care can be evaluated. A formal assessment of risk factors is difficult and not generally favoured. If infections are to be questioned and appraised, susceptibility has to be overtly recognized so that the ensuing plan of care and practices can be assessed (Fig. 11.3).

A simple identification, recording and discussion of each risk factor will form the basis of a systematic approach to informed care and can be a first step towards a desired outcome. Kingsley (1992) outlines the following elements for assessing patients and planning care:

- A risk assessment standard statement
- A written prompt on the nursing process assessment form
- Available written guidelines on appropriate infection control actions to take once risk has been identified.

Checking risk factors will enable the practitioner to:

- Plan the most appropriate care
- Counsel staff on methods of minimizing the risk of infection
- Counsel the patient about avoidance/prevention of infection
- Recognize the likelihood of infection occurring and spot the first signs as early as possible
- Consider the likelihood of an established infection progressing to a more serious form
- Understand the possible causation or contributory factors of an infective illness
- Give an informed opinion as to whether or not infection could have been prevented.

Isolation nursing for infected and susceptible patients

Specific precautions are required to prevent transmission of infectious agents from patient to patient, from patients to staff and from healthcare workers to patients. This might require separating the infected or vulnerable patient from other patients and from healthcare workers using barrier clothing such as plastic aprons, disposable gloves and masks.

The purpose of barrier clothing can be described as:

- The barrier prevents the infective agent from attaching to the skin or uniform so making the carer a means of transmission to other patients
- The barrier effectively blocks off the portal of entry into the carer.

Isolation measures are started to:

- Stop the spread of microorganisms from an infected patient to susceptible individuals (source isolation)
- Prevent severely immunocompromised patients from becoming infected (protective isolation).

Source isolation

The idea of containing infection at its source was first put forward by Florence Nightingale in 1863 (Jackson & Lynch 1987). Fever nursing, as it was called, related to the importance of contact transmission by body substances as opposed to environmental transmission. This idea of transmission by body substances has become the modern cornerstone for source isolation. Bagshawe et al (1978a,b,c,d) laid the foundation for source-specific precautions based on routes of infection; and the 1996 CDC standard precautions (Garner 1996) reflect this. Guidelines have recently been published by the DoH to reflect this approach (DoH 2001).

Protective isolation

Infection is a major cause of death in patients whose immune system is compromised either by a disease or its treatment or by thermal injury.

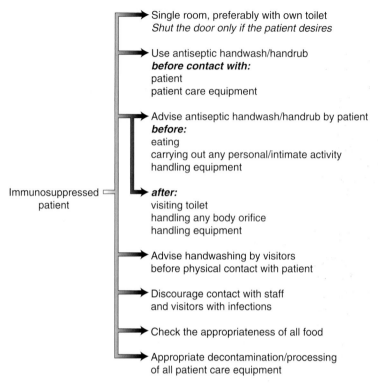

Figure 11.4 Trigger points when nursing a severely immunocompromised patient in a single room in a general ward.

They are vulnerable to infection from:

- their own endogenous microorganisms
- opportunistic microorganisms
- a much smaller dose of microorganisms than would be problematic for a non-immunocompromised person.

It is not always possible to control the patient's own body flora but certain measures can be used to eliminate or minimize the risk from exogenous organisms. Some healthcare establishments have purpose-built positive pressure facilities with high efficiency particulate (HEPA) filters to care for such patients. However, in many hospitals within the UK, a side room off a general ward is all that is available. In these circumstances, the hand hygiene of staff before contact with the patient and decontamination of patient care equipment is essential (Fig. 11.4).

Isolation nursing – a bitter, toxic, costly pill?

Coleman (1987) describes isolation as a bitter, toxic and costly pill:

- A bitter pill for the patient to swallow because isolation is an unpleasant experience
- Toxic because of its side-effects of depression and regression, which can interfere with recovery (Gammon 1998, Jackson & Lynch 1987). Patients

in isolation not only lose the support and companionship of fellow patients but also have reduced contact with staff members, who tend to visit them only during clinical procedures. This sense of alienation can be further exacerbated by the use of protective clothing by staff when providing care
- Costly because of the extra resources and time needed.

STAFF COMPLIANCE

The failure of staff to comply with the techniques prescribed has been described by Larson (1983) and Gould (1985a,b). They showed that many nurses were ignorant of modes of spread and how to prevent transmission of an infection. They were also unable to apply theoretical knowledge to nursing a patient with an infection. The following points are worth considering:

- Has the patient been given the reason for their isolation and encouraged to ask questions?
- Do all staff understand the disease?
- Do all staff know when to wear protective clothing and why?
- Does the door of the isolation room need to be kept closed at all times?
- Are staff able to explain to the patient, relatives and other patients who may be concerned, the reason for isolation, without creating panic?
- Do visitors need to wear aprons and gloves?
- Is there a reason why the patient cannot leave the room for brief walks?
- Do you encourage staff to enter the room as frequently as possible?
- Is the patient asked daily how and what they feel?
- Does anyone review daily whether isolation is still required?

ETHICAL COUNTERPOINT

In many district general hospitals single rooms are at a premium. Seriously ill patients are often nursed in single rooms to maintain their dignity and to allow relatives the opportunity to spend time with the patient. Often, there is a conflict of interest when the room is required for a patient with a possibly highly infectious condition. Whose needs are most important:

- the terminally ill patient and close relatives and friends, who need the privacy of a single room to express their emotions?
- the other patients on the ward, who could find it difficult to deal with having a very ill or dying patient in their midst?
- the patient with a suspected or confirmed infection who needs to be segregated to prevent the infection spreading to others?

REFERENCES

Atkin K, Parker G, Lunt N, Hirst M 1993 Practice nurses count: the new national census. Nursing Standard 8(5):21–24

Ayliffe GAJ 1986 Nosocomial infection – the irreducible minimum. Infection Control 7(2):92–95

Bagshawe KD, Blowers R, Lidwell OM 1978a Isolating patients in hospital to control infection. Part I – sources and routes. British Medical Journal 2:609–612

Bagshawe KD, Blowers R, Lidwell OM 1978b Isolating patients in hospital to control infection. Part II – who should be isolated, and where? British Medical Journal 2:684–686

Bagshawe KD, Blowers R, Lidwell OM 1978c Isolating patients in hospital to control infection. Part III – design and construction of isolation accommodations. British Medical Journal 2:744–748

Bagshawe KD, Blowers R, Lidwell OM 1978d Isolating patients in hospital to control infection. Part IV – nursing procedures. British Medical Journal 2:808–811

Ben-Yehuda A, Weksler ME 1992 Host resistance and the immune system. Clinics of Geriatric Medicine 8:701–711

Bowell B 1990 Assessing infection risks. Nursing 4(12):19–23

Bowell B 1992 Protecting the patient at risk. Nursing Times 88(3):32–35

British Dental Association (BDA) 1991 The control of cross-infection. Advice sheet A12. BDA Advisory Service, London

Choban PS, Heckler R, Burge J, Flancbaum L 1995 Increased risk of nosocomial infections in obese surgical patients. American Surgeon 61:1001–1005

Ciesielski C, Marianos D, Ou CY et al 1992 Transmission of human immunodeficiency virus in a dental practice. Annals of Internal Medicine 116:798–805

Coleman D 1987 The when and how of isolation. Registered Nurse 50(10):50–59

Creighton S, Pearce J, Stanton S 1991 Complications of caesarean section. In: Studd J (ed) Progress in obstetrics and gynaecology, vol. 9. Churchill Livingstone, London

Crossley KB, Peterson PK 1995 Infections in the elderly. In: Mandell GL, Bennett JE, Dolin R (eds) Principles and practice of infectious diseases, 4th edn. Churchill Livingstone, New York

Cruse PJE, Foord R 1980 The epidemiology of wound infection: a ten year prospective study of 62939 wounds. Surgical Clinics of North America 60:27–40

Davidson AIG, Clark C, Smith G 1971 Postoperative wound infection: a computer analysis. British Journal of Surgery 58:333–337

Department of Health (DoH) 1996 MRSA – what nursing and residential homes need to know. DoH, Wetherby

Department of Health (DoH) 2001 The epic project. Developing national evidence-based guidelines for preventing healthcare associated infections. Journal of Hospital Infection 47(suppl) S1–S82

Department of Health and Social Security (DHSS) 1986 The report of the Committee of Inquiry into an outbreak of food poisoning at Stanley Royd Hospital. HMSO, London

Donowitz GR 1987 The immunosuppressed patient. In: Farber BF (ed) Infection control in intensive care. Churchill Livingstone, Edinburgh

Duggan JM, Oldfield GS, Ghosh HK 1985 Septicaemia as a hospital hazard. Journal of Hospital Infection 6:406–412

Duke FM 1994 Blood disorders. In: Alexander MF, Fawcett JN, Runciman PJ (eds) Nursing practice: hospital and home: the adult. Churchill Livingstone, Edinburgh

Edmond MB, Wenzel RP, Pasculle AW 1996 Vancomycin-resistant *Staphylococcus aureus*: perspectives on measures needed for control. American College of Physicians 124(3):329–334

Farber BF, Wenzel RWP 1980 Postoperative wound infection rates: results of proactive statewide surveillance. American Journal of Surgery 140:343–346

Farrow SC, Kaul S, Littlepage BC 1988 Disinfection methods in general practice and health authority clinics: a telephone survey. Journal of the Royal College of General Practitioners 38:447–449

Fekety R 1995 Antibiotic-associated colitis. In: Mandell GL, Bennett JE, Dolin R (eds) Principles and practice of infectious diseases, 4th edn. Churchill Livingstone, New York

Fiore AE, Joshi M, Caplan ES 1995 Approach to infection in the multiply traumatized patient. In: Mandell GL, Bennett JE, Dolin R (eds) Principles and practice of infectious diseases, 4th edn. Churchill Livingstone, New York

Foy C, Gallagher M, Rhodes T et al 1990 HIV – measures to control infection in general practice. British Medical Journal 300:1048–1049

Gammon J 1998 Analysis of the stressful effects of hospitalisation and source isolation on coping and psychological constructs. International Journal of Nursing Practice 4(2):84–96

Garner J 1996 Guideline for isolation precautions in hospital. American Journal of Infection Control 24:24–52

Glenwright HD, Martin MV 1993 Infection control in dentistry – a practitioner's guide. Occasional paper, issue no. 2. British Dental Association, London

Gould D 1985a Don't spread that infection. Nursing Mirror 161(4):52–53

Gould D 1985b Isolation procedures in one health district. Occasional paper no. 7. Nursing Times 81(45):47–50

Hamilton D 1982 The nineteenth century surgical revolution – antisepsis or better nutrition. Bulletin of History of Medicine 56:30

Hillis DM, Huelsenback JP 1994 Support for dental HIV transmission. Nature 369:24–25

Hirsch MS 1995 Herpes simplex virus. In: Mandell GL, Bennett JE, Dolin R (eds) Principles and practice of infectious diseases, 4th edn. Churchill Livingstone, New York

Ho M 1995 Cytomegalovirus. In: Mandell GL, Bennett JE, Dolin R (eds) Principles and practice of infectious diseases, 4th edn. Churchill Livingstone, New York

Jackson MM, Lynch P 1987 An alternative to isolating patients. Body substance isolation (BSI) system. American Journal of Care for the Aging 8(6):308–311

Jarrett J 1985 The natural history and prognosis of diabetes. Medicine International 2(13):530–532

Jensen JRE, Benson RC, Bobak IM 1981 Maternity care – the nurse and the family. CV Mosby, St Louis

John JF, Ribner BS 1991 Antibiotic resistance in long-term care facilities. Infection Control and Hospital Epidemiology 12(4):245–250

Kingsley A 1992 First step towards a desired outcome. Preventing infection by risk recognition. Professional Nurse 7(11):725–729

Larson E 1983 Compliance with isolation technique. American Journal of Infection Control 11(6):221–225

Leigh DA 1981 An eight-year study of postoperative wound infection in two district general hospitals. Journal of Hospital Infection 2:207–217

Leigh DA, Emmanuel FXS, Sedgewick J, Dean R 1990 Post-operative urinary tract infection and wound infection in women undergoing caesarean section: a comparison of two study periods in 1985 and 1987. Journal of Hospital Infection 15:107–116

Levine DP, Sobel JD 1995 Infections in intravenous drug abusers. In: Mandell GL, Bennett JE, Dolin R (eds) Principles and practice of infectious diseases, 4th edn. Churchill Livingstone, New York

Macgowan AP, Brown I, Feeney R et al 1995 Clostridium difficile-associated diarrhoea and length of hospital stay. Journal of Hospital Infection 31(3):241–244

Mehtar S 1992 Action of antibiotics and the development of antibiotic resistance. In: Taylor EW (ed) Infection in surgical practice. Oxford University Press, Oxford

Mishriki SF, Law DJW, Jeffery P 1990 Factors influencing the incidence of postoperative wound infection. Journal of Hospital Infection 16:223–230

Mishriki SF, Jeffrey PJ, Law DJW 1992 Wound infection: the surgeon's responsibility. Journal of Wound Care 1(2):32–36

Morgan DR, Lamont TJ, Dawson JD, Booth C 1990 Decontamination of instruments and control of cross infection in general practice. British Medical Journal 297:34–37

Musher DM 1995 Streptococcus pneumonia. In: Mandell GL, Bennett JE, Dolin R (eds) Principles and practice of infectious diseases, 4th edn. Churchill Livingstone, New York

Nagachinta T, Stephens M, Reitz B 1987 Risk factors for surgical wound infection following cardiac surgery. Journal of Infectious Diseases 156:967–973

National Research Council of Medical Sciences 1964 Post operative wound infections. The influence of ultraviolet irradiation of the operating room and various other factors. Annals of Surgery 160(suppl 2):1–192

Nice C, Feeney A, Godwin P et al 1996 A prospective audit of wound infection rates after caesarean section in five West Yorkshire hospitals. Journal of Hospital Infection 33:55–61

Overend A, Hall WW, Godwin PGR 1992 Does earwax lose its pathogens on your auriscope overnight? British Medical Journal 305:1571–1573

Parrot T, Evans A, Lowes A, Dennis K 1989 Infection following caesarean section. Journal of Hospital Infection 13:349–354

Patterson TF, Andriole VT 1995 Bacteriuria during pregnancy. In: Mandell GL, Bennett JE, Dolin R (eds) Principles and practice of infectious diseases, 5th edn. Churchill Livingstone, New York

Porter SR, Scully C, El-Maayatah M 1996 Compliance with infection control procedures in dentistry. British Medical Journal 312:705

Public Health Medicine Environmental Group (PHMEG) 1996 Guidelines on the control of infection in residential and nursing homes. DoH, London

Rehu M, Nilsson C 1990 Risk factors for febrile morbidity associated with caesarean section. Obstetrics and Gynaecology 56:269–273

Reynolds HY 1995 Chronic bronchitis and acute infectious exacerbations. In: Mandell GL, Bennett JE, Dolin R (eds) Principles and practice of infectious diseases, 4th edn. Churchill Livingstone, New York

Riley TV 1994 The epidemiology of Clostridium difficile-associated diarrhoea. Review of Medical Microbiology 5:117–122

Saltzman RL, Peterson PK 1987 Immunodeficiency of the elderly. Review of Infectious Disease 9:1127–1139

Scully C, Cawson RA, Griffiths MJ 1990 Occupational hazards to dental staff. British Dental Journal

Scully C, Mortimer P 1994 Gnashings of HIV. Lancet 344:904

Scully C, Porter SR, Epstein JB 1992 Compliance with infection control procedures in a dental hospital clinic. British Dental Journal 17(3):406–412

Scully C, Haj M, Porter SR 1993 Infection control in dentistry. British Medical Journal 306:1754

Stamm WE, Martin SM, Bennett JV 1997 Epidemiology of nosocomial infections due to gram-negative bacilli: aspects relevant to development and use of vaccine. Journal of Infectious Diseases 136(suppl):S151–S160

Swartz MN 1995 Cellulitis and subcutaneous tissue infections: In: Mandell GL, Bennett JE, Dolin R (eds) Principles and practice of infectious diseases, 4th edn. Churchill Livingstone, New York

Tramont EC, Hoover DL 1995 General nonspecific defence mechanisms. In: Mandell GL, Bennett JE, Dolin R (eds) Principles and practice of infectious diseases, 4th edn. Churchill Livingstone, New York

Webster J 1988 Post-caesarean wound infections: a review of risk factors. Australian and New Zealand Journal of Obstetrics and Gynaecology 28:201–207

Webster O, Bowell B 1986 Thinking prevention. Nursing Times 82(28):68–74

Wrightson P 1996 Incidence of infection after caesarean section: a study. Nursing Standard 10(37):34–37

Safe care: reflective practice

12

■ CONTENTS

SUMMARY

Caring suggests that the needs of the patients, as well as those of the carers, have been considered. The carers require an understanding of patients' conditions, the actions that will help patients in their recovery and how to ensure that the act of caring does not affect patients adversely. Previous chapters examined the knowledge-base that will help carers provide safe and informed infection control care. The effectiveness of the science of care is often measured by a successful patient outcome but the art of infection control care is rarely examined. This chapter allows staff members, patients and their relatives to reflect upon the care given and received during a routine admission, and when a patient was affected by a methicillin-resistant *Staphylococcus aureus* (MRSA) infection.

INTRODUCTION

To progress along the road towards comprehensive, safe healthcare, we must acquire and assimilate the relevant knowledge. This process involves the questioning of actions, whether they are your own or those of other people, and the ability to learn from experience. A practice that is not questioned becomes a ritual, with mistakes rarely being rectified. Learning, on the other hand, brings with it added responsibility. Knowledge has to be shared; ensuing actions have to be informed by this learning and the effectiveness of its application assessed. Such examination is never value-free because a person's thoughts, feelings and behaviour are all governed by that person's beliefs, as well as by their knowledge. Such individuality creates an ideal platform for practitioners to question and evaluate care and outcome, as information can be gathered from many different viewpoints. An individual's reflections will also vary with their level of knowledge, grade and experience. Apprentices will measure their own practice and patient outcome against a set of rules or a code of practice. Skilled practitioners, on the other hand, are governed and influenced by the knowledge and intuition that result from experience (Benner et al 1996). All contributions provide a rich source of information that can facilitate a meaningful appraisal, both of continuous care and of the final outcome. This can take place only if health professionals are not afraid to reflect on their practice and are prepared to question and be questioned.

Another source of knowledge and wisdom is the patient. In the process of receiving care, patients observe, feel and form conclusions about their own treatment and outcome. The 'questioning' should include the points of view of patients, not only at the point of discharge but throughout their stay in care settings. Staff members who have sufficient professional detachment to allow their practices and decisions to be questioned, without considering this to be an attack on their professional ability, will enable patients to explore the care that they provide. Such high levels of communication encourage the development of mutual trust and so facilitate useful dialogue regarding the care received and delivered. Communication, therefore, is the best 'in-built' method of quality assurance.

Although much of the material contained in the following 'care evaluations' is based on observation, an interview and a questionnaire survey carried out during a research study (Horton 1993), personal experience and conversations with patients and staff have also contributed.

The reflections depicted here relate only to patients who developed infections. The majority of patient episodes are uncomplicated and the health professional's role in ensuring a satisfactory outcome should be recognized and commended. Furthermore, this chapter does not examine the complete care picture, but deals only and specifically with the infection control component. The aim is to trigger in readers a desire to examine and articulate the infection control elements in their own practice.

CASE PRESENTATIONS

Case study 12.1 Infection control in the care of a patient admitted for surgery

A 57-year-old female patient with osteoarthritis enters hospital for a total hip replacement. Her medical history suggests chronic obstructive pulmonary disease. The patient had previously worked as a nursing assistant. The following events occur:

- The patient is welcomed by a staff nurse, introduced to her 'room-mate' (due to undergo similar surgery) and familiarized with ward facilities

- An extensive social and medical history of the patient is obtained
- Information is given to the patient regarding pre- and postoperative procedures
- The operative site and surrounding areas are shaved
- Surgery is uncomplicated: blood transfusion and two vacuum drains in place, prophylactic and follow-up antibiotic therapy
- Postoperatively, the patient is unable to pass urine and so is catheterized; the catheter remains in place for 4 days
- The patient develops profuse diarrhoea on the fifth postoperative day; the cause is established to be *Clostridium difficile* toxin positive. She is treated with metronidazole. Her diarrhoea lasts for 4 days
- The remaining stay is uneventful.

The patient's impression

The twin-bedded room did not have a toilet but toilets were quite nearby. Both the doctor and the staff nurse took my medical history and explained the surgery to me. The nurse described the sequence of events I should expect.

The shaving of my middle and legs was not pleasant. It was a bit painful despite the baby powder that the nurse used. My hair must be tough, the nurse had to change the blade two or three times. My room-mate, who was having the same operation, was not shaved; I wonder why? By the time I went to theatre the next day the shaved skin was rough and itchy.

After the operation, the blood drip kept on blocking up and had to be frequently examined. A lot of the nurses were blowing their noses because they were suffering from colds. Should nurses with colds carry a small plastic bag in their pockets for used tissues? Nurses kept their scissors and dressing tapes in the pocket where used tissues were placed. I was worried in case these items would be contaminated with the cold bug. I did not want my bad chest complicated with a cold. I needed all my strength to get over the operation. Only one nurse washed her hands before she looked at my drip and my arm.

In the end, the nurse took the drip down. The doctor came to put it in the other arm. I don't think he washed his hands either. He did clean my arm though. I bled a bit and made a mess of the bedclothes. He was by himself and had come with just a needle, a spirit swab and the drip bag. He used a paper tissue from my box to press on the arm and left the bloody tissues and the needle on the table. The nurse took them away with her bare hands. Was this safe? And anyway, shouldn't someone talk to the doctor about this dangerous practice? He fixed my drip with a tape from his pocket.

I had to be catheterized because using a bedpan was so painful with my arthritis and the operation. It was left in for a few days. The nurse had difficulty inserting the catheter. The light in the room is not very bright and it must have been very dark around and between my thighs. I wondered if she was able to see. The catheter was connected to a bag and hooked on to a stand. The tube seemed to pull a lot.

The emptying of catheter bags was very meticulous during the day. At night though, both mine and the lady in the next bed's catheter bags were emptied at midnight. The nurse did not change her gloves or wash her hands when going from one to another. I was relieved when my catheter was removed!

I was given medication through a mini-nebulizer. It was interesting to see how practices varied. Many nurses washed their hands before and after helping with the treatment. They also rinsed, dried and wiped the nebulizer with a spirit swab. Others simply rinsed it and left it in a receiver. They did not wash their hands.

My room-mate was discharged before me. The nurses must have been very busy. They did not have time to clean the mattress before placing new sheets. The thermometer remained, as did the used oxygen mask.

I developed diarrhoea, which halted my recovery. Maybe I should have told the staff nurse about the chicken sandwich brought in by my daughter a couple of days ago. I suppose I was worried that I might be told off. I was relieved when the staff nurse said it was due to the antibiotics.

Having to use the commode was unpleasant! I also found it difficult to walk up to the washbasin to wash my hands after using the commode. I used my washcloth until my daughter brought in some 'wet-wipes'.

My daughter was asked to wear plastic aprons and gloves during this time, I wonder why?

The wound is healing well, the stitches are out and I am going home with my daughter.

I was looked after very well. Although very busy, the nurses were always kind and considerate and remained unhurried. I was very grateful.

The staff members' perspective

Patient placement

Infections of bones can be very serious. The infection control care on our ward is of high quality. Patients for total hip replacements are placed in single rooms or cohorted for 5 to 7 days to protect them from infected patients.

There is a likelihood of airborne transmission of bacteria, as well as a danger of staff inadvertently transferring infection from one patient to another.

So many staff are involved in the patients' care; there are the doctors and the therapy staff. Do they receive any training in infection control? We have to cover all eventualities. Separating these patients highlights their vulnerability to infections.

Collecting and giving information and patient education

The history obtained has to be comprehensive to help us devise a holistic care plan. The patients' involvement in their own care is encouraged but the possibility of them acquiring an infection is not discussed because this could create anxiety, and that has to be avoided.

If patients are in the habit of handwashing after visiting the toilet, they will ask for a bowl. But they may not take kindly to being asked to wash their hands. It may not be a normal practice for them and this has to be respected. Some of them are 70 years old and over and have managed to survive unharmed.

Making patients' intrinsic and extrinsic risk factors explicit

The risk factors are not specified in care plans or nursing notes. We are trying to reduce the time spent on report handovers so such things are not discussed in detail. But when devising care plans staff do consider the patient as a whole and the treatments and procedures carried out.

Preoperative shaving

Preoperative shaving is carried out to appease the consultant. It has to take place on the evening before surgery; there would be no time to shave patients immediately prior to or on the day of the surgery. At least this way everyone follows a set routine with no chance of missing anyone. Thankfully, only one orthopaedic consultant still insists on shaving.

Intravenous infusions

Handling of the i.v. sites, giving sets and solutions is aseptic.

The nursing staff are not always informed by the medical staff when they are due to perform certain procedures. A 'ready prepared' trolley with sterile strip dressings and a box for sharps disposal is always available. It is not often used. Most staff members have attended the acquired immunodeficiency syndrome (AIDS) lectures and are aware of dangers of handling sharps.

Urinary catheterization

Nurses follow a very strict code of practice when carrying out an aseptic procedure. Wound dressings, intravenous infusion care and catheterization are based on principles of asepsis.

Principles of asepsis

Asepsis is when only the sterile items and a non-touch technique are used.

Catheter bags are only emptied as needed. This eliminates the risk of reuse of gloves or jugs. Yes, the night staff total the intake and output at midnight. That is unavoidable because of the medical staff preference.

Mini-nebs are not shared between patients – there is no risk of 'cross-infection'.

Diarrhoeal disease

All diarrhoeas are treated as infectious and 'barrier nursed' until we receive the laboratory results. Standard precautions are implemented to avoid confusion. Visitors are quite happy to follow our advice.

Patient discharge

Many students tell us that washing of beds between patients is not considered necessary. The bedding and the used items are changed.

Reflections

We believe that the care we provide is safe. Infections are not a major problem and we receive more 'thank you' letters than complaints.

Infection control in a mental health setting – staff perspective

Infection control does not apply as much with us as it would on an acute general ward. Our patients are physically healthy. We concentrate more on the psychological and behavioural aspects of our patients.

Infection control in an obstetric setting – staff perspective

Our ladies are not ill. Having babies is a natural function, not a disease. And anyway, they are not in long enough for us to put infection control principles into action.

As can be seen, from Case 12.1 and above, numerous issues surround the delivery of infection control care. The responsibility often rests with the team leaders to ensure a safe code of practice for staff members working directly under their supervision. The points indicated in Reflective Practice 12.1 may prove helpful in providing a framework of reflective practice.

■ **REFLECTIVE PRACTICE 12.1   Important issues for the team leader/ primary nurse**

1. What is your ward philosophy with regard to infection control? Is it made explicit or felt to be implicit within the total care?
2. If 'implicit', how is it identified/defined when evaluating care?
3. What proportion of care delivery is in the form of physical intervention? And what is the level of risk associated with such interventions?
4. What level of responsibility for the infection control care of a patient is yours to 'own'? For example:
   (a) Have you been allocated and accepted the responsibility of ensuring that all individuals within your team and all others involved in the patient's care 'know' what is meant by safe practice?
   (b) Have you ever questioned the level of your own knowledge of the subject?
   (c) Do you make a point of continuously reiterating the risks associated with the 'type' and 'timing' of preoperative shaving, and urinary and vascular catheterization?
   (d) If the reason given for not discussing the intrinsic and extrinsic risk factors is a lack of time, have you ever analysed the content of your handovers? How efficient and sufficient is your ward handover procedure?

Infections caused by staphylococci are an important cause of morbidity and mortality. Staphylococcal infections, especially those associated with MRSA, are costly in terms of treatment as well as in the disruption they cause to hospital routine during outbreaks. MRSA are said to vary in their virulence and epidemic potential (Cox et al 1995). Some strains, known as epidemic methicillin-resistant *Staphylococcus aureus* (EMRSA), cause severe and life-threatening infections and require aggressive and costly measures to curtail the spread. According to Keane et al (1991), outbreaks of MRSA infections are very difficult to control and require 'draconian measures entailing considerable expense'. The authors identify a number of reasons for this:

- Asymptomatic carriage can often occur for long periods
- Current methods to detect colonization of patients are slow and insensitive and an outbreak could have been underway for some time before being recognized
- Carriage could be at a variety of sites, any one of which might be the dominant reservoir for spread
- The need for scrupulous handwashing is often underestimated
- Isolation facilities must be provided, although these might be insufficient if large numbers of people are involved in the outbreak.

The revised guidelines for the control of MRSA suggest care based on risk assessment in order to obviate the need for strict precautions for all MRSA-positive patients (British Society for Antimicrobial Chemotherapy, HIS, ICNA Working Party Report 1998). There are guidelines for MRSA-positive patients in nursing and residential homes (DoH 1996) but the control of MRSA elsewhere in the community is less well defined. There is a constant movement of patients between community and hospitals. Patients colonized with MRSA in hospital have been known to carry the organism for months or years afterwards (Frenay et al 1992, Hicks et al 1991). Nursing homes have also been affected by MRSA, with risks of infection higher in nursing home patients colonized with MRSA than in those colonized with methicillin-sensitive *Staphylococcus aureus* (MSSA). Health professionals caring for MRSA-positive patients are also at risk of becoming colonized with the organism and subsequently transmitting it to other patients. It is, therefore, necessary to try to eradicate the organism wherever possible.

Precautionary measures have to be instituted when the organism is first isolated. These measures can be modified if the organism is of a less aggressive strain and/or the carriage sites are found to be negative at screening. Case studies 12.2–12.4 provide an account of how various individuals view this condition.

Case study 12.2 The MRSA patient in hospital

The patient's impression

I was transferred from a four-bedded bay into a single room. The nurse told me that the bacteria causing infection in my wound were resistant to many antibiotics and, because they could spread, it was better for me not to come into contact with other patients.

Everyone except the doctors wore plastic aprons and gloves; even my visitors were asked to wear them. The nurse told me that the bacteria did not affect healthy people but that they could carry them to other vulnerable patients. I can understand that nurses have to 'dress up' but why do visitors?

The nurse said that they had to follow a regimen of taking different specimens and bathing me with antiseptic. I wish I understood it all a little better.

I wonder why the door is kept shut at all time. Nurses only come in when they have something to do. Even the domestic lady seems to rush through her cleaning.

It feels funny to be touched by the physiotherapist wearing plastic gloves.

I do miss seeing and talking to other patients and staff. Everyone is so busy! The nurse tells me that I may have to remain isolated for up to 1 month!

I have been told I can go home and the district nurse will take over the regimen. It has not been a pleasant experience. I hope I never get these bacteria again!

The nursing staff's perspective

We follow the policy laid down by the infection control department. The infection control nurse guides us through the regimen.

It is easier if everyone follows the same precautions; it avoids confusion and having to explain the infection to everyone. As long as correct precautions are taken, staff and other patients will be safe.

Patients become quite concerned about too many people finding out about their 'bug'. And anyway, we have to consider patient confidentiality!

As long as the bacteria do not spread to other patients we feel that we have done a good job.

The therapy staff's perspective

The sister said that Mrs B was now being barrier nursed and told us to wear plastic apron and gloves, to discard them in the room and to wash our hands thoroughly before leaving the room.

The ward staff either did not themselves know or were unwilling to give us more information on this MRSA. We have pregnant staff, staff with young babies and one person's husband has leukaemia. They were all worried in case they took these bacteria home with them.

The patient had to be X-rayed in the room. Should the machine have been covered with a plastic sheet? How safe is it to reuse the X-ray frame afterwards?

We go from patient to patient and ward to ward. What are the chances of our spreading the bacteria?

The patient was rather 'down' about being cooped up and was asking all kinds of questions which I could not answer.

I must read up more about this infection.

The domestic assistant's perspective

I don't think we should have to clean the rooms of people with dangerous infections. The nursing staff know and understand more and would know what to do.

The sister said that I did not need to know about the infection but that I would be safe as long I followed her instructions. The sister has talked about the domestic staff being part of her team, yet she did not trust us with the information, which would have put our minds at rest.

Anyway, the patient herself told me that she had resistant bacteria in her wound.

I have a cut on my hand. Will it become infected with these bacteria and will I take them home?

The ambulance personnel

We follow the guidelines developed by our headquarters personnel. Either the general practitioner (GP) or the ward staff inform us that the patient is infected. Although we take the same precautions for most infections, i.e. gown and gloves, it is useful to know the nature of the infection. It helps us to reassure any worried staff.

The ambulance is decontaminated with disinfectant and the linen and equipment changed after the patient has been transported.

The voluntary staff

We usually know that a patient in a single room is being barrier nursed because there is a trolley with aprons and gloves outside the room.

It depends on who is on as to whether we are allowed to go into the room. Some staff tell us that as long we wash our hands we are safe.

We would like to know more about the disease. I am not sure if the voluntary staff are protected in the same way as other staff.

Case study 12.3 The MRSA patient at home

The community nurse's perspective

The general practitioner was contacted by the hospital microbiologist with the results of Mrs B's leg ulcer swab; it was MRSA positive.

This was a second attack of MRSA for Mrs B. Last time she was in hospital and had to be isolated, and hence was apprehensive about how she might be looked after at home.

There are not the same concerns about its spread in the home.

The precautions were modified for two reasons: (i) Mrs B's carriage sites were negative; and (ii) the MRSA was not of the epidemic strain.

We used plastic aprons and gloves when 'dressing' the wound and used alcohol hand-rub.

Oral antibiotic and antiseptic nasal ointment were prescribed. The antiseptic wash was discontinued once the 'screening' results were received.

The small quantity of dressing material was double-bagged in small plastic bags and disposed of with the domestic waste.

The linen was processed through the 'hot' cycle of the washing machine.

Mrs B's movements were not restricted.

Although we were not able to reassure her daughter, who kept her young son away from his grandmother for 2 weeks, we wanted to take the 'drama' out of MRSA and I think we succeeded.

The relative's perspective

My mother had the same 'bug' when she was in hospital a year ago. She was barrier nursed and we had to put on plastic aprons and gloves.

I now have a small baby who has had to have many courses of antibiotics because of a bad chest. I don't want him to catch the bacteria.

I cannot understand why the same bug is less serious at home than in hospital. The nurse tells me that this bug is only dangerous for people who are already ill.

The nurse persuaded me to bring my son to visit my mother. The baby is all right!

Case study 12.4 The MRSA patient in a nursing home

Staff members' perspectives

We function mainly with non-qualified staff, who do not always receive the level of supervision that the hospital staff may receive. Precautions have to be relatively rigid to avoid confusion.

Everything used by the MRSA-positive patient has to be kept and dealt with separately.

The patient is confined to her room, which is a pity. She is not allowed visits by other patients either. I am not sure why this has to be because the MRSA was only isolated from her catheter specimen!

We decided to let her sit in the lounge after the first week. I hope we did the right thing. It has not spread to other residents so far. We hope we can contain it.

An important and often unrecognized source of infection are healthcare workers, who might be incubating a disease, infected or be asymptomatic carriers of an infectious organism. Case study 12.5 discusses one such episode of a staff-related outbreak.

Case study 12.5 Viral diarrhoea associated with an infected healthcare worker

Three care of the elderly wards reported a number of staff and patients to be affected by a diarrhoeal disease. A total of 40 patients and 25 staff developed symptoms of nausea, vomiting, diarrhoea and 'queasy' abdomen; symptoms were consistent with those associated with small round structured viruses (SRSVs). The condition proved very debilitating for many of the frail, elderly patients; there were four fatalities. Although not established to be the cause of deaths, the infection was thought to have contributed to their early demise.

The initial enquiry found that a physiotherapist, associated with all three wards, had been sent home 2 days before the first patient developed the disease. She had become ill the evening before but had reported for work and cared for patients on the three affected wards before going 'sick'.

Consequences

1. All three wards were closed to admissions for a total of 15 days.
2. Curtailment of staff movement became impractical. Staff members were 'borrowed' from non-affected wards and kept on the affected wards

until the end of the outbreak. 'Bank' and 'agency' staff were employed to staff the non-affected wards.

3. An outbreak control group, consisting of senior hospital personnel, was convened. The group met on five occasions.

4. A member of nursing staff from one of the affected wards continued to report for duty at a nursing home where she worked as a 'bank' nurse. She developed the disease whilst on duty. Consequently, six staff members and 13 patients in the nursing home developed the infection 48 h later. The nursing home also instigated outbreak control measures.

5. A number of secondary cases were reported. These included both visitors and family members of the affected patients and staff.

6. The media interest and the publicity surrounding the outbreak generated much anxiety amongst patients who were due to be admitted to the non-affected wards.

7. The cost of the outbreak in terms of ward closures, extended lengths of stay by affected patients, precautionary measures, employment of bank and agency staff is easy to determine. What is beyond calculation is the suffering and anxiety amongst patients and staff. There is also a 'nagging' doubt that some fatalities could have been prevented.

REFLECTIONS

In developing a reflective approach, it will help to provide all members of the care team with a platform from which to explore their own approach to infectious patients. The following questions could be useful for this purpose:

1. What is the individual practitioner's understanding of the presenting infection?
2. What are the concerns, worries and fears surrounding the infection?
3. How has an infected patient's care varied from that of non-infected patients?
4. What do the practitioners feel and think about the care provided?
5. Would the approach be different in future? If so, how?
6. Are affected patients ever allowed to explore their own feelings surrounding the episode?
7. Does every healthcare worker know the implication of transmitting an infection to vulnerable patients and colleagues?
8. Does every manager make it easy for his or her own staff to take time 'off sick' for something that might seem trivial?
9. Should the staff member thought to be the index case be told of his or her role in the outbreak?
10. Would you tell the affected patients, relatives and staff members how they might have contracted the disease?

FINAL CONCLUSION

People acquire infections in hospitals, in their own homes and in community care settings. Individuals encountered by healthcare personnel are already vulnerable to infection and the vulnerability increases with every treatment and care procedure. Very little control can be exercised over the person's own intrinsic susceptibility but risks associated with treatments and care procedures can be prevented or minimized. This book has addressed the theory and practice of care that can influence these risks.

Infection control affects every practice and concerns every discipline associated with care. The responsibility for developing a structured framework for infection control practice, however, rests with the infection control team, especially the infection control nurses (ICN). The role of the ICN is multidimensional and multifaceted, and demands a detailed and broad level of knowledge, expertise and skills. Invariably, these attributes are enhanced as the role develops from role identification (what the job entails) by staff members, through becoming a successful change agent to being accepted as a specialist expert.

Quality is the main focus for delivering infection control service. The new NHS demands quality care from all healthcare workers, with the commitment from chief executives to enable a quality service by all. The mechanisms for ensuring quality are embedded risk management, clinical governance (NHSE 1995a) and controls assurance (NHSE 1995b). Infection control is now becoming a powerful tool since it can contribute positively to these issues and help the NHS achieve its objectives.

REFERENCES

Benner P, Tanner CA, Chelsa CA 1996 Expertise in Nursing Practice: caring, clinical judgement and ethics. Springer Publishing Company, New York

British Society for Antimicrobial Chemotherapy, HIS, ICNA Working Party Report 1998 Revised guidelines for the control of methicillin-resistant *Staphylococcus aureus* infection in hospitals. Journal of Hospital Infection 39:253–290

Cox RA, Conquest C, Mallaghan C, Marples RR 1995 A major outbreak of methicillin resistant *Staphylococcus aureus* caused by a new phage type (EMRSA-16). Journal of Hospital Infection 29:87–106

Department of Health (DoH) 1996 MRSA. What nursing and residential homes need to know. DoH, London

Frenay HME, Vandenbroucke-Grauls CMJE, Verhoef J 1992 Long-term carriage and transmission of methicillin resistant *Staphylococcus aureus* after discharge from hospital. Journal of Hospital Infection 22:207–215

Hicks NR, Moore EP, Williams EW 1991 Carriage and community treatment of methicillin resistant *Staphylococcus aureus*; what happens to colonised patients after discharge? Journal of Hospital Infection 19:17–24

Horton R 1993 Infection control in nurse education and practice. MPhil Thesis, University of Bradford, Bradford

Keane CT, Coleman DC, Cafferkey MT 1991 Methicillin resistant *Staphylococcus aureus* – a reappraisal. Journal of Hospital Infection 19(3):147–152

National Health Service Executive (NHSE) 1995a Clinical governance in the new NHS (HSC1995/065). NHSE, London

National Health Service Executive (NHSE) 1995b Corporate governance in the NHS: Controls assurance statements (HSG(97)17). NHSE, London

Index